Illustrated Obstetrics and Gynecology Problems

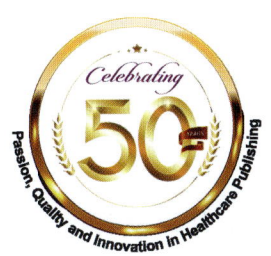

Disclaimer

The purpose of this resource is providing a clinical decision pathway with a survey of treatment options, to accommodate the educational interests of trainees and practitioners in addressing the scope of options that might be considered in their clinical practice. There is no assurance that the scope of clinical decision-making and treatment options outlined for any particular condition and/or individual clinical presentation is comprehensive. The publisher and authors of this publication disclaim any liability, loss, injury or damage incurred as a consequence, directly or indirectly, of the use and application of any of the contents of this learning material.

Illustrated Obstetrics and Gynecology Problems

Sireesha Y Reddy MD
Professor
Department of Obstetrics and Gynecology
Paul L Foster School of Medicine
Texas Tech University Health Sciences Center (TTUHSC) El Paso
El Paso, Texas, USA

Melissa D Mendez MD
Associate Professor
Department of Obstetrics and Gynecology
Paul L Foster School of Medicine
Texas Tech University Health Sciences Center (TTUHSC) El Paso
El Paso, Texas, USA

Sanja Kupesic Plavsic MD PhD
Professor
Department of Obstetrics and Gynecology
Associate Dean of Faculty Development
Director, Center for Advanced Teaching and Assessment in Clinical Simulation (ATACS)
Paul L Foster School of Medicine
Texas Tech University Health Sciences Center (TTUHSC) El Paso
El Paso, Texas, USA

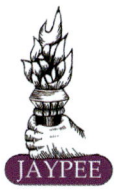

JAYPEE BROTHERS MEDICAL PUBLISHERS
The Health Sciences Publisher
New Delhi | London

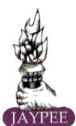 **Jaypee Brothers Medical Publishers (P) Ltd**

Headquarters
Jaypee Brothers Medical Publishers (P) Ltd
4838/24, Ansari Road, Daryaganj
New Delhi 110 002, India
Phone: +91-11-43574357
Fax: +91-11-43574314
Email: jaypee@jaypeebrothers.com

Overseas Office
J.P. Medical Ltd
83 Victoria Street, London
SW1H 0HW (UK)
Phone: +44 20 3170 8910
Fax: +44 (0)20 3008 6180
Email: info@jpmedpub.com

Website: www.jaypeebrothers.com
Website: www.jaypeedigital.com

© 2020, Jaypee Brothers Medical Publishers

The views and opinions expressed in this book are solely those of the original contributor(s)/author(s) and do not necessarily represent those of editor(s) of the book.

All rights reserved. No part of this publication may be reproduced, stored or transmitted in any form or by any means, electronic, mechanical, photocopying, recording or otherwise, without the prior permission in writing of the publishers.

All brand names and product names used in this book are trade names, service marks, trademarks or registered trademarks of their respective owners. The publisher is not associated with any product or vendor mentioned in this book.

Medical knowledge and practice change constantly. This book is designed to provide accurate, authoritative information about the subject matter in question. However, readers are advised to check the most current information available on procedures included and check information from the manufacturer of each product to be administered, to verify the recommended dose, formula, method and duration of administration, adverse effects and contraindications. It is the responsibility of the practitioner to take all appropriate safety precautions. Neither the publisher nor the author(s)/editor(s) assume any liability for any injury and/or damage to persons or property arising from or related to use of material in this book.

This book is sold on the understanding that the publisher is not engaged in providing professional medical services. If such advice or services are required, the services of a competent medical professional should be sought.

Every effort has been made where necessary to contact holders of copyright to obtain permission to reproduce copyright material. If any have been inadvertently overlooked, the publisher will be pleased to make the necessary arrangements at the first opportunity. The **CD/DVD-ROM** (if any) provided in the sealed envelope with this book is complimentary and free of cost. **Not meant for sale.**

Inquiries for bulk sales may be solicited at: jaypee@jaypeebrothers.com

Illustrated Obstetrics and Gynecology Problems

First Edition: **2020**

ISBN: 978-93-5270-495-8

Printed at: Samrat Offset Pvt. Ltd.

Dedicated to

Sanja
Always patient, professional, and poised
All the authors confirm "When we grow up, we want to be just like her."

Sireesha Y Reddy

My husband, partner and co-parent, for all your patience.

Melissa D Mendez

My loving boys, Branko, Ivor and Hobbes.

Sanja Kupesic Plavsic

Contributors

Ann M Dobry DO
Resident
Department of Obstetrics and Gynecology
Paul L Foster School of Medicine
TTUHSC El Paso
El Paso, Texas, USA

Carla Martinez MD
Assistant Professor
Department of Obstetrics and Gynecology
Paul L Foster School of Medicine
TTUHSC El Paso
El Paso, Texas, USA

Christopher Ortiz DO
Resident
Department of Obstetrics and Gynecology
Paul L Foster School of Medicine
TTUHSC El Paso
El Paso, Texas, USA

Dhyana Velasco MD
Resident
Department of Obstetrics and Gynecology
Paul L Foster School of Medicine
TTUHSC El Paso
El Paso, Texas, USA

Diego Ramirez MD
Resident
Department of Obstetrics and Gynecology
Paul L Foster School of Medicine
TTUHSC El Paso
El Paso, Texas, USA

Heather Pugmire MD
Department of Obstetrics and Gynecology
Bingham Memorial Hospital
Blackfoot, Idaho, USA

Humera Chaudhary MD
Assistant Professor
Department of Radiology
Paul L Foster School of Medicine
TTUHSC El Paso
El Paso, Texas, USA

Kathleen Green MD
Assistant Professor
Department of Obstetrics and Gynecology
University of Florida
Gainesville, Florida, USA

Luis S Noble MD
Clinical Professor
Department of Obstetrics and Gynecology
Paul L Foster School of Medicine
TTUHSC El Paso
El Paso, Texas, USA

Mary Traci Groening MD
Instructor
Department of Obstetrics and Gynecology
Paul L Foster School of Medicine
TTUHSC El Paso
El Paso, Texas, USA

Melissa D Mendez MD
Associate Professor
Department of Obstetrics and Gynecology
Paul L Foster School of Medicine
TTUHSC El Paso
El Paso, Texas, USA

Naima Khamsi MD
Instructor
Department of Obstetrics and Gynecology
Paul L Foster School of Medicine
TTUHSC El Paso
El Paso, Texas, USA

Osvaldo Padilla MD
Assistant Professor
Department of Pathology
Paul L Foster School of Medicine
TTUHSC El Paso
El Paso, Texas, USA

Robert W Vera MD
Associate Professor
Department of Obstetrics and Gynecology
Paul L Foster School of Medicine
TTUHSC El Paso
El Paso, Texas, USA

Safa Farrag MD
Assistant Professor
Department of Internal Medicine
Paul L Foster School of Medicine
TTUHSC El Paso
El Paso, Texas, USA

Sanja Kupesic Plavsic MD PhD
Professor
Department of Obstetrics and Gynecology
Associate Dean of Faculty Development
Director, Center for Advanced Teaching and Assessment in Clinical Simulation (ATACS)
Paul L Foster School of Medicine
TTUHSC El Paso
El Paso, Texas, USA

Shaked Laks MD
Assistant Professor
Department of Radiology
Paul L Foster School of Medicine
TTUHSC El Paso
El Paso, Texas, USA

Sireesha Y Reddy MD
Professor
Department of Obstetrics and Gynecology
Paul L Foster School of Medicine
TTUHSC El Paso
El Paso, Texas, USA

Sushila Arya MD
Assistant Professor
Department of Obstetrics and Gynecology
Paul L Foster School of Medicine
TTUHSC El Paso
El Paso, Texas, USA

Ulrich Honemeyer MD PhD
Professor
Fetal Medicine and Genetics Center
Dubai, UAE

Vladimir Sparac MD PhD
Assistant Professor
Dubrovnik International University
Split, Croatia, EU

Wael El-Mallah MD
Assistant Professor
Department of Internal Medicine
Paul L Foster School of Medicine
TTUHSC El Paso
El Paso, Texas, USA

Preface

Illustrated Obstetrics and Gynecology Problems provides an opportunity to the physicians in training and practicing and medical students, to go through common scenarios in obstetrics and gynecology practice and gain longitudinal experience with 60 virtual patients. This book addresses wide differential diagnosis concerns and workups for common presentations of obstetrics and gynecology patients.

The use of consistent formatting enables easy assessment of patients' chief complaints, history and investigations. Clinical questions section aims to provide answers for optimal diagnostic, treatment and care management strategies. Each case discussion ends with Take-home messages, summarizing important case-specific concepts in a succinct format. All case studies contain a short list of most relevant up-to-date references.

We believe that the use of this book will allow different levels of learners to improve their clinical knowledge and reasoning, as well as update their diagnostic and management skills. We hope that this book will assist medical students, residents and practicing physicians to more efficiently master the learning material for their boards and recertification examinations.

Good luck for your examinations and practice!

Sireesha Y Reddy
Melissa D Mendez
Sanja Kupesic Plavsic

Acknowledgments

We would like to thank all of our students, residents and fellows who challenged and pushed us ever forward. Special thanks to Dr Osvaldo Padilla who provided histopathology images for this project.

We would also like to thank the dedicated staff of M/s Jaypee Brothers Medical Publishers (P) Ltd, New Delhi, India who were willing to dedicate their time and energy to this project. The team has always provided excellent technical support.

Contents

Section 1
GYNECOLOGY

1. **Well-woman Examination** — 3
   Melissa D Mendez, Osvaldo Padilla
2. **Infertility Assessment** — 7
   Dhyana Velasco, Sireesha Y Reddy, Sanja Kupesic Plavsic
3. **Polycystic Ovary Syndrome** — 13
   Sanja Kupesic Plavsic
4. **Intrauterine Adhesions** — 18
   Sanja Kupesic Plavsic, Osvaldo Padilla
5. **Septate Uterus** — 23
   Sanja Kupesic Plavsic, Osvaldo Padilla
6. **Submucosal Uterine Fibroid** — 29
   Sanja Kupesic Plavsic, Vladimir Sparac
7. **Chlamydia Salpingitis** — 35
   Ulrich Honemeyer, Sanja Kupesic Plavsic
8. **Chronic Pelvic Pain and Pelvic Adhesions** — 41
   Dhyana Velasco, Sireesha Y Reddy
9. **Pelvic Inflammatory Disease and Tubo-ovarian Abscess** — 45
   Sushila Arya, Sanja Kupesic Plavsic
10. **Ovarian Hyperstimulation Syndrome** — 51
    Sushila Arya, Sanja Kupesic Plavsic
11. **Preconceptional Ultrasound** — 56
    Sanja Kupesic Plavsic
12. **Menopause** — 60
    Sanja Kupesic Plavsic
13. **Postmenopausal Bleeding** — 65
    Sanja Kupesic Plavsic, Osvaldo Padilla
14. **Endometrial Polyp** — 73
    Melissa D Mendez, Sireesha Y Reddy, Osvaldo Padilla, Sanja Kupesic Plavsic
15. **Hematometra in a Postmenopausal Patient** — 79
    Sushila Arya, Sanja Kupesic Plavsic

16. Endometrial Carcinoma *Sanja Kupesic Plavsic, Osvaldo Padilla*	84
17. Leiomyosarcoma *Christopher Ortiz, Melissa D Mendez, Osvaldo Padilla, Sanja Kupesic Plavsic*	90
18. Ovarian Cystadenocarcinoma *Sanja Kupesic Plavsic, Osvaldo Padilla*	95
19. Borderline Ovarian Tumor *Sanja Kupesic Plavsic, Osvaldo Padilla*	102
20. Ovarian Dermoid *Sireesha Y Reddy, Osvaldo Padilla, Sanja Kupesic Plavsic*	107
21. Hemorrhagic Cyst *Sanja Kupesic Plavsic, Osvaldo Padilla*	111
22. Ectopic Pregnancy *Sushila Arya, Sireesha Y Reddy, Sanja Kupesic Plavsic*	117
23. Ovarian Torsion *Sanja Kupesic Plavsic, Sireesha Y Reddy*	122
24. Pelvic Congestion Syndrome *Sanja Kupesic Plavsic*	127
25. Incisional Endometriosis *Sireesha Y Reddy, Sanja Kupesic Plavsic*	132
26. Secondary Dysmenorrhea *Sushila Arya, Luis S Noble, Sanja Kupesic Plavsic*	136
27. Uterine Fibroid *Sanja Kupesic Plavsic, Osvaldo Padilla*	141
28. Pedunculated Uterine Fibroid and Endometriosis *Ulrich Honemeyer, Sanja Kupesic Plavsic*	147
29. Intrauterine Device Complications *Sanja Kupesic Plavsic*	153
30. Abnormal Pap Smear and Cervical Dysplasia *Sushila Arya, Osvaldo Padilla, Heather Pugmire, Sanja Kupesic Plavsic*	158
31. Condylomata Acuminata *Sushila Arya, Sireesha Y Reddy, Sanja Kupesic Plavsic*	164
32. Primary Amenorrhea *Sushila Arya, Sireesha Y Reddy, Sanja Kupesic Plavsic*	169
33. Labia Minora Hypertrophy *Ann M Dobry, Sireesha Y Reddy*	174
34. Lichen Sclerosus *Sushila Arya, Sireesha Y Reddy, Sanja Kupesic Plavsic*	178

Section 2
OBSTETRICS

35. Early Pregnancy Loss — 185
Melissa D Mendez

36. Residual Products of Conception — 190
Sanja Kupesic Plavsic, Osvaldo Padilla

37. Preterm Labor — 195
Melissa D Mendez, Naima Khamsi, Diego Ramirez, Sanja Kupesic Plavsic

38. Cervical Insufficiency — 200
Diego Ramirez, Melissa D Mendez, Sireesha Y Reddy

39. Multifetal Gestation — 205
Melissa D Mendez, Carla Martinez

40. Intrauterine Growth Restriction — 210
Melissa D Mendez, Carla Martinez, Osvaldo Padilla

41. Oligohydramnios — 216
Melissa D Mendez, Sanja Kupesic Plavsic

42. Placenta Previa — 221
Melissa D Mendez

43. Placenta Percreta — 224
Melissa D Mendez, Shaked Laks, Osvaldo Padilla, Sanja Kupesic Plavsic

44. Fetal Malpresentation — 230
Melissa D Mendez

45. Gestational Hypertensive Disorders — 234
Melissa D Mendez, Sanja Kupesic Plavsic

46. Operative Delivery — 241
Melissa D Mendez, Sushila Arva

47. Cesarean Section — 245
Mary Traci Groening

48. Caudal Regression Syndrome — 252
Ulrich Honemeyer, Sanja Kupesic Plavsic

49. Fetal Hydronephrosis — 257
Ulrich Honemeyer, Sanja Kupesic Plavsic

50. Asymptomatic Adnexal Mass in Pregnancy — 262
Sanja Kupesic Plavsic

51. Adnexal Mass and Pelvic Pain in Pregnancy — 266
Sanja Kupesic Plavsic, Ulrich Honemeyer

52. Appendicitis in Pregnancy *Safa Farrag, Humera Chaudhary, Sanja Kupesic Plavsic*	272
53. Congenital Heart Disease in Pregnancy *Safa Farrag, Wael El-Mallah, Sanja Kupesic Plavsic*	276
54. Deep Venous Thrombosis in Pregnancy *Safa Farrag, Humera Chaudhary, Sanja Kupesic Plavsic*	280
55. Gallstones in Pregnancy *Safa Farrag, Humera Chaudhary, Padilla Osvaldo, Sanja Kupesic Plavsic*	284
56. Liver Disease in Pregnancy *Safa Farrag, Humera Chaudhary, Sanja Kupesic Plavsic*	289
57. Kidney Stones in Pregnancy *Safa Farrag, Humera Chaudhary, Sanja Kupesic Plavsic*	293
58. Thyroid Nodule in Pregnancy *Safa Farrag, Humera Chaudhary, Sanja Kupesic Plavsic*	297
59. Gestational Trophoblastic Disease *Sanja Kupesic Plavsic*	301
60. Postpartum Tubal Ligation *Melissa D Mendez, Kathleen Green, Robert W Vera*	307
Index	*313*

Abbreviations

ACC	American College of Cardiology
ACOG	American College of Obstetricians and Gynecologists
ADHD	Attention deficit hyperactivity disorder
AFC	Antral follicle count
AFLP	Acute fatty liver of pregnancy
AFP	Alpha fetoprotein
AHA	American Heart Association
ALT	Alanine transaminase
AMH	Anti-Müllerian hormone
ANCS	Antenatal corticosteroids
ARDS	Adult respiratory distress syndrome
ART	Assisted reproductive technology
ASCCP	American Society for Colposcopy and Cervical Pathology
ASCUS	Atypical cells of undetermined significance
ASRM	American Society for Reproductive Medicine
AST	Aspartate transaminase
BMD	Bone mineral density
BMI	Body mass index
BOT	Borderline ovarian tumors
BP	Blood pressure
BPP	Biophysical profile
BTL	Bilateral tubal ligation
CA-125	Cancer antigen 125
CBC	Complete blood count
CBD	Common bile duct
CC	Clomiphene citrate
CDC	Center for Disease Control and Prevention
CEA	Carcinoembryonic antigen
CGD	Complicated gallstone disease
CIN	Cervical intraepithelial neoplasia
CKC	Cold knife cone biopsy
CL	Cervical length
CMP	Comprehensive metabolic panel
CO_2	Carbon dioxide
COS	Controlled ovarian stimulation
CREST	Collaborative Review of Sterilization Study
CRL	Crown rump length
CRP	C-reactive protein
CRS	Caudal regression syndrome
CS	Cesarean section
CT	Computed tomography

CTA	Computed tomographic angiography
CUS	Compression ultrasonography
CV	Cardiovascular
CVA	Costo-vertebral angle
CXR	Chest X-ray
D&C	Dilatation and curettage
DIC	Disseminated intravascular coagulopathy
DM	Diabetes mellitus
D5NS	Dextrose 5% in normal saline (0.9%)
DVT	Deep venous thrombosis
DXA	Dual energy X-ray absorptiometry
E2	Estradiol
EGF	Epidermal growth factor
EM	Emergency medicine
EOMI	Extraocular movement intact
ER	Emergency room
ERCP	Endoscopic retrograde cholangiopancreatogram
ESR	Erythrocyte sedimentation rate
ETOH	Ethanol or ethyl alcohol
EUS	Endoscopic ultrasound
FDA	Food and Drug Administration
FHT	Fetal heart tracing
FNA	Fine needle aspiration
FRAX	Fracture risk assessment tool
FSH	Follicle stimulating hormone
G	Gram
GGT	Gamma-glutamyl transpeptidase
GI	Gastrointestinal
GIS	Gel instillation sonography
GnRH agonists	Gonadotropin releasing hormone agonists
G/P	Gravida/para
GTD	Gestational trophoblastic disease
GU	Genito-urinary
Hb	Hemoglobin
HCG	Human chorionic gonadotropin
HCT	Hematocrit
HD	High definition
HDL	High density lipoproteins
HEENT	Head, Eyes, Ears, Nose and Throat
HELLP	Hemolysis (H), elevated liver enzymes (EL), low platelet count (LP)
HIT	Heparin induced thrombocytopenia
HIV	Human immunodeficiency virus
HPV	Human papilloma virus
Hr	High-risk
HRT	Hormonal replacement therapy
HSG	Hysterosalpingogram
ICP	Intrahepatic cholestasis of pregnancy

ICSI	Intracytoplasmatic sperm injection
IGF	Insulin like growth factor
IL-6	Interleukin-6
IM	Intramuscularly
IV	Intravenous
IVF/ET	*In vitro* fertilization/Embryo transfer
IU	International unit
IUCD	Intrauterine contraceptive device
IUD	Intrauterine device
IUGR	Intrauterine growth restriction
IUI	Intrauterine insemination
IUP	Intrauterine pregnancy
LDL	Low density lipoproteins
LEEP	Loop electrosurgical excision procedure
LFT	Liver function tests
LH	Luteinizing hormone
LLETZ	Large loop excision of the transformation zone
LLQ	Left lower quadrant
LMP	Last menstrual bleeding
LMWH	Lower molecular weight heparin
LNG-IUD	Levonorgestrel IUD
LOD	Laparoscopic ovarian drilling
LS	Lichen sclerosus
LTCS	Low transverse cesarean section
LUQ	Left upper quadrant
MC	Menstrual cycle
MMR	Measles, Mumps, Rubella
MPA	Medroxyprogesterone acetate
MRI	Magnetic resonance imaging
MRV	Magnetic resonance venogram
MTX	Methotrexate
NKDA	Not known drug allergies
NOF	National Osteoporosis Foundation
NPO	Nothing per os
NSAIDs	Nonsteroidal anti-inflammatory drugs
NST	Non-stress test
NSVD	Normal spontaneous vaginal delivery
NYHA	New York Heart Association
OB	Obstetrical
OCP	Oral contraceptive pills
OHSS	Ovarian hyperstimulation syndrome
OR	Operating room
P	Pulse
PCOS	Polycystic ovarian syndrome
PCS	Pelvic congestion syndrome
PDGF	Platelet derived growth factor
PE	Pulmonary embolism

PE	Physical exam
PEP	Persistent ectopic pregnancy
PET	Positron emission tomography
PID	Pelvic inflammatory disease
PNV	Prenatal vitamins
PPROM	Preterm premature rupture of membranes
PROM	Premature rupture of membranes
PTH	Parathyroid hormone
RAI	Radioactive iodine
RLQ	Right lower quadrant
ROS	Review of systems
RPD	Renal pelvic diameter
RPOC	Retained products of conception
RR	Respiratory rate
RUQ	Right upper quadrant
SAb	Spontaneous abortion
SERM	Selective estrogen receptor modulator
SIS	Saline infusion sonohysterography
SOB	Shortness of breath
STD	Sexually transmitted disease
STI	Sexually transmitted infection
SVD	Spontaneous vaginal delivery
SVE	Sterile vaginal exam
3D	Three-dimensional
T	Temperature
TCE	Transcatheter embolization
TGF	Transforming growth factor
TOA	Tubo-ovarian abscess
TSH	Thyroid stimulating hormone
TV US	Transvaginal ultrasound
UAE	Uterine artery embolization
UDCA	Ursodeoxycholic acid
US	Ultrasound
US	The United States
USPTF	United States Preventive Services Task Force
UTI	Urinary tract infection
VACTERL	Disorder consisting of vertebral defects, anal atresia, cardiac defects, tracheo-esophageal fistula, renal anomalies and limb abnormalities
VEGF	Vascular endothelial growth factor
V/Q	Ventilation-perfusion scan
VTE	Venous thromboembolism
WBC	White blood cell counts
WHO	World Health Organization
WNL	Within normal limits

SECTION 1

GYNECOLOGY

Section Outline

1. Well-woman Examination
2. Infertility Assessment
3. Polycystic Ovary Syndrome
4. Intrauterine Adhesions
5. Septate Uterus
6. Submucosal Uterine Fibroid
7. Chlamydia Salpingitis
8. Chronic Pelvic Pain and Pelvic Adhesions
9. Pelvic Inflammatory Disease and Tubo-ovarian Abscess
10. Ovarian Hyperstimulation Syndrome
11. Preconceptional Ultrasound
12. Menopause
13. Postmenopausal Bleeding
14. Endometrial Polyp
15. Hematometra in a Postmenopausal Patient
16. Endometrial Carcinoma
17. Leiomyosarcoma
18. Ovarian Cystadenocarcinoma
19. Borderline Ovarian Tumor
20. Ovarian Dermoid
21. Hemorrhagic Cyst
22. Ectopic Pregnancy
23. Ovarian Torsion
24. Pelvic Congestion Syndrome
25. Incisional Endometriosis
26. Secondary Dysmenorrhea
27. Uterine Fibroid
28. Pedunculated Uterine Fibroid and Endometriosis
29. IUD Complications
30. Abnormal Pap Smear and Cervical Dysplasia
31. Condylomata Acuminata
32. Primary Amenorrhea
33. Labia Minora Hypertrophy
34. Lichen Sclerosus

CHAPTER 1

Well-woman Examination

Melissa D Mendez, Osvaldo Padilla

■ CLINICAL CASE

KB is a 30-year-old G3P2 who presents to your office for a well-woman examination. She states that her periods were previously regular, every month and now she has not had a period in 6 months. She uses a Mirena IUD for contraception which you placed last year after the birth of her last baby and she is happy with the result. Her last Pap smear was 2 years ago and it was negative. She did not have an HPV test at that time. She was vaccinated against HPV about 5 years ago. She has not needed a mammogram or breast ultrasound for any reason. She has not had her cholesterol or thyroid checked. Her last HIV examination was last year, during her last pregnancy.

Menarche: Age 13.

Menses: 28/5.

LMP: 6 months ago.

Pregnancy: One miscarriage at 8 weeks requiring dilation and curettage. Two full term spontaneous vaginal deliveries, the last one complicated by preeclampsia without severe features.

Sexual history: In a monogamous relationship with her husband of 6 years. She denies a history of sexually transmitted diseases.

Contraception: Mirena IUD.

Review of Systems
- No chest pain or shortness of breath
- No diarrhea or constipation
- No urinary frequency, no hematuria or dysuria.

Past medical history: Noncontributory.

Past surgical history: Noncontributory.

Vaccines: Up to date.

Current medications: Multivitamin.

Allergies: No known drug allergies.

Social history: She does not smoke, no drug use, and no alcohol use.

Family history: Noncontributory.

Physical Examination

Vital signs: T 37.2°C oral, BP 123/73, P 83, BMI 25.

Cardiac examination: Regular rate and rhythm.

Chest examination: Lungs clear to auscultation bilaterally.

Abdomen: Nondistended, non-tender, no hepatosplenomegaly.

Extremities: No edema, 2+ pulses felt bilateral lower extremities.

Vaginal examination: Vaginal walls appear pink with rugae. Cervix appears normal, no discharge, no strings seen at os.

Bimanual examination: Uterus anteverted 8 weeks size, nontender, mobile. Adnexa have no masses, are nontender.

Pap smear results: Normal, as shown in Figure 1.1, and a negative human papillomavirus test.

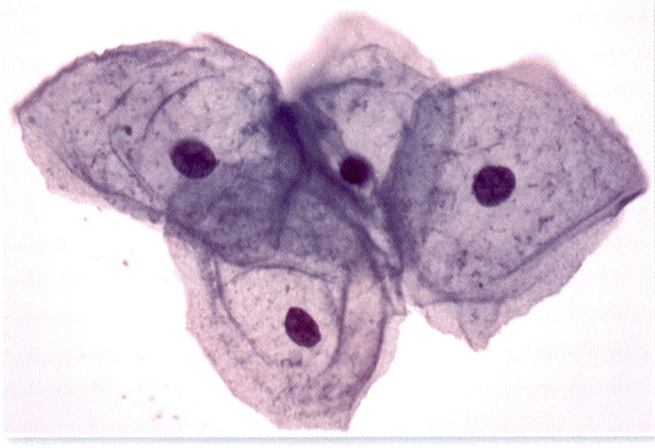

Figure 1.1: A normal Pap smear

■ CLINICAL QUESTIONS

1. What screening examinations are appropriate during a well woman examination?

Ans. Well women care guidelines are based on age. The age groups are: adolescents (13–18 years); reproductive-aged women (19–45 years); mature women (46–64 years), and women older than age 64. The American College of Obstetrics and Gynecology (ACOG) most recently updated their guidelines for well women care in 2015.[1] Patients should have a blood pressure and weight or body mass index (BMI) assessed. Patients aged 21 and older should have a pelvic examination if they have menstrual disorders, vaginal discharge, infertility or pelvic pain.[1] A bimanual examination is indicated for any procedures, such as an endometrial biopsy or IUD insertion. The decision to perform a full pelvic examination in asymptomatic women should be determined between the patient and her physician. A clinical breast examination is recommended to be performed every 1–3 years.[2] The patient can be offered cholesterol screening as needed. A discussion about diet and exercise to prevent obesity and cardiovascular disease should also take place.[3]

2. What are the current guidelines to screen for cervical cancer?

Ans. The current guidelines set forth by ACOG and American Society for Colposcopy and Cervical Pathology (ASCCP) are to begin screening for cervical cancer with Pap smears at age 21. A screening Pap smear should be obtained every 3 years through age 29.[2] A screening Pap smear test can be obtained at 5-year intervals in women who are age 30–65 with both a negative Pap smear and negative HPV test.[2]

3. What vaccines are appropriate during a well woman examination?

Ans. Each patient should be offered the appropriate vaccines based on risk factors and age group. If you choose not to stock all vaccines, you should be able to refer the patient to another provider or the local health department for the appropriate vaccines. The influenza vaccine should be given to all persons six months and older on a yearly basis.[4] Adults should also receive the tetanus, diphtheria, and pertussis vaccine at least once during their adulthood and during pregnancy after 28 weeks. A tetanus booster should be given every 10 years. Measles, mumps, rubella booster should be given in the preconception period at least three months prior to conception if the original vaccine has been shown to no longer be effective. Based on risk factors, the patient may also qualify for meningococcal, hepatitis A and hepatitis B vaccines.[5]

4. What is the management of a lost IUD?

Ans. One study suggests there is about a 10% rate of malpositioning of an IUD once placed. Symptoms associated with a malpositioned IUD are pain, irregular bleeding, pregnancy and suspected adenomyosis.[6] Once you suspect an IUD is misplaced, you may choose to visualize with either 2D or 3D ultrasound. 3D ultrasound has been shown to better visualize the IUD arms in the coronal view.[7] Retraction of the strings is the most common cause of missing strings. You can attempt to locate retracted IUD strings with a cytobrush or hook placed gently into the cervical os to sweep the strings from the endocervix.[8]

■ TAKE-HOME MESSAGES

- Guidelines for well women screening are grouped according to age. These age groups are: adolescents (13–18 years); reproductive-aged women (19–45 years); mature women (46–64 years), and women older than age 64.[1]
- Patients should have a blood pressure and weight or BMI assessed. Patients aged 21 and older should have a pelvic examination if they have menstrual disorders, vaginal discharge, infertility or pelvic pain.[1]
- A clinical breast examination is recommended to be performed every 1–3 years.[2]
- The patient can be offered cholesterol screening as needed.[2] Diet and exercise to prevent obesity and cardiovascular disease should also be discussed.[3]
- Cervical cancer screening with Pap smears should begin at age 21. A screening Pap smear should be obtained every 3 years through age 29.[2]

- A screening Pap smear test can be obtained at 5-year intervals in women who are age 30–65 with both a negative Pap smear and negative HPV test.[2]
- The influenza vaccine should be given to all persons six months and older on a yearly basis.[4]
- Adults should also receive the tetanus, diphtheria, pertussis vaccine at least once during their adulthood and during a pregnancy after 28 weeks.[4] A tetanus booster should be given every 10 years.[4]
- Measles, mumps, rubella booster should be given in the preconception period at least three months prior to conception if the original vaccine is shown to be ineffective.[4]

REFERENCES

1. Conry JA, Brown H. Well-Woman Task Force-components of the Well-woman Examination. Obstet Gynecol. 2015;126(4): 697-701.
2. The American College of Obstetricians and Gynecologists Committee Opinion Number 534. Well-woman visit. Obstet Gynecol. 2012.
3. Smith SC, Grundy SM 2013 ACC/AHA guideline recommends fixed-dose strategies instead of targeted goals to lower blood cholesterol. J Am Coll Cardiol. 2014;64(6):601-12.
4. The American College of Obstetricians and Gynecologists Committee Opinion number Integrating immunizations into practice. Obstet Gynecol. 2013;121(4):897-903.
5. Adult Immunization Schedules. Cdc.gov.vaccines/schedules/hcp/imz/adult.html accessed. 2015.
6. Braaten KP, Bensen CB, Maurer R, Goldberg AB. Malpositioned intrauterine contraceptive devices. Obstet Gynecol. 2011;118(5):1014-20.
7. Benacerraf BR, Shipp TD, Bromley B. Three-dimensional ultrasound detection of abnormally located intrauterine contraceptive devices which are a source of pelvic pain and abnormal bleeding. Ultrasound Obstet Gynecol. 2009; 34:110-5.
8. Prabhakaran S, Chuang A. In office retrieval of intrauterine contraceptive devices with missing strings. Contraception. 2011;83(2):102-6.

CHAPTER 2

Infertility Assessment

Dhyana Velasco, Sireesha Y Reddy, Sanja Kupesic Plavsic

■ CLINICAL CASE

BR is a 32-year G1P0 who presents with a history of secondary infertility for 8 years. She also has complaints of oligomenorrhea, with a recent diagnosis of polycystic ovarian syndrome (PCOS). She is taking metformin. She also has complaints of dysmenorrhea, pelvic pain, dyspareunia, postcoital bleeding, and heavy menses. On initial evaluation, she was diagnosed with a sexually transmitted disease. Subsequently, she and her partner received treatment. Test of cure was negative. Six months later, on a follow-up visit, patient was still complaining of dyspareunia, dysmenorrhea, and postcoital bleeding. Patient's abnormal bleeding pattern was initially treated with OCPs, but now patient is attempting pregnancy. Partner has children from a previous marriage; all his children are healthy and the youngest is 12 years old. Patient desires to have children.

Menses: Irregular intervals every 2–12 months.

LMP: 6 months ago; Urine pregnancy test negative.

Sexual history: Single male partner, history of *Chlamydia* and *Trichomonas*, both treated. Contraception: Attempting pregnancy. History of OCP use.

Review of Systems
- Denies weight loss or weight gain. Denies diabetes.
- Denies nausea, vomiting, indigestion, and constipation.
- Complains of abnormal and painful periods, pelvic pain, painful intercourse, and abnormal bleeding. Denies any abnormal vaginal discharge, vaginal itching or burning, urinary incontinence, urinary urgency, urinary frequency, vaginal dryness, or painful urination.

Past medical history: Significant for missed abortion 10 years ago and D and C.

Past surgical history: None.

Current medications: Sprintec and Glucophage.

Allergies: No known drug allergies.
Social history: Denies alcohol use.
Family history: Noncontributory.

Physical Examination

Alert and in no acute distress.

Vital signs: BP 105/63, HR 98.

Height: 60 in. Weight: 178 lbs.

Skin: No rashes.
Good dentition, no erythema, no exudates.

Neck: No masses, thyroid normal size.

Cardiac: Regular rate and rhythm; peripheral pulses intact, no edema.

Pulmonary: No respiratory distress.

Abdominal: Non-distended, non-tender.

Neuro: Cranial nerves II-XII intact.

Psych: Oriented to all spheres.

Pelvic Examination

- *Vulva:* Normal appearance
- *Urethra:* Normal
- *Vaginal examination:* Normal appearance of the vaginal walls
- *Cervix:* Tender
- *Uterus:* Tender, retroverted, and normal size
- *Adnexa:* No masses bilaterally
- *Rectum:* No presence of hemorrhoids.

Laboratory Tests

Pap smear negative for intraepithelial lesions or malignancy.

Pelvic ultrasound: Transvaginal ultrasound demonstrates enlarged ovaries with more than 10 follicles scattered at the periphery of enlarged ovarian stroma (Fig. 2.1). Color Doppler reveals increased intraovarian vascularity (Fig. 2.2). Saline infusion sonography (SIS) reveals partial intrauterine adhesion (Fig. 2.3).

Patient was scheduled for diagnostic laparoscopy/hysteroscopy/chromopertubation for her history of infertility (Figs 2.4 to 2.6).

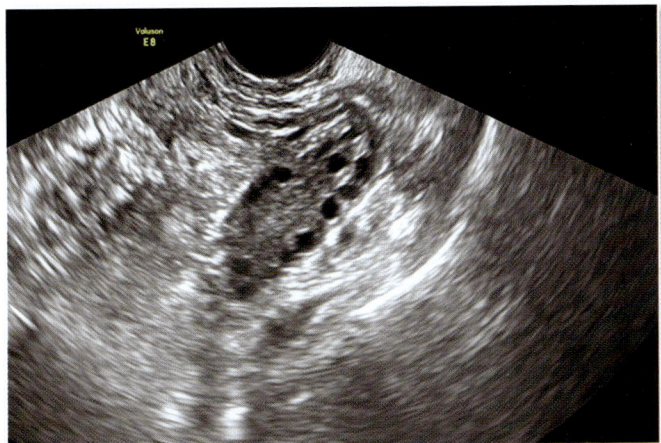

Figure 2.1: Polycystic ovarian appearance by transvaginal B mode ultrasound

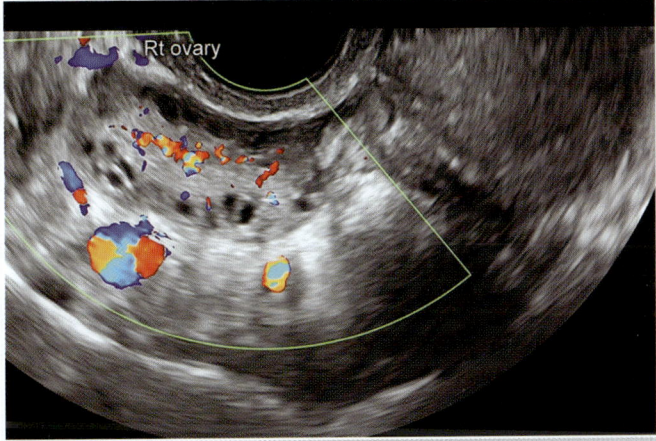

Figure 2.2: Color Doppler ultrasound illustrating increased intraovarian vascularity

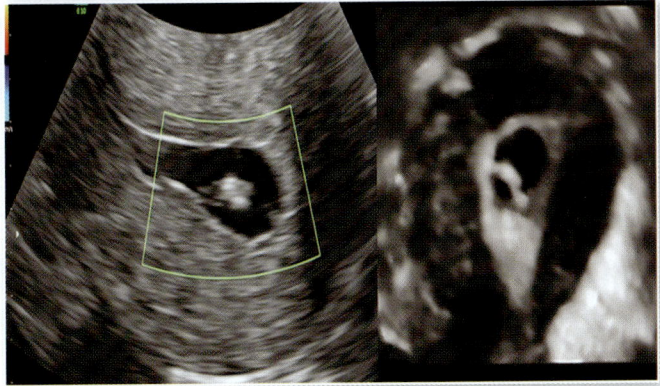

Figure 2.3: 2D and 3D saline infusion sonography illustrating thick partial intrauterine adhesions. Color Doppler reveals no blood flow

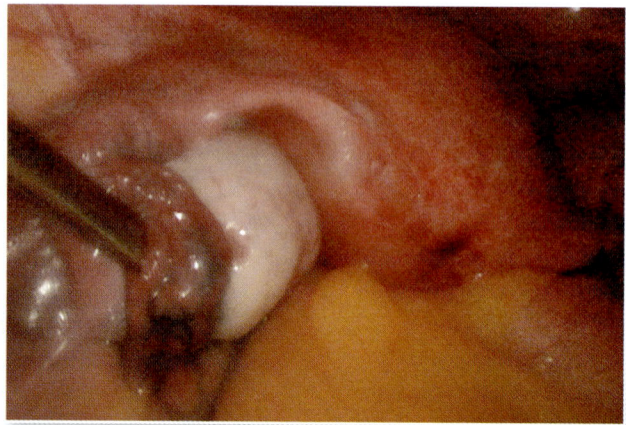

Figure 2.4: Laparoscopic chromopertubation reveals that methylene blue dye can be seen from the end of the fallopian tube spilling into the abdominal cavity indicating tubal patency

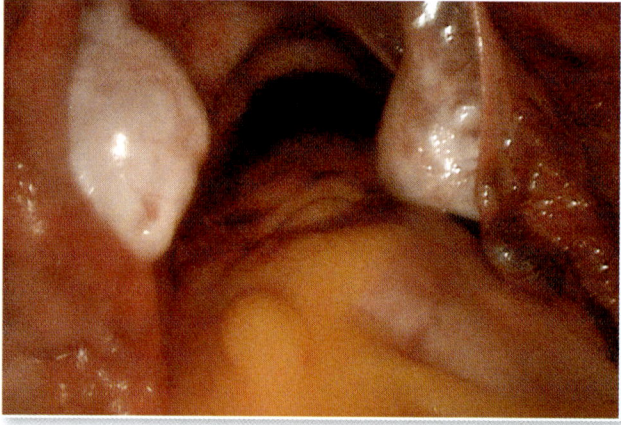

Figure 2.5: Laparoscopic chromopertubation shows the left fallopian tube patency with spillage of methylene blue dye into the abdominal cavity

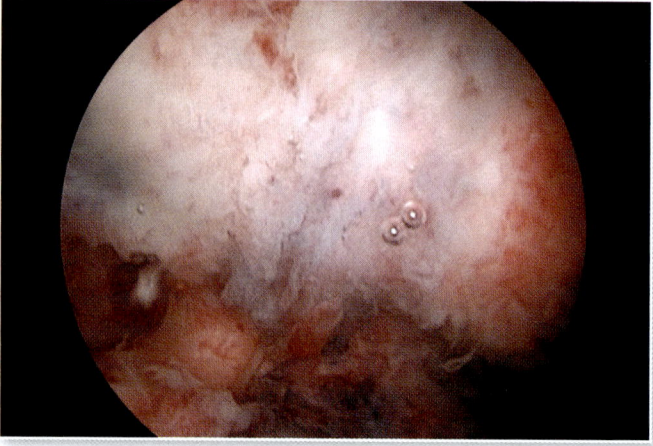

Figure 2.6: Hysteroscopy reveals an intrauterine adhesion at the right uterine fundus. Methylene blue can be seen staining the endometrium

CLINICAL QUESTIONS

1. This patient asks you why she cannot get pregnant? Based on her history, what might you tell her?

Ans. Infertility has many causes. Female factor infertility attributes to 37% of all infertility couples, male factor infertility about 8%, both male and female factor in 35%, unexplained in 5% and remainder get pregnant.[1] The most common male factors are hypogonadism and post-testicular defects, and the most common female factors are ovulatory dysfunction, tubal causes, endometriosis, coital issues, and cervical factor.[1]

2. What are the risk factors for infertility in general population of female patients? What are the risk factors for infertility in this patient?

Ans. It is estimated that 27% of cases of infertility are attributed to ovarian causes, whereas 22% are attributed to tubal or uterine causes.[2] The greatest risk factors for this patient's infertility are a history of PID, PCOS, and D and C. PID is a risk factor for infertility because it can cause tubal obstruction and widespread adhesions.[3] PCOS is a risk factor because it causes anovulatory cycles.[4]

3. She would like to know if she needs to see a reproductive infertility specialist first?

Ans. You tell her that it is appropriate for primary care physicians to initiate the infertility evaluation. When there are abnormal findings, the patient should be referred to an infertility specialist. Fertility specialists provide expertise and cost efficient care while meeting the emotional, experiential and diagnostic needs of the patient.[5] American Society for Reproductive Medicine (ASRM) provides the guidelines for referrals to infertility specialists.[6]

4. She would like to know what tests you will be ordering to evaluate her infertility.

Ans. You will let her know that both she and her partner have a high likelihood of having a diagnosis that may lead to a cause of her infertility. So, both individuals should be evaluated. Semen analysis to assess male factors, day 3 FSH and estradiol levels, hysterosalpingography to assess tubal patency and uterine anomalies, endocrine causes, such as thyroid or pituitary prolactinomas, ovarian reserve evaluation using an antral follicle count, sonogram, and possibly a laparoscopy.[7]

She had a sonogram which revealed thickened endometrial lining. A saline infusion sonohysterography (SIS) revealed intrauterine adhesions. She was told to have a diagnostic laparoscopy with chromopertubation and a hysteroscopy to remove the adhesions. Figures 2.4 and 2.5 reveal that both fallopian tubes are patent using methylene blue dye test. Figure 2.6 reveals an intrauterine pathology. There is an intrauterine fundal adhesion that was incised with the resectoscope.

TAKE-HOME MESSAGES

- Male factor and ovulatory dysfunction are the two most common causes of infertility.[1-4]
- An infertility specialist evaluation is generally most cost effective and patient centered.
- A majority of the cases of female infertility are due to ovarian and tubal causes.[3]
- PID can cause intrinsic tubal disease and lead to tubal obstruction. A hysterosalpingogram can aid in the diagnosis of tubal factor as a cause for female infertility.[5,6]

- Fertility evaluation should take place if a couple unable to conceive after one year of unprotected intercourse and if the woman is over 35.[5-7]
- Basic infertility evaluation includes history, physical, semen analysis, menstrual history, hysterosalpingogram and sonography.[7]
- Laparoscopic chromopertubation with methylene blue dye can assist in assessing tubal patency. Spillage into the abdomen reveals tubal patency.[7]

REFERENCES

1. WHO Technical Report Series. Recent Advances in Medically Assisted Conception. 1992;820:1-111.
2. Hoffman BL, Schorge JO, Schaffer JI, et al. Chapter 19. Evaluation of the Infertile Couple. Williams Gynecology, 2nd edn. New York, NY: McGraw-Hill; 2012.
3. Hou H Y, et al. Related factors associated with pelvic adhesion and its influence on fallopian tube recanalization in infertile patients. Zhonghua Fu Chan Ke Za Zhi. 2012;47(11):823-8.
4. Gordon P, Treasure JL, King EA, et al. Prevalence of polycystic ovaries in women with anovulation and idiopathinc hirsutism. British Medical Journal. 1986;293(6543):355-9.
5. Vander Laan B, Karande V, Krohm C, et al. Cost considerations with infertility therapy: outcome and cost comparison between health maintenance organization and preferred provider organization care based on physician and facility cost. Hum Reprod. 1998;12(5):1200.
6. Practice Committee of the American Society for Reproductive Medicine. Revised minimum standards for practices offering assisted reproductive technologies: a committee opinion. Fertil Steril. 2014;102(3):682.
7. Practice Committee of American Society for Reproductive Medicine. Diagnostic Evaluation of the infertile female: a committee opinion. Fertil Steril. 2012;98(2):302.

CHAPTER

Polycystic Ovary Syndrome

3

Sanja Kupesic Plavsic

■ CLINICAL CASE

SC is a 28-year-old oligomenorrheic and hirsute female who failed to conceive despite two years of normal sexual activity. Her family history is significant for type 2 diabetes mellitus. Her pregnancy test is negative. Elevated testosterone and decreased progesterone levels were detected. Her FSH was normal, but her LH was elevated. Her TSH, prolactin, chemistry panel, cholesterol, triglycerides, HDL, and LDL were all within normal limits. Her fasting insulin level and fasting glucose were elevated (38 IU/mL and 140 mg/dL respectively) and the 2-hour value on glucose tolerance test was 250 mg/dL. Results of her transvaginal ultrasound examination are presented on Figures 3.1 to 3.4.

Menarche: Age 13.

Menses: 45–90 days/5–7 days.

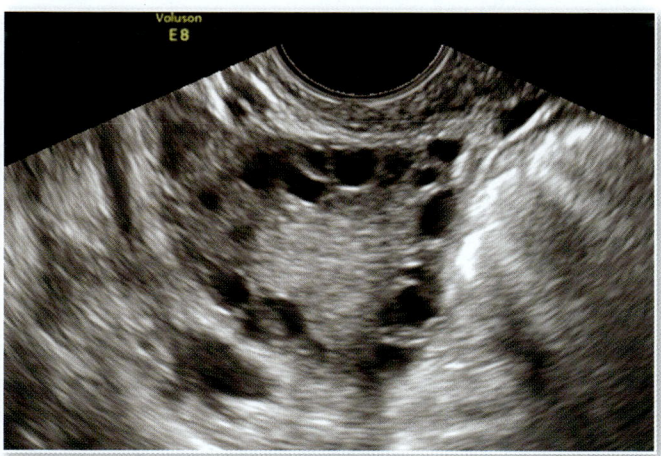

Figure 3.1: Transvaginal ultrasound demonstrates bilaterally enlarged ovaries (right ovary 12 cm³ and left ovary 15 cm³), multiple small peripheral cysts measuring between 2 and 10 mm (15 cysts on the right, and 18 cysts on the left ovary), around a dense core of stroma

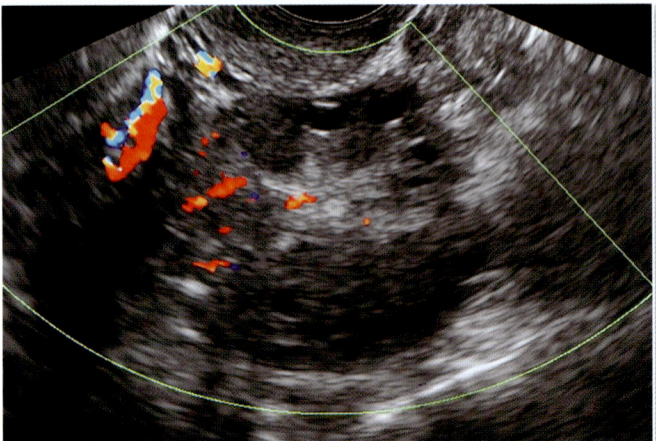

Figure 3.2: Transvaginal color Doppler imaging shows increased intraovarian vascularity

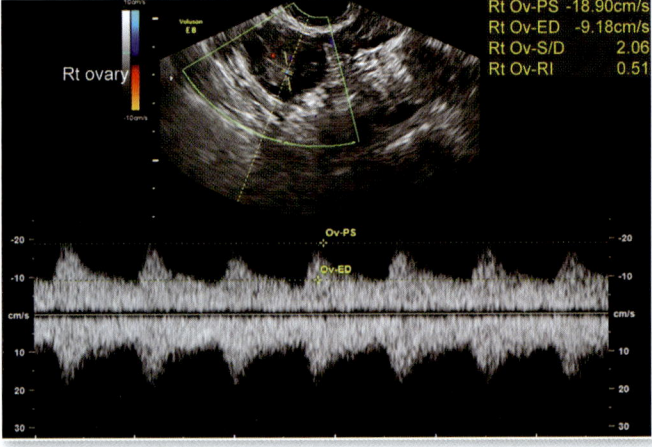

Figure 3.3: Pulsed Doppler waveform analysis reveals moderate vascular impedance (RI 0.51) in the ovarian stromal vessels

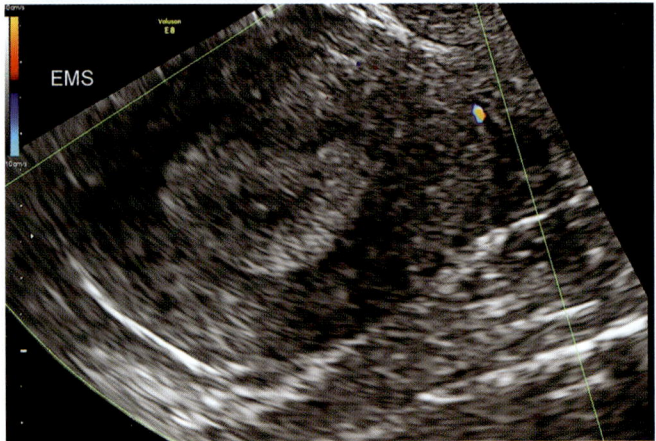

Figure 3.4: Transvaginal color Doppler image of the uterus demonstrates thick avascular endometrium (maximal thickness of 16 mm)

LMP: 4 months ago.

Pregnancies: None.

Sexual history: Two male partners over her lifetime. *Chlamydia* test and Pap smear were performed 4 months ago; both were normal.

Contraception: None.

Review of Systems

- No headaches, no problems with vision
- No history of blood clots DVT or PE
- No heart palpitations, no shortness of breath
- No abdominal/pelvic pain
- No nausea, vomiting, constipation and/or diarrhea
- Normal urination; no symptoms of UTI.

Past medical history: None; no hospitalizations.

Past surgical history: None.

Vaccines: Up to date.

Medications: None.

Allergies: None known drug allergies.

Social history: SC is a librarian. She drinks alcohol occasionally and in moderation. She does not smoke, and reports no history of substance abuse.

Family history: Mother: 64 years; history of type 2 diabetes mellitus. Father: 68 years, history of hypertension and type 2 diabetes mellitus. No family history of uterine, breast, ovarian or colon cancer.

Physical Examination

- *Vital signs:* T 36.7°C; BP 140/90; P 72; BMI 32.
- Coarse hair was noticed on the face, chest, upper arms and legs. Acne noted over face, chest, and back. Evidence of thinning hair. Darkened skin was noted on the neck, in the armpits and inner thighs. Skin tags were visualized in the armpits.
- Normal heart, lungs and thyroid examination.
- Pelvic examination was unremarkable, including no evidence of clitoromegaly. Uterus and adnexa were very difficult to assess secondary to the patient's obesity.
- Because the patient has amenorrhea for 4 months, an endometrial aspiration was performed. The uterus sounded to 7 cm and there was a good amount of tissue retrieved, that was sent for histologic evaluation. The endometrial aspirate showed proliferative endometrium without hyperplasia or neoplasia.

■ CLINICAL QUESTIONS

1. What is the most likely diagnosis?

Ans. The clinical, laboratory, and imaging results are consistent with PCOS.

2. What is the most appropriate therapeutic choice for this patient?

Ans. Because SC desires a pregnancy, she is a good candidate for metformin, not only for the control of her blood sugar, but also for regulation of her menstrual cycle.[1] 1,500–2,000 mg of metformin per day, divided in two to three doses should be prescribed to stimulate resumption of normal menses and ovulation. The patient also requires change of her lifestyle, including low caloric diet and exercise program for weight loss. At the time of her follow up visit in three months the blood sugar needs to be reassessed.[2]

3. The patient comes for follow-up examination 3 months later and you find that she lost 5 kg and that her blood sugars responded well. What is the next step in the management of this patient?

Ans. Ovulation induction with clomiphene citrate.[2]

4. What should be done if the patient conceives?

Ans. Once the patient conceives, metformin should be discontinued, because its use is not FDA approved during pregnancy.

■ TAKE-HOME MESSAGES

- PCOS is one of the most common female endocrinopathies, with an incidence of 5–10% in women of reproductive age.[1,2]
- Polycystic ovaries are characterized with enlarged ovarian volumes (>10 cm³), presence of multiple small follicles measuring less than 10 mm. Because these small follicles are incapable to ovulate, the hormonal levels became imbalanced: estrogen, androgen and LH levels are typically elevated, while progesterone level is decreased.[1,3]
- Women with PCOS have less than 6–8 menstrual periods per year (oligomenorrhea). Irregular or absent menstrual periods increase their risk of endometrial overgrowth or even endometrial cancer.[3,4]
- Most, but not all patients with PCOS are overweight or obese, with insulin resistance and at increased risk of developing diabetes, heart disease and sleep apnea.[5]
- A significant proportion of PCOS patients are infertile and infertility evaluation is recommended after 12 months of trying to get pregnant.[1,2]
- OCPs are the first treatment option for patients who do not want to conceive. OCPs protect from endometrial overgrowth, and alleviate acne and hirsutism symptoms.[6]
- Lifestyle changes consisting of low calories diet, weight loss and exercises improve body composition, hyperandrogenism, and insulin resistance in women with PCOS.[7]
- In women with PCOS metformin treatment reduces hyperinsulinemia and hyperandrogenemia, independently of changes in body weight. In a large number of subjects these changes are associated with striking, sustained improvements in menstrual abnormalities and resumption of ovulation.[8]
- There are many controversies regarding the treatment of infertile women with PCSOS. The first line treatment for ovulation induction of PCOS patients is the antiestrogen, clomiphene citrate (CC). Should CC fail, the second line intervention is administration of exogenous gonadotropins and laparoscopic ovarian surgery.[9] The use of gonadotropins is associated with increased chances for multiple pregnancy, and therefore, intense sonographic monitoring of ovarian response is required. Recommended third line treatment is in vitro fertilization and embryo transfer (IVF/ET).[9]
- Laparoscopic ovarian drilling (LOD) may reduce the need for gonadotropins or may facilitate their use. The procedure is performed on an outpatient basis, and reports from the literature indicate a high rate of spontaneous ovulation and conception.[10] Major advantage of LOD is reduction in multiple pregnancy rates. The major ongoing concern of LOD is a possible negative effect on the ovarian reserve.

REFERENCES

1. Pannill M. Polycystic Ovary Syndrome: an Overview. Medscape. http://www.medscape.com/viewarticle/438597_5. Updated November 14, 2015.
2. Legro RS, Barnhart HX, Schlaff WD, et al. Clomiphene, metformin, or both for infertility in the polycystic ovary syndrome. N Engl J Med 2007; 356(6):551-66.
3. Rotterdam ESHRE/ASRM-Sponsored PCOS consensus workshop group. Revised 2003 consensus on diagnostic criteria and long-term health risks related to polycystic ovary syndrome (PCOS). Hum Reprod 2004; 19(1):41-7.
4. Dumesic DA, Lobo RA. Cancer risk and PCOS. Steroids 2013; 78(8):782-5.
5. Randeva HS, Tan BK, Weickert MO, et al. Cardiometabolic aspects of the polycystic ovary syndrome. Endocr Rev 2012; 33(5):812-41.
6. Legro RS, Arslanian SA, Ehrmann DA, et al. Diagnosis and treatment of polycystic ovary syndrome: an Endocrine Society clinical practice guideline. J Clin Endocrinol Metab 2013; 98(12):4565-92.
7. Pasquali R, Gambineri A, Cavazza C, et al. Heterogeneity in the responsiveness to long-term lifestyle intervention and predictability in obese women with polycystic ovary syndrome. Eur J Endocrinol 2011; 164(1):53-60.
8. Moghetti P, Castello R, Negri C, et al. Metformin effects on clinical features, endocrine and metabolic profiles, and insulin sensitivity in polycystic ovary syndrome: a randomized, double-blind, placebo-controlled 6-month trial, followed by open, long-term clinical evaluation. J Clin Endocrinol Metab 2000; 85(1):139-46.
9. Thessaloniki ESHRE/ASRM-Sponsored PCOS Consensus Workshop Group. Consensus on infertility treatment related to polycystic ovary syndrome. Fertil Steril 2008; 89(3):505-22.
10. Farquhar C, LIlford RJ, Marjribanks J, Vandekerckhove P. Laparoscopic "drilling" by diathermy or laser for ovulation induction in anovulatory polycystic ovary syndrome. Cochrane Database Syst Rev 2005; 20(3):CD001122.

CHAPTER

Intrauterine Adhesions

4

Sanja Kupesic Plavsic, Osvaldo Padilla

■ CLINICAL CASE

DM is a 33-year-old G1P0 who was referred to a gynecologist because of secondary amenorrhea. Ten months ago she was diagnosed with missed abortion at 8 weeks gestation. Due to retained products of conception she underwent D and C. Since then she reports extremely light menstrual flow.

Menarche: Age 13.

Menses: Amenorrheic for one year.

LMP: 1 year ago.

Pregnancies: One missed abortion at 8 weeks gestation.

Sexual history: Has had three male partners over her lifetime. *Chlamydia* test and Pap smear were performed 6 months ago both were normal.

Review of Systems

- No headaches, no problems with vision
- No history of blood clots DVT or PE
- No heart palpitations, no shortness of breath
- No abdominal/pelvic pain
- No nausea, vomiting, constipation and/or diarrhea
- Normal urination; no symptoms of UTI.

Past medical history: None; no hospitalizations.

Past surgical history: None.

Vaccines: Up to date.

Medications: None.

Allergies: None known drug allergies.

Social history: DM is a secretary. She drinks alcohol occasionally and in moderation. She does not smoke, and reports no history of substance abuse.

Family history: Mother: 55 years, no medical problems. Father: 58 years, controlled hypertension. No family history of uterine, breast, ovarian or colon cancer.

Physical Examination

- *Vital signs*: BP 120/80; P 62; BMI 19
- Normal heart, lungs, thyroid and neck
- Abdominal examination and pelvic examination: Normal.

Investigations

- Pregnancy test is negative. Estrogen–progestin withdrawal test was negative
- FSH, LH, and estradiol levels were normal
- Orders were placed for pelvic ultrasound and saline infusion sonohysterography (SIS). The results are presented in Figures 4.1 to 4.4. Based on sonographic findings, the patient was scheduled for therapeutic hysteroscopy for lysis of intrauterine adhesions.

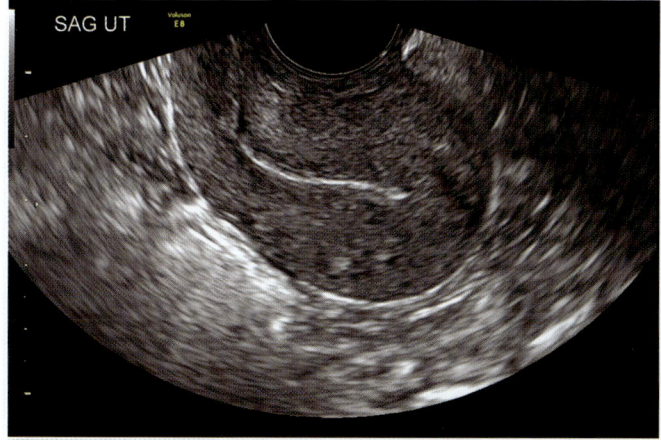

Figure 4.1: Transvaginal scan of the patient presenting with hypomenorrhea. The endometrium is hyperechogenic and thin (3 mm)

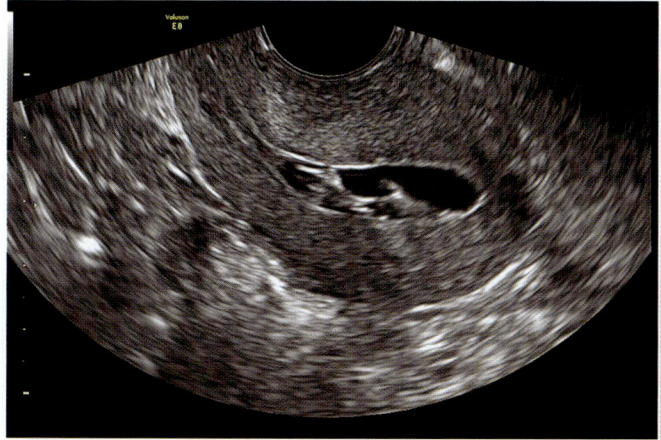

Figure 4.2: Saline infusion sonography of the same patient. Following distension of the uterine cavity with saline a fibrotic band, typical for intrauterine adhesion is clearly visualized

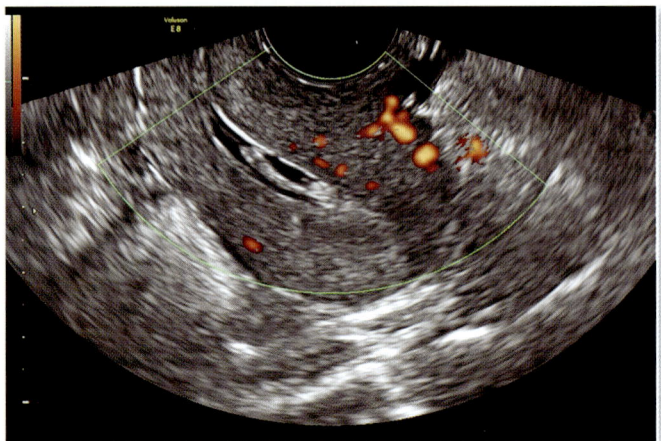

Figure 4.3: The same patient evaluated by color Doppler ultrasound. Note avascular intrauterine adhesions

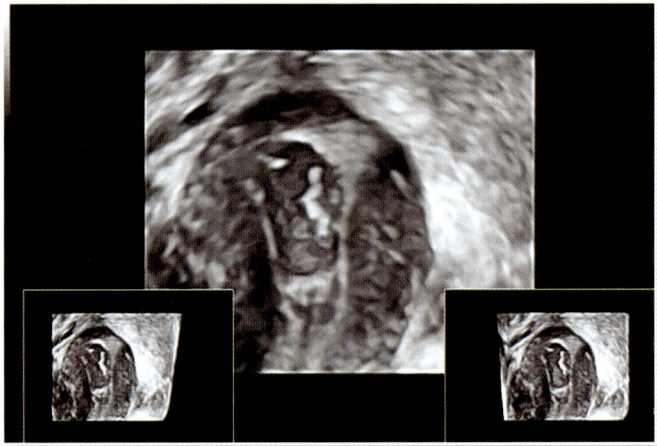

Figure 4.4: Three-dimensional ultrasound (surface rendering mode) clearly outlines two intrauterine adhesions

■ CLINICAL QUESTIONS

1. What is Asherman's syndrome?

Ans. Asherman's syndrome is defined as secondary amenorrhea, occurring in patients with normal endocrine function, due to intrauterine adhesions. Intrauterine adhesions or synechia may form due to endometrial trauma from D and C for treatment of pregnancy complications, such as incomplete abortion, postpartum hemorrhage or retained products of conception. In developing countries with relatively high prevalence of tuberculosis, genital tuberculosis may also lead to formation of avascular or hypovascular fibrous strands within the uterine cavity (Fig. 4.5). Intrauterine adhesions can also develop as a result of endometrial trauma following myomectomy or D and C for indications not related to pregnancy.

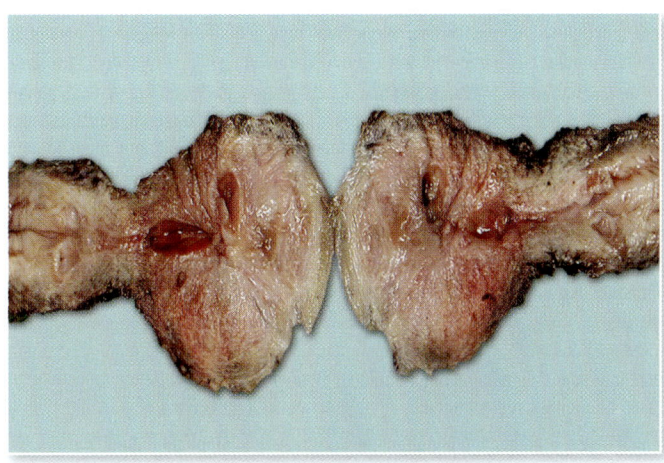

Figure 4.5: Intrauterine adhesions typically demonstrate "loose" fibrous connective tissue with variable vascularity and inflammation

2. What is used for prevention of intrauterine adhesions?

Ans. Expectant management of spontaneous abortion and medical management of spontaneous or induced abortion may potentially reduce the prevalence of Asherman syndrome. Routine use of estrogen following D and C has been suggested for postpartum patients (due to their hypoestrogenic state). However, a final recommendation cannot be made because of insufficient data in evidence based literature.

3. What is the gold standard for management of intrauterine adhesions?

Ans. Hysteroscopy is the gold standard for diagnosis and lysis of intrauterine adhesions/synechiae. It allows direct visualization of the uterine cavity and differentiation between partial and diffuse intrauterine adhesions. Adhesions are surgically resected under direct visualization, decreasing the likelihood of trauma to the surrounding endometrium. To reduce the risk of formation of postoperative intrauterine adhesions gynecologist may place an intrauterine bladder catheter with a 5 cc balloon for 10 days, introduce an IUD for three months or prescribe postoperative estrogen therapy for women with no contraindications. Based on the available data, the outcomes are better with the use of catheter and postoperative estrogen therapy. Estrogen (2.5 mg of conjugated equine estrogen or 4 mg of estradiol) is given twice daily for 30 days, followed with 10 days of progestin therapy. Patients should be followed three months after hysteroscopy with SIS, hysterosalpingogram or office hysteroscopy to reassess the anatomy of the uterine cavity.

■ TAKE-HOME MESSAGES

- Clinical symptoms of intrauterine adhesions/synechiae are secondary amenorrhea, hypomenorrhea, infertility and recurrent pregnancy loss. Some patients may refer cyclic pelvic pain due to obstruction of menstrual flow and hematometra.[1,2]
- Diagnostic assessment consists of the medical history (focusing on the history of uterine procedures, such as D and C related to pregnancy), surgical history (e.g. myomectomy, endometrial ablation), and history of pelvic inflammatory disease (endometritis).[1-6]

- If progestin and/or estrogen-progesteron withdrawal test does not result in uterine bleeding, the patient should be evaluated by pelvic ultrasound and SIS. Alternatively, X-ray hysterosalpingogram (HSG) or office hysteroscopy can be performed.[1,2] Hysteroscopy is performed in an office or operative room setting.
- According to the American Society for Reproductive Medicine, intrauterine adhesions are classified based upon the extent of the uterine cavity involvement (adhesions involving less than 1/3rd of the uterine cavity, adhesions involving from 1/3rd to 2/3rd of the uterine cavity, adhesions involving more than 2/3rd of the uterine cavity), the type of adhesions (filmy, filmy and dense, dense), and the patient's menstrual pattern (normal, hypomenorrhea, amenorrhea).[1,2]
- Therapeutic hysteroscopy begins by placing the hysteroscope at the level of the internal cervical os and lysis of the most proximal adhesions with sharp dissection by rigid scissors. Alternatively, the surgeon can use bipolar electrosurgery to vaporize the intrauterine fibrotic bands. The final goal of operative hysteroscopy is to restore the uterine cavity.[1,2]
- Ultrasound guided hysteroscopy may be beneficial in patients with complete obliteration of the uterine cavity.[7]
- The recurrence rate following hysteroscopic lysis of intrauterine adhesions is 33% in patients with mild-to-moderate intrauterine adhesions, and up to 66% in patients with severe adhesions.[8]
- The recurrence of intrauterine adhesions can be reduced by reducing the mechanical barrier (e.g. inserting an intrauterine bladder catheter or IUD) with or without pharmacological therapy. For women with no contraindications for estrogen therapy, postoperative estrogen treatment for 30 days, followed with 10 days of progestin therapy is recommended. [9,10]
- Reassessment of the uterine cavity with office hysteroscopy, SIS or HSG should be performed three months after the procedure.[1,2]

■ REFERENCES

1. Hooker AB, Lemmers M, Thurkow AL, et al. Systematic review and meta-analysis of intrauterine adhesions after miscarriage: prevalence, risk factors and long-term reproductive outcome. Hum Reprod Update. 2014;20(2):262-78.
2. Cedars MI, Anaya T. Intrauterine adhesions. UpToDate. http://www.uptodate.com/contents/intrauterine-adhesions. Accessed February 20, 2015.
3. Rasheed SM, Amin MM, Abd Ellah AH, et al. Reproductive performance after conservative surgical treatment of postpartum hemorrhage. Int J Gynaecol Obstet. 2014;124(3):248-52.
4. Di Spiezio Sardo A, Mazzon I, Bramante S, et al. Hysteroscopic myomectomy: a comprehensive review of surgical techniques. Hum Reprod Update. 2008;14(2):101-19.
5. Taskin O, Sadik S, Onoglu A, et al. Role of endometrial suppression on the frequency of intrauterine adhesions after resectoscopic surgery. J Am Assoc Gynecol Laparosc. 2000;7(3):351-4.
6. Mazzon I, Favilli A, Cocco P, et al. Does cold loop hysteroscopic myomectomy reduce intrauterine adhesions? A retrospective study. Fertil Steril. 2014;101(1):294-8.
7. Fedele L, Bianchi S, Dorta M, Vignali M. Intrauterine adhesions: detection with transvaginal US. Radiology. 1996;199(3):757-9.
8. AAGL Advancing Minimally Invasive Gynecology Worldwide. AAGL practice report: practice guidelines for management of intrauterine synechiae. J Minim Invasive Gynecol. 2010;17(1):1-7.
9. Chen Y, Chang Y, Yao S. Role of angiogenesis in endometrial repair of patients with severe intrauterine adhesion. Int J Clin Exp Pathol. 2013;6(7):1343-50.
10. Roy KK, Negi N, Subbaiah M, et al. Effectiveness of estrogen in the prevention of intrauterine adhesions after hysteroscopic septal resection: a prospective, randomized study. J Obstet Gynaecol Res. 2014;40(4):1085-8.

CHAPTER 5

Septate Uterus

Sanja Kupesic Plavsic, Osvaldo Padilla

■ CLINICAL CASE

AH is a 35-year-old G3P0 who is referred to a gynecologist because of secondary infertility. Her LMP started three weeks ago. Her cycles are regular, every 28 days and periods last about 5 days. Her obstetrical history is significant for three missed abortions: 5 years ago at 7 weeks gestation, three years ago at 8 weeks gestation and one year ago at 9 weeks gestation. Pap smear, wet mount, Chlamydia and gonorrhea tests performed three months ago were within normal limits. Sperm analysis of her husband is normal.

Menarche: Age 13.

Menstrual cycle: 28/5 days.

LMP: 3 weeks ago.

Obstetric history: Three miscarriages (7, 8, and 9 weeks) five, three and one year ago.

Sexual history: In monogamous relationship with her husband; no history of sexually transmitted disease (STD).

Contraception: None.

Review of Systems

- No chest pain or shortness of breath
- No diarrhea or constipation
- No urinary frequency, hematuria or dysuria.

Past medical history: Dysmenorrhea.

Past surgical history: Tonsillectomy.

Vaccines: Up to date (hepatitis B vaccine series, MMR booster, and flu shot).

Current medications: None.

Allergies: No known drug allergies.

Social history: AH is a secretary; she does not smoke, drinks alcohol occasionally, and reports no history of substance abuse.

Family history: Unremarkable.

Physical Examination

Vital signs: T 36.8°C oral; BP 110/80; P 74; BMI 21.

Cardiac examination: No heart murmur was detected.

Chest examination: Clear lungs, breathing sound was clear.

Abdominal examination: Within normal limits.

Pelvic examination: External genitalia and cervix with no visible abnormalities. The uterus of normal, non-gravid size is in AVF, and is without nodularity. There are no palpable adnexal masses.

■ CLINICAL QUESTIONS

1. What is the first line of investigation for this patient?

Ans. The first line investigation for this patient is three-dimensional (3D) transvaginal ultrasound (Figs 5.1 and 5.2).

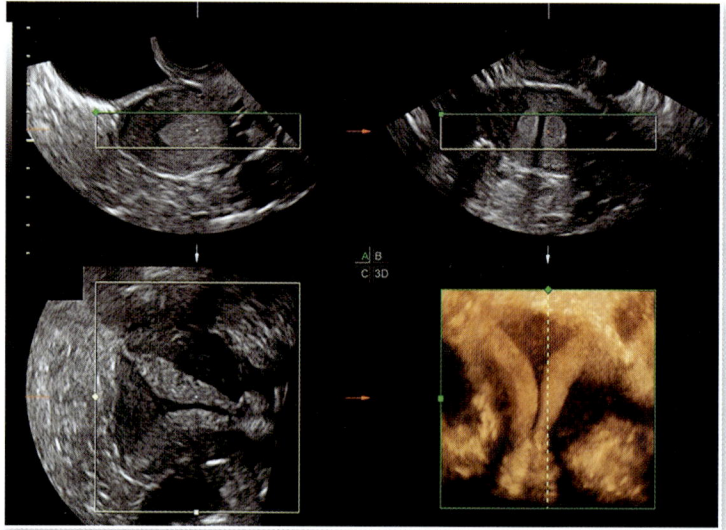

Figure 5.1: Three-dimensional transvaginal ultrasound demonstrates clear division of the uterine cavity in coronal plane (lower left image, C) and by surface reconstruction (lower right image, D). Divided uterine cavity and convex fundus are typical for septate uterus, and distinguish this anomaly from a bicornuate uterus, which has a typical heart shape fundal cleft

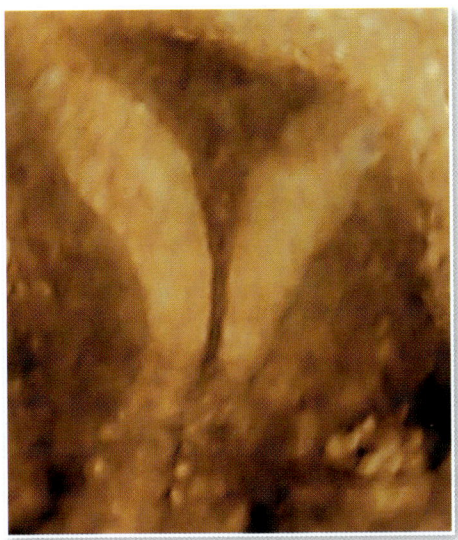

Figure 5.2: Three-dimensional reconstruction of the uterine cavity. Note a division of the uterine cavity and endocervical canal. Note that pelvic examination did not reveal abnormal cervical morphology, indicating that there is a single external orifice

2. **What are the advantages of 3D ultrasound for the assessment of uterine anomalies?**

Ans. Three-dimensional ultrasound displays the images in longitudinal (A), transverse (B) and coronal (C) planes (Fig. 5.1). The longitudinal (A) and transverse (B) planes are available with conventional 2D ultrasound scanning, but are not demonstrated simultaneously. Coronal plane (C) is a digital reconstruction of the plane orthogonal to the transducer (Fig. 5.1), and is not available on conventional 2D imaging. Coronal plane (C) and surface reconstruction (D) are especially useful for demonstration of uterine anomalies and/or confirmation of normality.[1-6]

3. **What is the difference in clinical and imaging findings between septate, bicornuate, and didelphys uterus?**

Ans. Septate uterus involves a partial or full midline septum between the two uterine horns, which is composed of the myometrium and fibrous tissue.[1-6] The external contour of septate uterus is convex or flat (Fig. 5.3). Embryologically, this anomaly results from an abnormality of the midline septal regression (similar to the development of the arcuate uterus) after complete fusion of the Müllerian ducts.[7]

Bicornuate uterus (commonly referred as "heart shaped" uterus) results from a partial non-fusion of the Müllerian ducts. In complete bicornuate uterus the central myometrium may extend to the level of the internal cervical os (bicornuate unicollis), or external cervical os (bicornuate bicollis). The latter is distinguished from the uterus didelphys because it demonstrates some degree of fusion between the two horns, while in classic didelphys uterus, the two horns and cervices are completely separated. Another difference between dydelphys and bicornuate uterus is that the horns of the bicornuate uteri are not fully developed; typically, they are smaller than those of the didelphys uterus.[6,7] Clinically, the

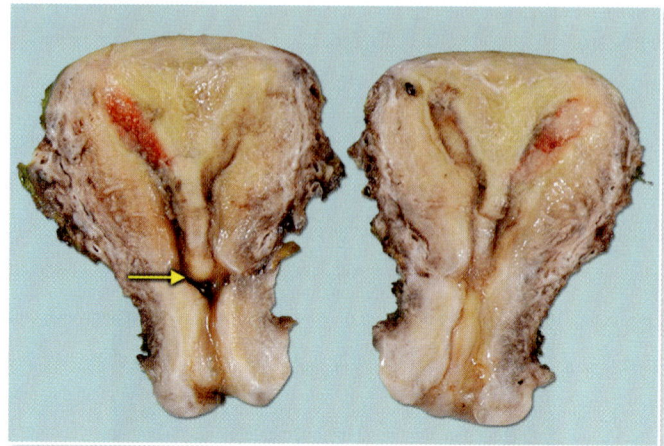

Figure 5.3: Gross anatomy image of a septate uterus in which the uterine cavity is partitioned into two. Note that the septal tip (yellow arrow) only extends to the lower uterine area with only one cervical os identified. The outer uterine surface is grossly unremarkable

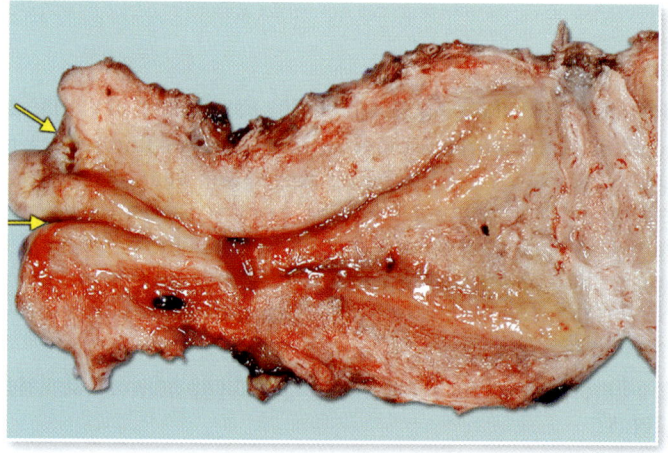

Figure 5.4: Gross anatomy of uterus didelphys. Note complete uterine septum that partitions the uterus into two distinct uterine cavities, endocervical canals and cervices (demarcated by two separate yellow arrows)

pregnancy rates of patients with bicornuate uterus are similar to the general population, so surgery is not usually indicated. It is an option if the patient has a history of recurrent pregnancy loss, reunification of the uterus may be attempted via laparoscopy or laparotomy.[6]

Uterus didelphys is comprised of two separate, fully developed uterine horns with two cervices (Fig. 5.4). It has a high association with transverse vaginal septa. This may lead to difficulties in intercourse or vaginal delivery.[6] Clinically, patients may present with preterm births, recurrent pregnancy loss, and pelvic pain. Patients may opt to have the septum resected and/or have metroplasty performed. These patients have good reproductive outcomes and they have full-term pregnancies because each horn is technically a fully developed uterus. Surgical treatment is not indicated if a patient has recurrent pregnancy loss because it is generally believed that it would not improve pregnancy outcomes.

Embryologically, didelphys uterus has a similar etiology as bicornuate uterus (failure of fusion of the paramesonephric ducts during the seventh to ninth weeks of development).[7]

4. List the advantages and disadvantages of different diagnostic procedures used for detection of congenital uterine anomalies.

Ans. Table 5.1 presents the advantages and disadvantages of X-ray hysterosalpingography (HSG), 2D ultrasound, 3D ultrasound, SIS, MRI, hysteroscopy, and laparoscopy in the assessment of congenital uterine anomalies (From reference 6, with permission).

Table 5.1 Diagnostic procedures for detection of congenital uterine anomalies (from reference 6, with permission)

Diagnostic method	Advantages	Disadvantages
X-ray HSG	• Provides a good outline of the uterine cavity • Simultaneous demonstration of tubal patency	• Invasive • Exposure to radiation • Lack of visualization of the uterine fundus • Impossible distinction between different types of fusion and resorption disorders • Patients' discomfort
2D ultrasound	• Noninvasive • Uterine cavity can be visualized in longitudinal and transverse planes • Detection of the two endometrial echoes in the upper portion of the uterine cavity in transverse plane indicates duplication anomaly of the uterus • Good screening tool	• Does not visualize the coronal plane • Morphology of the uterus cannot be objectively analyzed
3D ultrasound	• Noninvasive • Visualization of the coronal plane • Assessment of planar reformatted sections through the uterus • Coronal plane and surface rendering of the uterine cavity • Simultaneous assessment of the fundal shape	• Operator dependent • Requires technical competence • Limitations: shadowing caused by the uterine fibroids, irregular endometrial lining and decreased volume of the uterine cavity (in cases of intrauterine adhesions)
Saline infusion sonography	• Invasive • Simultaneous demonstration of tubal patency	• Minimally invasive • Operator dependent • Avoids radiation exposure • Patients' discomfort
MRI	• Noninvasive • Simultaneous visualization of the uterine cavity and fundal shape • High diagnostic precision and accuracy	• Expensive
Hysteroscopy	• Direct visualization of the uterine cavity • Allows concurrent diagnosis and treatment	• Invasive • Cannot accurately differentiate between the different subtypes of congenital uterine anomalies (does not visualize the fundal shape)
Hysteroscopy + laparoscopy	• Allows concurrent diagnosis and treatment	• Invasive • Direct visualization of the uterine cavity (hysteroscopy) and uterine surface/serosa (laparoscopy)

■ TAKE-HOME MESSAGES

- The reported prevalence of congenital uterine anomalies in the general population of reproductive age women is between 3 and 4%[8]. A recent 3D ultrasound study reported that the rate of congenital uterine anomalies is 13.3% in the subfertile female population.[8] Noninvasive ultrasound studies confirmed that congenital uterine anomalies are highly prevalent in women seeking assisted reproductive treatment, and apparently the most common types of the uterine anomaly are arcuate and septate uterus.[1,5,8]
- A number of imaging techniques can be used to diagnose and differentiate among congenital uterine anomalies (Table 5.1).[6] 2D ultrasound has low accuracy rates, but can be efficiently used as a screening tool.
- X-ray HSG and SIS are highly accurate for the assessment of the uterine cavity, but are invasive and do not clearly demonstrate the shape of the uterine fundus.
- 3D ultrasound is highly accurate diagnostic modality for detection of the congenital uterine anomalies due to its ability to simultaneously visualize the uterine cavity and external contours of the uterine myometrium and fundus. Because of multiplanar imaging and surface rendering, 3D ultrasound can detect uterine anomalies that are more inconspicuous, such as arcuate uterus, which can be overlooked by invasive procedures like hysteroscopy. Another advantage is that the 3D ultrasound can group the congenital uterine anomalies into subclassifications. In a study which was performed to investigate the diagnostic accuracy and precision of this novel imaging technique, a 93% positive and 100% negative predictive values were confirmed.[9]
- Due to high cost MRI is not accepted as a screening or diagnostic tool for detection of congenital uterine anomalies. More studies are required to determine its diagnostic accuracy.
- By many specialists, hysteroscopy and laparoscopy is considered the "gold standard" which allows direct visualization of the uterine cavity and uterine serosa, and surgical treatment of the uterine defect.
- In patients with recurrent abortions and septate uterus, reproductive outcome is significantly improved after hysteroscopy metroplasty.[10-12]
- Higher risk of miscarriage was reported among patients incidentally diagnosed with septate uterus who conceived after medically assisted reproduction. In this respect, infertile patients undergoing ART should undergo detailed assessment of uterine morphology by 3D ultrasound.[13]

■ REFERENCES

1. Kupesic S, Kurjak A. Diagnosis and treatment outcome of the septate uterus. Croatian Med J 1998; 39(2):185-90.
2. Kupesic S. Clinical implications of sonographic detection of uterine anomalies for reproductive outcome. Ultrasound Obstet Gynecol 2001;18(4):387-400.
3. Kupesic S, Kurjak A. Role of three-dimensional ultrasound in diagnosis of congenital uterine anomalies. Ultrasound Rev Obstet Gynecol 2005; 5:194-201.
4. Sparac V, Kurjak A, Kupesic S, Goldenberg M, Ilijas M, Skenderovic S, Jukic S. Histological architecture and vascularization of intrauterine septa excised during hysteroscopic procedure. Gynecol Perinatol 1996;5:101-3.
5. Kupesic S, Kurjak A, Skenderovic S, Bjelos D. Screening for uterine abnormalities by three-dimensional ultrasound improves perinatal outcome. J Prenat Med 2002;30(1): 9-17.
6. Tabi S, Kupesic Plavsic S. The role of 3D ultrasound in the assessment of congenital uterine anomalies. Donald School J Ultrasound Obstet Gynecol. 2012;6(4):415-23.
7. Healey A. Imaging of Gynecological Disorders in Infants and Children. Embryology of the Female Reproductive Tract. Berlin: Springer-Verlag: Berlin Heidelberg 2012.
8. Jayaprakasan J, Chan YY. Sur S, et al. Prevalence of uterine anomalies and their impact on early pregnancy in women conceiving after assisted reproduction treatment. Ultrasound Obstet Gynecol 2011;37(6):727-32.
9. Bermejo C, Martinez TP, Cantarero R, et al. Three-dimensional ultrasound in the diagnosis of Mullerian duct anomalies and concordance with magnetic resonance imaging. Ultrasound Obstet Gynecol 2010; 35(5):593-601.
10. Chan YY, Jayaprakasan K, Tan A, et al. Reproductive outcome in women with congenital uterine anomalies: a systematic review. Ultrasound Obstet Gynecol 2011;38(4):371-82.
11. Mollo A, De Franciscis P, Colacurci N, et al. Hysteroscopic resection of the septum improves the pregnancy rate of women with unexplained infertility: a prospective controlled trial. Fertil Steril 2009;91(6):2628-31.
12. Pabuccu R, Gomel V. Reproductive outcome after hysteroscopic metroplasty in women with septate uterus and otherwise unexplained infertility. Fertil Steril 2004;81(6):1675-8.
13. Ghi T, De Musso F, Maroni E, Youssef A, Savelli L, Farina A, Casadio P, Filicori M, Pilu G, Rizzo N. The pregnancy outcome in women with incidental diagnosis of septate uterus at first trimester scan. Hum Reprod 2012;27(9):2671-5.

CHAPTER 6

Submucosal Uterine Fibroid

Sanja Kupesic Plavsic, Vladimir Sparac

■ CLINICAL CASE

HS is a 34-year-old G3P0, presenting with heavy bleeding—gushing and prolonged menstrual periods. Her last menstrual period started 3 weeks ago. Her cycles are regular, every 28 days and periods last between 7 and 10 days, but this month she is bleeding on and off for nearly 3 weeks.

Laboratory studies are typical for iron deficiency anemia. No abnormalities are detected in WBC and platelet counts, and blood coagulation. Liver and renal function tests are normal. Pap smear, wet mount, *Chlamydia* and *Gonorrhea* tests performed 10 months ago were within normal limits. Pelvic ultrasound revealed a well-defined 4 × 3 cm solid mass with a whorled appearance, distorting the surrounding endometrium (Fig. 6.1).

Menarche: Age 13.

Menses: 28/10 days, prolonged, in clots.

LMP: 3 weeks ago.

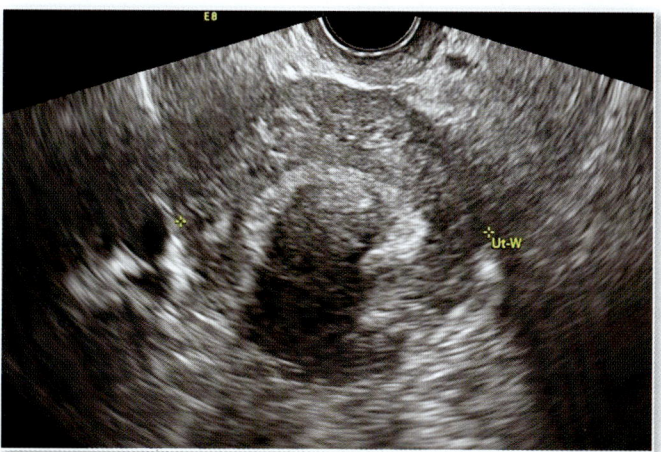

Figure 6.1: Transvaginal ultrasound demonstrates enlarged uterus with a well-defined 4 × 3 cm solid mass with a whorled appearance, distorting the surrounding endometrium

Obstetric history: Three miscarriages (8, 9, and 10 weeks) four, two and one year ago.

Sexual history: In monogamous relationship with her husband of 5 years. No history of sexually transmitted disease (STD).

Contraception: None.

Review of Systems

- No chest pain or shortness of breath
- Patient complains of premenstrual headache and dysmenorrhea
- No diarrhea or constipation
- Patient also complains of urinary frequency; no hematuria or dysuria.

Past medical history: Noncontributory.

Past surgical history: Appendectomy.

Vaccines: Up to date (hepatitis B vaccine series, MMR booster and flu shot).

Current medications: Ibuprofen over the counter.

Allergies: No known drug allergies.

Social history: HS is a dentist; she does not smoke, social ETOH, no drug abuse.

Family history: Mother: 65 years, with no health issues. Father: 67 years, history of stomach cancer.

Physical Examination

Vital signs: T 36.7°C oral, BP 120/70, P 80, BMI 25.

Cardiac examination: No heart murmur was detected.

Chest examination: Clear lungs, breathing sound was clear.

Abdominal examination: Within normal limits.

Pelvic examination: External genitalia with no abnormalities. Soft and slightly enlarged uterus by palpation. No adnexal masses are appreciated.

■ CLINICAL QUESTIONS

1. What is the best next step in evaluation of this patient?

Ans. The best next step in evaluation of this patient is to perform SIS, an adjunct imaging modality used for characterization of focal uterine cavity masses diagnosed on B mode ultrasound. Our patient is presenting with recurrent pregnancy loss (defined as three consecutive pregnancy losses), which increases the likelihood of an intrauterine abnormality. SIS was performed and Figure 6.2 illustrates the findings. Submucosal/ intracavitary fibroid projecting into the uterine cavity is clearly visualized. The fibroid

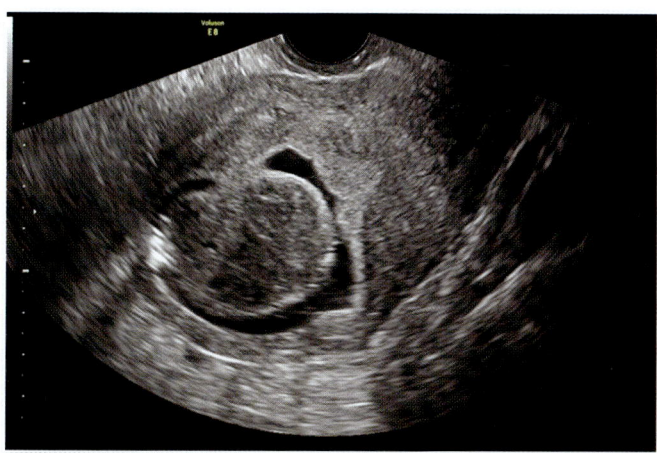

Figure 6.2: Saline infusion sonography of the same patient. Fibroid is located completely in the uterine cavity, and is attached to the uterine wall with a very narrow base

is attached to the uterine wall with a very narrow basis which allows hysteroscopic resection.

2. What are the advantages of SIS?

Ans. SIS is a valuable test in the evaluation of the uterine cavity and evaluation of female infertility. It offers several advantages over the traditional HSG. This well tolerated minimally invasive procedure does not use ionizing radiation and iodinated contrast medium. It provides excellent anatomic assessment of the uterine cavity together with visualization of the entire uterus. It can establish the location of the fibroid(s) with respect to the endometrial lining and is very helpful in directing subsequent intervention.[1]

3. How submucosal fibroids are differentiated from endometrial polyps on SIS?

Ans. Submucosal fibroids appear as hypoechoic masses, isoechogenic to the myometrium, in contrast to endometrial polyps which are typically hyperechogenic with respect to the myometrium (Fig. 6.3). Absence of endometrial–myometrial interface is commonly seen in submucosal fibroids, while polyps usually have an intact underlying endometrial–myometrial interface. The position of the fibroid within the uterine cavity is not a reliable factor for differentiation between endometrial polyps and intracavitary/submucosal fibroids, because some fibroids (like in our case) may appear polypoid as they are entirely contained within the cavity.[1]

Color Doppler assessment of the vascular pattern is another differentiating factor between submucosal fibroids and endometrial polyps. Endometrial polyps typically demonstrate single feeding artery in the pedicle, while submucosal fibroids presents with arborized vessels and/or multiple vascular pattern (Figs 6.3 and 6.4).

Section 1: Gynecology

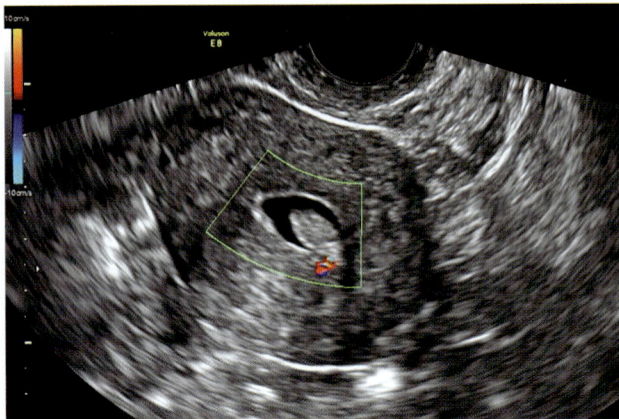

Figure 6.3: Saline infusion sonography with color flow imaging. Note hyperechogenic focal lesion with single feeding vessel. Sonographic and Doppler findings are suggestive of an endometrial polyp

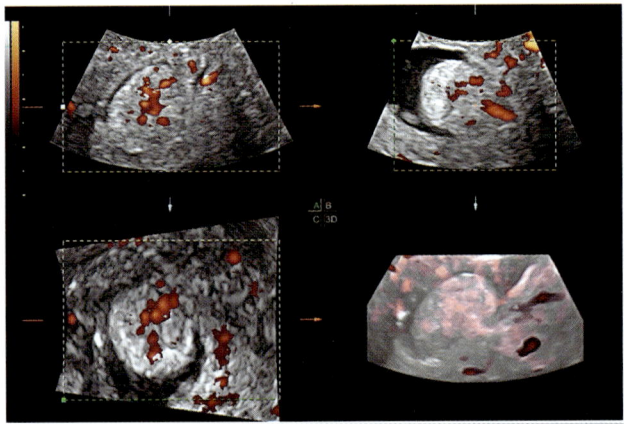

Figure 6.4: 3D saline infusion sonography with power Doppler imaging reveals isoechoic lesion with multiple vascular pattern, suggestive of a submucosal fibroid

4. **What are the sonographic/SIS criteria for submucosal/intracavitary fibroid to be successfully resected by hysteroscopy?**

Ans. The extent to which the fibroid projects into the lumen of the uterine cavity is of clinical importance. Fibroid projecting into the lumen by more than 50% of its surface can be resected by hysteroscopy (Fig. 6.5).[1] Maximal size of the fibroids suitable for resection is not precisely established. Hysteroscopic resection is a viable option for fibroids measuring less than 5 cm, but resection also depends on fibroid's position. If located at easily approachable position, even fibroids measuring 6 cm may be successfully removed by hysteroscopy. Fibroids located at the anterior and posterior uterine wall are the easiest for resection, while those located at side walls and fundal region are more complicated. The most complicated location is the cornual region due to thin wall and limited space for resection.[2]

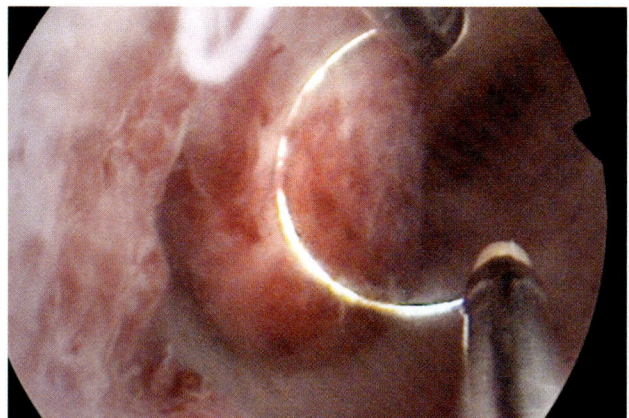

Figure 6.5: Hysteroscopic image of a fibroid protruding into the lumen before hysteroscopic resection. *From*: Sparac V, Kurjak A, Bekavac I, Kupesic Plavsic S. Endoscopic surgery in gynecology. Kupesic Plavsic S (Ed). Color Doppler, 3D and 4D Ultrasound in Gynecology, Infertility and Obstetrics, 2nd edition. New Delhi: Jaypee Publisher 2011, Figure 8.16, p 107

■ TAKE-HOME MESSAGES

- Submucosal fibroids may cause heavy and prolonged bleeding leading to anemia. The prevalence of uterine fibroids increases with age, which becomes significant as more women are delaying childbearing. Therefore, fibroids and infertility frequently occur together.[3]
- In women with infertility, an effort should be made to adequately evaluate and classify fibroids, particularly those impinging on the endometrial cavity, using transvaginal ultrasound, SIS, hysteroscopy or MRI.[4]
- Preoperative assessment of submucosal fibroids should include the assessment of the fibroid size and location within the uterine cavity, and evaluation of the degree of invasion of the cavity and assessment of the thickness of the residual myometrium to the serosa.[4]
- The use of 2D and 3D transvaginal ultrasound, with saline infusion is an integral part of preoperative evaluation of patients with submucosal fibroids.[5]
- A combination of sonographic features, such as echogenicity, endometrial–myometrial interface and vascular pattern are used for differentiation between submucosal/intracavitary fibroids and endometrial polyps.[6]
- In infertile patients submucosal fibroids should be removed hysteroscopically to improve pregnancy rates.
- Submucosal fibroids are successfully treated with therapeutic hysteroscopy. Best results are achieved with the fibroid size <5 cm, although even larger fibroids may be successfully managed hysteroscopically, but repeat procedures are often necessary.[2]
- Hysteroscopic resection of submucosal uterine fibroids is a simple, well tolerated and effective procedure. Fertility outcome and menorrhagia are both enhanced by hysteroscopic myomectomy.[7]
- In patients with thin myometrium, in whom when the margin between the deepest part of the fibroid and the serosa is less than 5–8 mm intraoperative ultrasound should be performed to prevent bowel lesion.[7]
- For monopolar resection, glycine is used as distension medium and a high frequency current is required. The bipolar system is a newer electrosurgical system in therapeutic hysteroscopy, with similar safety and efficacy as the monopolar system. The advantage of this system is reduced risk of metabolic complications due to the use of isotonic saline as a distension medium.[7]
- Innovations to the existing hysteroscopic techniques and the development of the hysteroscopic morcellator will hopefully result in a greater number of gynecologic surgeons being able to safely perform hysteroscopic resection of submucosal uterine fibroids.[5,7]

- New minimally invasive therapeutic techniques for treatment of submucosal fibroids include high intensity focused ultrasound (HIFU) [8] and ultrasound guided percutaneous microwave ablation (PMWA).[9]
- The use of uterine artery embolization (UAE) in fertile women has not been studied extensively for the management of submucosal fibroids. Recent study reported an increase in adverse pregnancy outcomes after UAE compared with myomectomy.[10]

REFERENCES

1. Berridge DL, Winter TC. Saline Infusion Sonohysterography: Technique, indications and imaging findings. J Ultrasound Med. 2004;23(1):97-112.
2. Sparac V, Kurjak A, Bekavac I, Kupesic Plavsic S. Endoscopic surgery in gynecology. Kupesic Plavsic S (Ed). Color Doppler, 3D and 4D Ultrasound in Gynecology, Infertility and Obstetrics, 2nd edition. New Delhi: Jaypee Publisher. 2011, p 96-111.
3. Van Heertum K, Barmat L. Uterine fibroids associated with infertility. Womens Health. 2014;10(6):645-53.
4. Caranza –Mamne B, Havelock J, Hemmings R, et al. The management of uterine fibroids in women with otherwise unexplained infertility. J Obstet Gynaecol Can. 2015;37(3):277-88.
5. Pakrashi T. New hysteroscopic techniques for submucosal uterine fibroids. Curr Opin Obstet Gynecol. 2014;26(4):308-13.
6. Bhaduri M, Tmlinson G, Glanc P. Likelihood of sonohysterographic findings for discriminating endometrial polyps from submucosal fibroids. J Ultrasound Med. 2014;33(1):149-54.
7. Capmas P, Levaillant JM, Fernandez H. Surgical techniques and outcome in the management of submucous fibroids. Curr Opin Obstet Gynecol. 2013;25(4):332-8.
8. Wang W, Wang Y, Wang T, et al. Safety and efficacy of US guided high intensity focused ultrasound for treatment of submucosal fibroids. Eur Radiol. 2012;22(11):2553-8.
9. Yang Y, Zhang J, Han ZY, et al. Ultrasound guided percutaneous microwave ablation for submucosal uterine fibroids. J Minim Invasive Gynecol. 2014;21(3):436-41.
10. Van der Kooji SM, Ankum WM, Hehenkamp WJ. Review of nonsurgical/minimally invasive treatments for uterine fibroids. Curr Opin Obstet Gynecol. 2012;24(6):368-75.

CHAPTER

Chlamydia Salpingitis

7

Ulrich Honemeyer, Sanja Kupesic Plavsic

■ CLINICAL CASE

MS is a 33-year-old nulliparous patient (G0P0) who presents to ER with severe right-sided abdominal and pelvic pain, nausea, and vomiting. Pelvic examination revealed right adnexal fullness, and palpable mass in the right posterior fornix associated with tenderness. Transvaginal ultrasound detected right adnexal mass measuring 7 × 3 cm (Fig. 7.1). Uterus and left ovary were normal.

Menarche: Age 13.

Menses: 28/5 days.

LMP: 7 days ago.

Pregnancies: None.

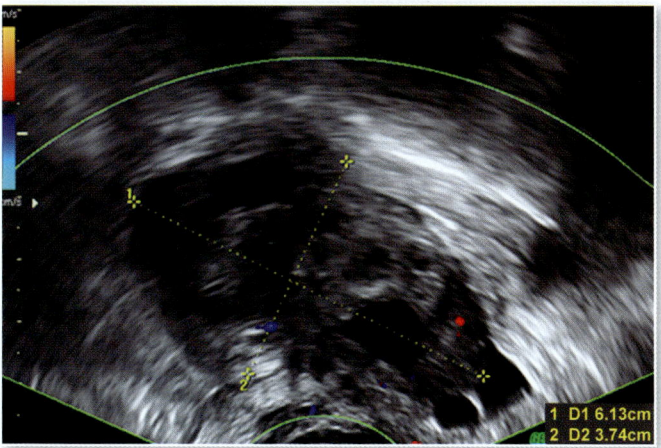

Figure 7.1: Transvaginal color Doppler ultrasound demonstrates right adnexal mass measuring 7 × 3 cm with increased perfusion. Sonographic findings are suggestive of acute pelvic inflammatory disease

Sexual history: Seven male partners over her lifetime. Patient is currently in a monogamous relationship with her husband but is unable to conceive after two years of regular, unprotected intercourse.

Contraception: None

Review of Systems

- No headaches, no problems with vision
- No history of blood clots, DVT or PE
- No heart palpitations, no shortness of breath
- Right-sided abdominal/pelvic pain; Sharp right upper and lower quadrant pelvic pain; Intensity: 8–9/10. History of nausea and vomiting; no constipation or diarrhea.
- Patient complains of symptoms consistent with urinary tract infection. Urinalysis is within normal limits.

Past medical history: None; no hospitalizations.

Past surgical history: None.

Vaccines: Up to date.

Current medications: None.

Allergies: None.

Social history: MS is an architect. She drinks alcohol occasionally and in moderation. She does not smoke, and reports no history of substance abuse.

Family history: Mother 61 years, history of hypertension; Father 72 years, history of type 2 diabetes mellitus. No family history of uterine, breast, ovarian or colon cancer.

Physical Examination

- *Vital signs:* T 37.5°C; BP 110/70; P 82; BMI 25
- Normal heart, lungs, and thyroid examinations
- Pelvic examination revealed cervical motion tenderness and right adnexal fullness. Palpable mass in the right posterior fornix was associated with tenderness.

Laboratory tests were performed:

- Blood group   "O" Rh positive
- Preoperative Hb   13.4 g%
- RBC   5.7 mmol/L
- Renal function tests   WNL
- Liver function tests   WNL
- HBsAg/HIV   Negative
- Platelet count   282 K/µL (WNL)
- ESR   19 mm/1st hour
- CRP   9.53 mg/L (elevated)
- AFP   1 ng/L (WNL)
- CA-125   152 U/mL (elevated)
- CEA   1.6 ng/mL (WNL)

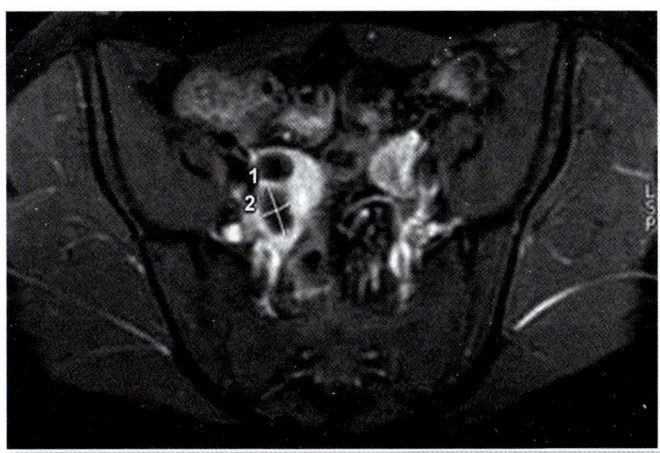

Figure 7.2: MRI of the pelvis revealed 6 × 3.4 cm complex right adnexal mass, suspicious of ovarian malignancy

Complex adnexal mass on ultrasound and elevated CA-125 (152 IU/mL) indicated further investigations, including MRI. MRI of the pelvis revealed 6 × 3.4 cm complex right adnexal mass, with thick septations (Fig. 7.2).

CLINICAL QUESTIONS

1. What is the most appropriate next step in management of this patient?
Ans. This patient should be planned for laparoscopic surgery.

2. Based on the assessment of patient's history and imaging, what is the possible risk of minimally invasive surgery in this patient?
Ans. Ureteral injury is potential complication of laparoscopic surgery in this patient. In patients with pelvic inflammatory disease (PID), adhesions, endometriosis and pelvic tumors ureters are likely to be displaced into an abnormal location, which substantially increases the risk for ureteral injury. Some experts suggest the prophylactic placement of ureteral stents in selected cases to aid in intraoperative ureteral identification.[1]

3. What are the indications for preoperative ureteral catheter (stent) placement?
Ans. Iatrogenic ureteral injury is a serious complication that can occur during abdominal and/or pelvic surgery, occurring at a rate of 0.3–1.5%.[2] Despite the low incidence rate, ureteral injuries can lead to significant morbidity. Studies identified resections of large pelvic masses, malignant neoplasms, PID, infiltrative endometriosis of the pelvic floor, frozen pelvis, total laparoscopic hysterectomy, (laparoscopic) dissection of iliac lymphatic nodes, previous surgery, cervical fibroids, or radiation therapy as risk factors for ureteral injury.[3]

4. What is the standard of preoperative patient counseling regarding her surgery and fertility potential?
Ans. The patient should give an informed consent for laparoscopic procedure. The indications, possible findings (PID vs. ovarian malignancy), and complications should be discussed in detail. The course and extent of surgery should be also explained (Figs 7.3 to 7.7). Patient and her husband stated that they are interested to proceed with infertility treatment and

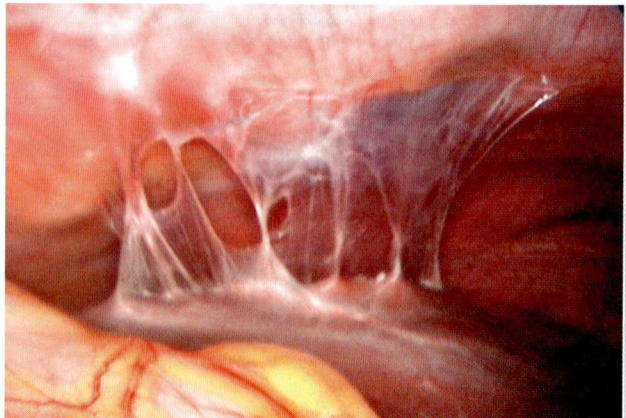

Figure 7.3: Laparoscopy revealed perihepatic adhesions, typical for Fitz–Hugh–Curtis syndrome. "Violin string" adhesions are stretching from the peritoneum to the anterior surface of the liver

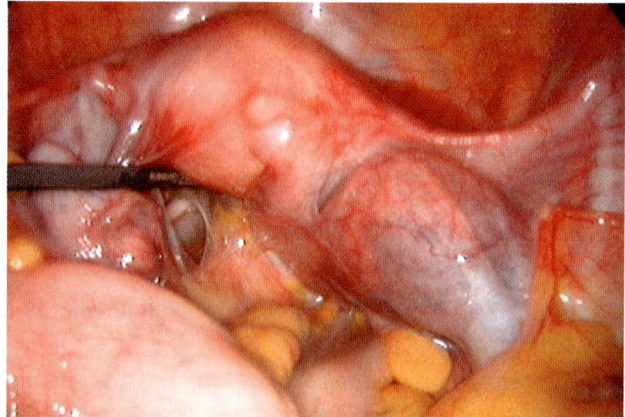

Figure 7.4: Laparoscopy revealed dilated fallopian tubes, consistent with distal tubal occlusion and severe peritubal and periovarian adhesions

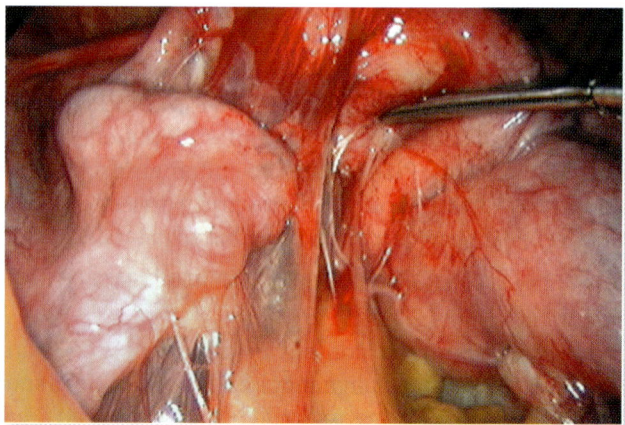

Figure 7.5: Severe adhesions were visualized in cul-de-sac. Adhesiolysis was performed

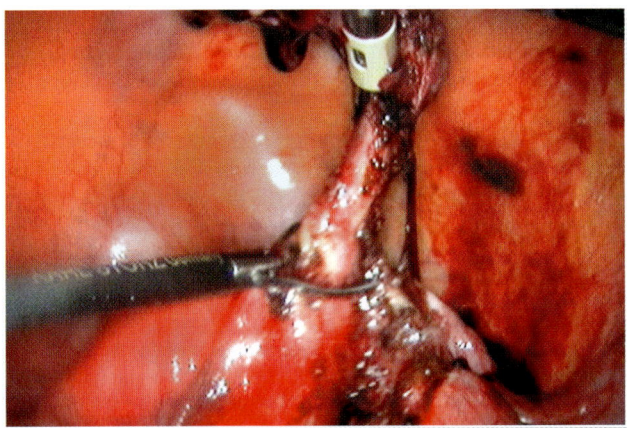

Figure 7.6: Due to severe tubal damage, salpingectomy without leaving tubal stump was performed bilaterally[7]

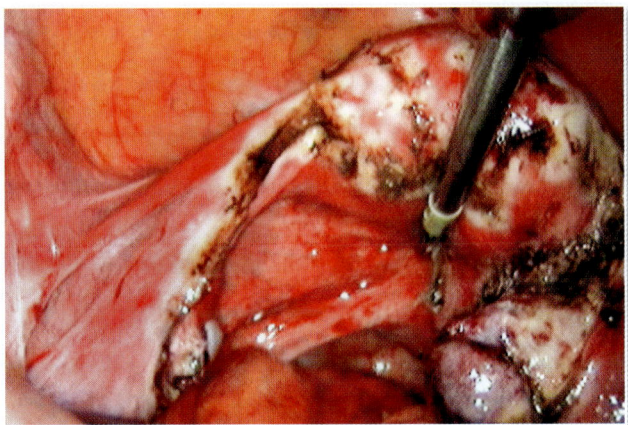

Figure 7.7: Laparoscopic image after adhesiolysis and bilateral salpingectomy

IVF/ET. They should be educated about negative effect of hydrosalpinges on outcome of IVF/ET.[4-6] The surgeon should obtain patient's consent to perform salpingectomy (if intraoperative findings prove irreversible tubal damage) and/or extensive surgery (if intraoperative findings show adnexal malignancy). The physician who does not comply with patient's agreement to a particular procedure may be found liable for failing to do so.

■ TAKE-HOME MESSAGES

- Many retrospective studies have shown that hydrosalpinges are associated with poor IVF outcomes. The live birth rate achieved with IVF/ET among patients with hydrosalpinges is approximately 50% that observed in patients without hydrosalpinges.[5,6]
- Hydrosalpinx fluid is suggested to act on two different target systems: directly on the transferred embryos (embryo- and gametotoxicity) and endometrial receptivity (direct effect on the endometrium due to intrauterine fluid accumulation and alterations in endometrial receptivity markers).[6]

- When performing salpingectomy it is common practice to leave a long tubal stump to minimize the risk of bleeding from the isthmic portion of the fallopian tube. Given the risk of future ectopic pregnancy in the tubal remnant, it is important to minimize the length of a tubal stump to prevent the occurrence of future ectopic pregnancy.[7,8]
- Data from the literature indicate that laparoscopic salpingectomy and/or proximal tubal occlusion improve subsequent pregnancy and live birth rates achieved with IVF/ET.[5,6,9]
- Data are insufficient to permit recommendations regarding the effectiveness of alternative treatments, such as transvaginal aspiration of hydrosalpingeal fluid and/or hysteroscopic tubal occlusion.[10-12]

REFERENCES

1. Tanaka Y, Asada H, Kuji N, Yoshimura Y. Ureteral catheter placement for prevention of ureteral injury during laparoscopic hysterectomy. J Obstet Gynaecol Res. 2008;34(1):67-72.
2. Parpala-Spårman T, Paananen I, Santala M, et al. Increasing numbers of ureteric injuries after the introduction of laparoscopic surgery. Scand J Urol Nephrol. 2008;42(5):422-7.
3. Liapis A, Bakas P, Giannopoulos V, Creatsas G. Ureteral injuries during gynecological surgery. Int Urogynecol J Pelvic Floor Dysfunct. 2001;12(6):391-3.
4. Strandell A, LIdhard A. Hydrosalpinx and ART. Salpingectomy prior to IVF can be recommended to a well-defined subgroup of patients. Hum Reprod. 2000;15(10):2072-4.
5. Putemans P, Campo R, Gordts R, et al. Hydrosalpinx and ART: hydrosalpinx—functional surgery or salpingectomy. Hum Reprod. 2000;15(7):1427-30.
6. Parihar M, MIrge A, Hasabe R. Hydrosalpinx functional surgery or salpingectomy? The importance of hydrosalpinx fluid in assisted reproductive technologies. J Genecol Endosc Surg. 2009;1(1):12-6.
7. Al-Inizi S. Recurrent ectopic pregnancy following ipsilateral proximal salpingectomy. J Clin Gynecol Obstet. 2015;4(1):188-190.
8. Yano T, Ishida H, Kinoshita T. Spontaneous ectopic pregnancy occurring in the remnant tube after ipsilateral salpingectomy: a report of two cases. Reprod Med Biol. 2009;8(4):177-9.
9. Practice Committee of the American Society for Reproductive Medicine in collaboration with Society of Reproductive Surgeons. Salpingectomy for hydrosalpinx prior to in vitro fertilization. Fertil Steril. 2008;90:S66-8.
10. Hammadieh N, Coomarasamy A, Ola B, et al. Ultrasound guided hydrosalpinx aspiration during oocyte collection improves pregnancy outcome in IVF: a randomized control trial. Hum Reprod. 2008;23(5):1113-7.
11. Hitkari JA, Singh SS, Shapiro HM, Leyland N. Essure treatment of hydrosalpinges. Fertil Steril. 2007;88:1663-6.
12. Hurst BS, Tucker KE, Awoniyi CA, Schlaff WD. Hydrodsalpinx treated with extended doxycycline does not compromise the success of IVF. Fertil Steril. 2001;75:1017-9.

CHAPTER 8

Chronic Pelvic Pain and Pelvic Adhesions

Dhyana Velasco, Sireesha Y Reddy

CLINICAL CASE

ME is a 32-year-old female G0P0 who presents with two-year history of pelvic pain.

She has been attempting pregnancy for one year. She reports pain for the last two years that is intermittent, dull in nature, diffuse in the abdomen and increases with intercourse. She recalls that her pain began after the infection. ME reports that she has been missing work and interfering with her daily life activities. She reports a history of *Chlamydial* infection about three years ago. All subsequent sexually transmitted infection testing was negative. She reports taking antibiotics after receiving the results. She denies any urinary or gastrointestinal symptoms. Her periods are regular. She denies that her husband has fathered any children.

Review of Systems

- Denies fever, anorexia, nausea, diarrhea, or vomiting
- Denies any epigastric pain
- Denies any heart palpitations or shortness of breath
- Denies any vaginal discharge and urinary symptoms
- Past gynecological history: Menses began age 12 with intervals every 26–28 days lasting about 4–5 days. She reports Chlamydial infection 2–3 years prior. All Pap smears normal. Last HIV, syphilis testing negative.

Past obstetrical history: Denies.

Past medical history: Denies.

Past surgical history: Denies.

Social history: Lives with her husband; married for 2 years; reports remote history of tobacco use. She denies any alcohol or drug use.

Family history: Mother: History of hypertension. Father: History of depression.

Physical Examination

Vital signs: T 36.8°C; P 60; RR 16; BP 90/60.

Abdomen: Normal bowel sounds; no distension; no guarding; no rebound; tenderness to palpation below the umbilicus; no masses palpated.

Genitourinary: Normal external genitalia; normal rectum; speculum examination: normal vaginal mucosa; normal cervix; normal physiologic clear mucous discharge seen. Manual examination elicits pain when the cervix is moved, uterine and adnexal tenderness bilaterally. No pain on rectal examination.

Pelvic ultrasound: Normal size uterus, normal size bilateral ovaries, minimal fluid in the cul-de-sac.

All laboratory values normal; *Chlamydia* and gonorrhea cultures are negative.

■ CLINICAL QUESTIONS

1. **This patient has a two-year history of pelvic pain. How would you categorize and differentiate her pain?**

Ans. Her pain should be categorized as chronic pain since it is at least six months duration, causes her some dysfunction in ability to perform routine activities and may or may not be associated with the menstrual cycle. Chronic pelvic pain can be difficult to differentiate. Gynecologic causes comprise of one-fifth of the causes for chronic pelvic pain. These can be PID, endometriosis, adenomyosis, adhesive disease, leiomyomas, dysmenorrhea, and pelvic congestion. One must consider urologic, gastrointestinal, musculoskeletal, neurological, and psychological issues.[1]

2. **How would you approach the evaluation of this patient given the chronic nature of her pain?**

Ans. International Pelvic Pain Society has designed a specific history and physical form that contains specific questions related to the history (including physical and sexual abuse, in addition to psychological symptoms that may be the cause or exacerbate the pain). The form contains specific aspects of the physical examination that may point to the localized or generalized tenderness. It attempts to quantify and map the pain. One must take a pain history with a thorough review of systems relating to the specific organ systems outlined above that contribute to pain syndromes. A physical examination that is done with sensitivity since it may reproduce the pain paying attention to referred pain, mobility of organs, areas of tenderness, size, and shape of organs. A psychological assessment may be used as well.[2]

3. **What risk factors does she exhibit that may be playing a role in her infertility?**

Ans. She has a history of *Chlamydia*. In general, risk factors for infertility in this setting of an STD can be the *Chlamydial* infection, most likely a delay in treatment of the *Chlamydial* infection, severity of infection and multiple episodic STD infections. A majority of the time this leads to a permanent injury to the endosalpinx, causing tubal dysfunction.[3]

4. **Given the chronic nature of her pain, what might be your next approach with this patient?**

Ans. For chronic pain patients, treating empirically while considering the diagnostic possibilities is preferable.[4] If one is considering endometriosis, a trial of oral contraceptive pills may be initiated. This patient was counseled and underwent a diagnostic laparoscopy to assist the physician in her evaluation of pelvic pain.[5] Figure 8.1 depicts the intraperitoneal view with the aid of diagnostic laparoscopy.

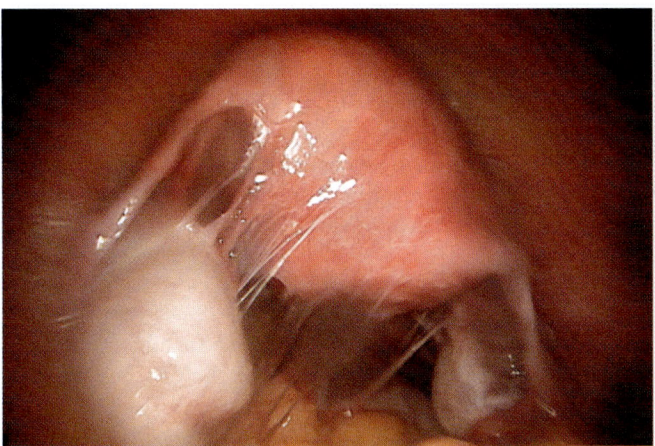

Figure 8.1: Filmy adhesions can be seen in the posterior cul-de-sac from the posterior surface of the uterus toe the left ovary, bowel. Adhesions from right ovary to bowel are also noted

5. How would you counsel this patient on her adhesions and chronic pelvic pain?

Ans. The association of pain and adhesions is not well understood. One postulation is that adhesive disease limits the mobility of organs and thereby causes visceral pain. Studies from laparoscopic conscious mapping showed that adhesive disease may account for some aspects of pain.[6] Adhesiolysis has not shown to be of long-term benefit and may increase risk of surgical complications.[7] Figure 8.2 shows the laparoscopic findings in the right upper quadrant. There are adhesions involving the liver and the anterior abdominal wall.

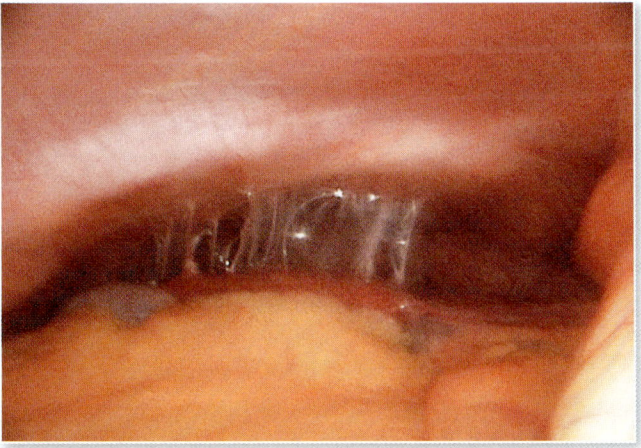

Figure 8.2: The adhesions in the right upper quadrant involving the liver and the anterior abdominal wall. A perihepatitis can occur in 10% of patients affected with *Chlamydia*. This can result in epigastric and right upper quadrant pain that can be confused with cholecystitis. The infection in this setting generally does not involve the stromal or parenchymal elements of the liver. These adhesions are often referred to as "violin strings"

TAKE-HOME MESSAGES

- Multiple pelvic sources like gastrointestinal, urologic, gynecologic, musculoskeletal, neurologic, psychological sources should be considered in the evaluation of a chronic pelvic pain patient.
- Laparoscopy can be a tool to aid in the diagnosis of the etiology of pelvic pain but this should be customized to the patient depending on her history and pelvic examination after empiric therapy has been used.
- Evaluation of the chronic pelvic pain patient can be complicated. Using the history and physical examination and questionnaire forms from the International Pelvic Pain Society can aid in the evaluation of the chronic pelvic pain patient.
- Adhesiolysis may not be beneficial in the long-term relief of chronic pelvic pain.[7]
- PID is generally an acute condition characterized by pelvic pain with pelvic organ tenderness on examination.[5] PID can lead to adhesive disease that can result in infertility related to tubal factor involving the endosalpinx.
- Long-term sequelae of PID can be adhesive disease, chronic pelvic pain, and infertility.
- *Chlamydial* infections carry the greatest risk for infertility.[3]
- Perihepatitis can occur in some patients characterized by right upper quadrant pain.[6]

REFERENCES

1. Haggerty CL, Peipert JF, Weitzen S, et al. Predictors of chronic pelvic pain in an urban population of women with symptoms and signs of pelvic inflammatory disease. Sex Transm Dis. 2005;32:293.
2. Hornstein MD, Thomas PP, Sober AJ, Wyshak G, et al. Association between endometriosis, dysplastic naevi and history of melanoma in women of reproductive age. Hum Reprod. 1997;12(1):143.
3. Cates W, Joesoef MR, Goldman MB. Atypical pelvic inflammatory disease: can we identify clinical predictors? Am J Obstet Gynecol. 1993;169(2 Pt 1):341.
4. Lentz GM, Bavendam T, Stenchever MA, et al. Hormonal manipulation in women with chronic, cyclic irritable bladder symptoms and pelvic pain. Am J Obstet Gynecol. 2002;186 (6):1268.
5. Westrom L, Joesoef R, Reynolds G, et al. Pelvic inflammatory disease and infertility. Sex Transm Dis. 1992;19(4):185.
6. Howard FM, El-Minawi AM, Sanchez RA. Conscious pain mapping by laparoscopy in women with chronic pelvic pain. Obstet Gynecol. 2000;96(6):934.
7. Swank DJ, Swank-Bordewijk SC, Hop WC, et al. Lancet. Laparoscopic adhesiolysis in patients with chronic abdominal pain: a blinded randomized controlled multi-center trial. 2003;361(9365):1247.

CHAPTER

Pelvic Inflammatory Disease and Tubo-ovarian Abscess

9

Sushila Arya, Sanja Kupesic Plavsic

■ CLINICAL CASE

NW is a 29-year-old G3P2, who presents to ER with lower abdominal pain and fever. Pain started 3 days ago but has gradually increased in intensity. Pain is constant, bilaterally in lower abdomen and pelvis, more toward left adnexa, with no aggravating or relieving symptoms. Patient reports fever with chills since last 4 hours and does not complain of urinary symptoms. She reports nausea, but no vomiting. Last menstrual period was 10 days ago. She has not been using any contraceptive. Her history is significant for right ectopic pregnancy about 2 years ago, which was treated with methotrexate (MTX).

Menarche: Age 11.

Menstrual periods: 28–20 days/5–7 days

Past obstetric history: 2 normal spontaneous vaginal deliveries (NSVD); 1 ectopic pregnancy, medically treated.

Gynecologic history: 7 male partners over her lifetime. History of *Chlamydia* infection at age of 16 years. Recent STD testing and Pap smear were normal as per patient, no records available.

Contraception: None.

Past medical history: None, no hospitalizations.

Past surgical history: None.

Current medications: None.

Allergies: No known drug allergies.

Social history: NW is a housekeeper. She drinks alcohol occasionally and in moderation. She denies tobacco and drug use.

Family history: Significant for father with heart disease, mother with diabetes mellitus Type 2. No hereditary cancers in the family.

Review of Systems

Positive for lower abdominal and pelvic pain, nausea, fever with chills and dizziness. All other ROS is negative.

Physical Examination

Vital signs: T 38.7°C; BP 104/61; P109; BMI 33.2.

General: Alert, oriented to time, place and person. In mild distress related to pain.

Neck, heart and lungs examination is unremarkable.

Abdomen: Soft, lower abdomen is tender, guarding +, no mass palpable.

Pelvic examination: Normal external genitalia. On speculum examination cervix is slightly erythematous, vaginal mucosa is unremarkable and copious mucopurulent discharge is noted. On bimanual examination uterine and left adnexal tenderness; difficult to assess uterine and adnexal size secondary to guarding and patient discomfort from tenderness. There is ill-defined adenexal fullness on left side.

- Urine pregnancy test is negative
- *CBC:* WBC is slightly elevated, 12,000/dL; H/H, chemistry panel, and urine analyses are within normal limits
- Wet mount swab is positive for bacterial vaginosis
- Results of her transvaginal ultrasound examination are presented in Figures 9.1 to 9.3. Sonographic and Doppler findings are suggestive of acute pelvic inflammatory disease (PID) and tubo-ovarian abscess (TOA).

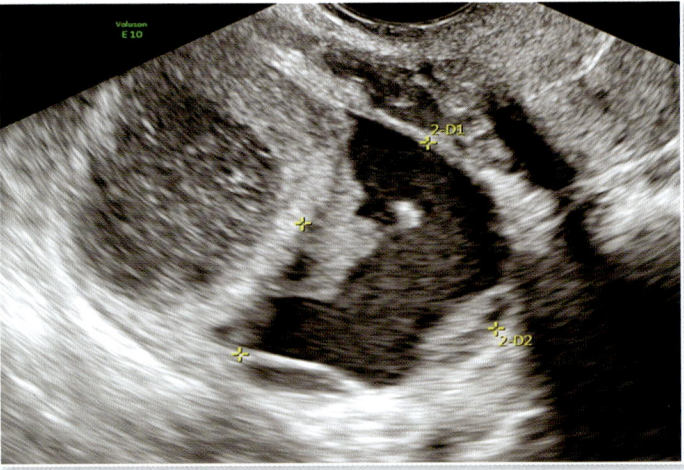

Figure 9.1: Transvaginal B mode imaging of the left adnexa. Note complex adnexal mass with thick incomplete septations and pseudopapillomatous structures

Chapter 9: Pelvic Inflammatory Disease and Tubo-ovarian Abscess 47

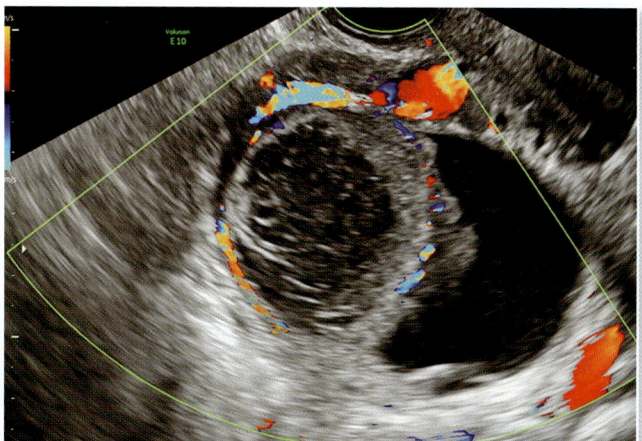

Figure 9.2: Color Doppler ultrasound of the same patient. Prominent color signals are identified in thick cystic wall and within septations

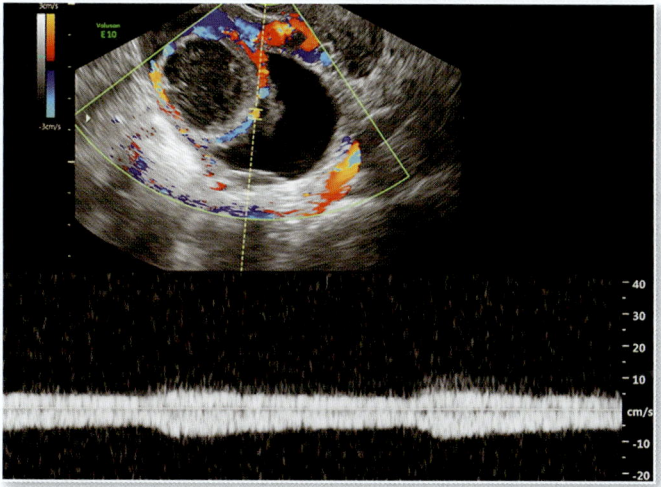

Figure 9.3: Pulsed Doppler waveform analysis reveals low vascular impedance blood flow signals

■ CLINICAL QUESTIONS

1. What are the common clinical features of PID and TOA?
Ans. Immediate clinical manifestations of acute PID are lower abdominal and/or pelvic pain, abnormal vaginal bleeding (postcoital, intermenstrual, and menorrhagia), deep dyspareunia, lower abdominal tenderness, cervical motion tenderness and fever.[1]

2. **What are late sequelae of PID?**

Ans. Late-term consequences of PID can be severe and a delay in diagnosis and treatment increases the chance of impaired fertility. With PID, 10–20% women become infertile, 40% develop chronic pelvic pain and 10–20% of those who conceive will have an ectopic pregnancy. Recurrent PID is experienced by 25% of women.[2]

3. **How is diagnosis of PID established?**

Ans. Diagnosis of PID is imprecise, lacks sensitivity and specificity because of wide variation in sign and symptoms. Clinical diagnosis of acute PID has 65–90% positive predictive value compared to laparoscopic diagnosis.[1] Most common criteria to start empiric treatment for PID is pelvic or lower abdominal pain in a young sexually active women where no other cause has been identified, with one or more signs: cervical motion or uterine and/or adnexal tenderness. Following criteria increase the specificity of diagnosis but can compromise sensitivity: elevated temperature >38.3°C, predominance of leukocytes in vaginal or cervical exudates, cervical friability, mucopurulent cervical or vaginal discharge, elevated ESR or CRP rate, presence of *Neisseria gonorrheae* and *Chlamydia trachomatis* on laboratory testing.[3] Most specific criteria for PID are: (i) histopathology evidence of endometritis on endometrial biopsy; (ii) demonstration of thickened, fluid-filled tubes with or without free pelvic fluid or tubo-ovarian complex on transvaginal ultrasound or MRI, and color Doppler findings of tubal hyperemia; (iii) laparoscopic findings consistent with PID. Laparoscopy is more accurate to diagnose acute salpingitis but might not detect subtle inflammation of the fallopian tubes. Therefore, its use is not justifiable when symptoms are mild or vague.[4]

4. **What are the most common organisms causing PID and TOA?**

Ans. *Neisseria gonorrhea* and *Chlamydia trachomatis* are implicated in many PID cases, though isolated in <50% of the times.[2,3] *Mycoplasma genitalium* is emerging as a cause of PID. Microorganisms implicated in TOA usually are the normal microflora of genital tract such as *Bacteroides, Peptostreptococcus,* streptococcal species, *Escherichia coli,* and other, gram-negative enteric organisms.[3] All patients diagnosed with PID should be tested for HIV, *N. gonorrhea* and *Chlamydia,* using nucleic acid amplification test, NAAT.

5. **What is the treatment for PID?**

Ans. Empiric regimen should provide coverage for likely pathogen. Treatment should be started as soon as diagnosis is made to minimize late-term sequelae. Hospitalization is required in cases with diagnostic uncertainty, severe signs and symptoms, potential TOA, failure with outpatient treatment, intolerance to oral treatment and pregnancy.[1] Parenteral treatment should continue for at least 24 hours after clinical improvement. Treatment of acute PID resolves acute symptoms in 90–95%, but there is a poor correlation between short-term response and long-term sequelae such as infertility.[5] Recommended parenteral regimens are cefotetan plus doxycycline or cefoxitin plus doxycycline or gentamycin plus clindamycin. Doxycycline should be given orally if possible due to pain with intravenous use.

Outpatient regimen for PID is a single dose of intravenous ceftriaxone and doxycycline plus metronidazole for 14 days. Centers for Disease Control and Prevention (CDC) recommend metronidazole when TOA is diagnosed and optional use of metronidazole in PID cases due to uncertainty of the importance of treating anaerobes. For alternate treatment options and details of each regimen please refer to the CDC website.

6. What is the treatment of TOA?

Ans. TOA is one of the late complications of PID, and represents encapsulation of the affected adnexa (fallopian tube and the ovary) with defined boundaries. Majority of TOA respond to antibiotics so medical management is considered first line. In 25% of cases medical management fails and surgical intervention or drainage become necessary. Commonly done surgical procedures are laparotomy or laparoscopic drainage of the abscess, and salpingo-oophorectomy with or without hysterectomy. Surgery for TOA is complicated and technically difficult. Combined data from various studies reported imaging guided drainage and antibiotics as safe and effective alternatives.[6]

Clindamycin penetrates neutrophils which facilitates its levels in the abscess. Clindamycin plus aminoglycoside should be standard for at least 24 hours followed by doxycycline and clindamycin or metronidazole for 14 days. This combination does not cover *Enterococcus* so addition of ampicillin or cephalosporin is recommended if *Enterococcus* be suspected.

Transvaginal or transabdominal aspiration should be performed under ultrasound or CT guidance. Drainage is critical if there is no response to parenteral broad-spectrum antibiotics. Gjelland et al. reported 93% patients avoided surgery when they were treated with antibiotics and transvaginal drainage with no major procedure related complications.[7] In a study by DeWitt Jason et al. the mean size of abscess requiring surgery or drainage was 7.3 cm. Larger TOA (>8 cm) abscesses had longer hospitalization, more complications and increased need of drainage compared with smaller abscesses.[6]

■ TAKE-HOME MESSAGES

- PID is infection of the upper genital tract, not associated with pregnancy or intraperitoneal operation. PID and salpingitis are interchangeable terms, because infection of the oviduct is the most common. Most long-term sequelae of PID are due to tubal lumen destruction. [1]with an estimated 18.9 million persons acquiring a new STD each year.[1]
- According to CDC, PID is the most common reason of gynecological indications for hospitalization.[1]
- Acute PID results from the ascending infection from the vagina and cervix microflora. Rarely PID can be due to transperitoneal spread like perforated appendicitis and abdominal abcess.[8]
- TOA is reported in 18–34% of PID patients.[6]
- Before the era of antibiotic therapy the mortality rate associated with PID was 1%. Even with current medical and surgical management the mortality from ruptured TOA is 5–10%.[8]
- Patient with PID should be treated aggressively due to devastating sequelae associated with no or late treatment. 85% of PID occur spontaneous, while 15% of patients report previous procedures, such as endometrial biopsy, IUD insertion, hysteroscopy and hysterosalpingogram.[9] Acute PID in the presence of IUD is commonly associated with anaerobic bacteria. Outpatient treatment can be offered to a compliant patient; if pelvic infection worsens or does not resolve then IUD removal is recommended.[9]
- Postmenopausal women should have appropriate work up to rule out other concurrent diseases especially malignancy.
- Latest information on various antibacterial regimens should be looked up at CDC website (http://www.cdc.gov).

REFERENCES

1. Workowski KA, Berman SM. Centers for disease control and prevention sexually transmitted disease treatment guidelines. Clin Infect Dis. 2011;53(Suppl. 3). doi:10.1093/cid/cir694.
2. Ness RB, Trautmann G, Richter HE, et al. Effectiveness of treatment strategies of some women with pelvic inflammatory disease: a randomized trial. ObstetGynecol. 2005;106(3):573-80.
3. 2015 Sexually Transmitted Diseases Treatment Guidelines. Pelvic inflammatory Disease. CDC Centers for Disease Control and Pevention; http://www.cdc.gov/std/tg2015/pid.htm
4. Gaitan H, Angel E, Diaz R, Parada A, Sanchez L, Vargas C. Accuracy of five different diagnostic techniques in mild-to-moderate pelvic inflammatory disease. Infect Dis Obstet Gynecol. 2002;10(4):171-180. http://ovidsp.ovid.com/ovidweb.cgi?T=JS&PAGE=reference&D=emed5&NEWS=N&AN=2003078754.
5. Madden T, Hladky K, Allsworth J, Houston L, Despotovic J, Schaecher C. "Predicting long-term PID sequelae with treatment markers" by Trautmann et al. Am J Obstet Gynecol. 2008;198(1):143-4. doi:10.1016/j.ajog.2007.11.063.
6. Dewitt J, Reining A, Allsworth JE, Peipert JF. Tuboovarian abscesses: is size associated with duration of hospitalization & complications? Obstet Gynecol Int. 2010;2010:847041. doi:10.1155/2010/847041.
7. Gjelland K, Ekerhovd E, Granberg S. Transvaginal ultrasound-guided aspiration for treatment of tubo-ovarian abscess: A study of 302 cases. Am J Obstet Gynecol. 2005;193(4):1323-30. doi:10.1016/j.ajog.2005.06.019.
8. Duarte R, Fuhrich D, Ross JDC. A review of antibiotic therapy for pelvic inflammatory disease. Int J Antimicrob Agents. 2015;46(3):272-7. doi:10.1016/j.ijantimicag.2015.05.004.
9. Linda O. Eckert; Gretchen M. Lentz; Chapter23: Infections of lower and upper genital tracts; vulva, vagina, cervix, toxic shock syndrome, endometritis, and salpingitis. Comprehensive Gynecology. 6th edition, Atlanta, GA: Elsevier Mosby 2012.2012.

CHAPTER 10

Ovarian Hyperstimulation Syndrome

Sushila Arya, Sanja Kupesic Plavsic

■ CLINICAL CASE

SD is a 30-year-old G0P0 who presents to ER with abdominal pain and distension, nausea, reduced appetite and dizziness, which started yesterday. Patient reports that she had 28 oocytes retrieved last week for an IVF/ET attempt. Her symptoms developed gradually but since last night it became severe enough to bring her to ER. Her history is significant for polycystic ovarian syndrome (PCOS), infertility for 4 years and right ectopic pregnancy about 5 years ago, which was treated with methotrexate (MTX).

Menarche: Age 10.

Menstrual periods: Irregular, 3–4 periods in a year.

Past obstetric history: 1 ectopic pregnancy, medically treated.

Gynecologic history: Two male partners over her lifetime. Recent STD testing and Pap smear were performed 6 months ago, and were normal. History of secondary infertility and PCOS.

Contraception: None, desires pregnancy.

Past medical history: PCOS; no hospitalizations.

Past surgical history: None.

Current medications: Ovulation induction, vaginal progesterone.

Allergies: No known drug allergies.

Social history: SD is a school teacher. She drinks alcohol occasionally and in moderation. She reports no history of tobacco or substance abuse.

Family history: Significant for mother with thyroid disease, and father with DM and heart disease who died at age 64 years.

Review of Systems

Positive for abdominal/pelvic pain, distension, nausea, and dizziness. All other review of systems is negative.

Physical Examination

Vital signs: T 36.9°C; BP 98/61; P 101; RR 22; O2 saturation 96% on room air; BMI 33.

General: Alert, oriented to time, place, and person. In mild distress due to abdominal pain and distension.

Neck, heart, and lungs examination are unremarkable.

Abdomen: Soft, distended; lower abdomen is tender, guarding +, no masses by palpation.

Pelvic examination: Normal external genitalia. On speculum examination cervix and vagina are unremarkable. Bimanual examination is deferred in lieu of ultrasound findings suggestive of ovarian hyperstimulation syndrome (OHSS) (Fig. 10.1).

Laboratory values: Her pregnancy test is negative; Hb/Hct is 11.5/34, WBC 7,000/dL, chemistry panel is unremarkable except slightly elevated AST/ALT 65/73. A urine analysis is within normal limits.

Large ascites was noted on ultrasound (Fig. 10.2). Due to pain and respiratory distress from ascites, the decision was made to perform paracentesis. Ultrasound guided paracentesis was done, and 1.5 L of ascites was drained. Patient was admitted for close monitoring. Rapid initial hydration was accomplished using bolus of IV 1 D5NS, followed by maintenance fluid; strict intake and output was monitored. Frequent laboratory (CBC, comprehensive panel), vitals and clinical status were monitored. Ambulation and intermittent compression devices were used to minimize thromboembolism risk. Patient improved with conservative management and was discharged home in 48 hours. She was advised to follow up with her infertility specialist. Embryo transfer was planned in next nonstimulated cycle.

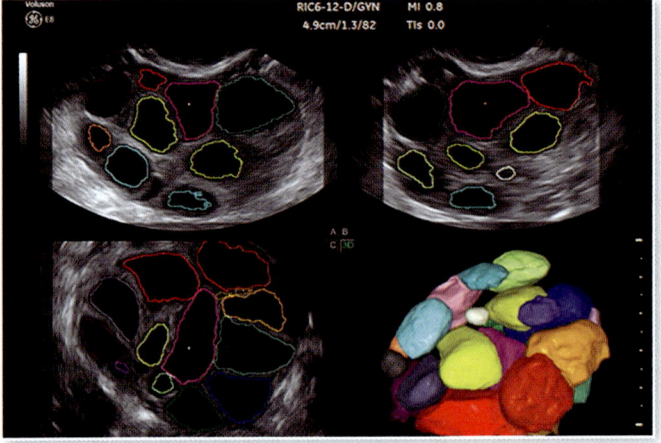

Figure 10.1: Three-dimensional ultrasound of the ovarian hyperstimulation syndrome after gonadotropin therapy

Chapter 10: Ovarian Hyperstimulation Syndrome

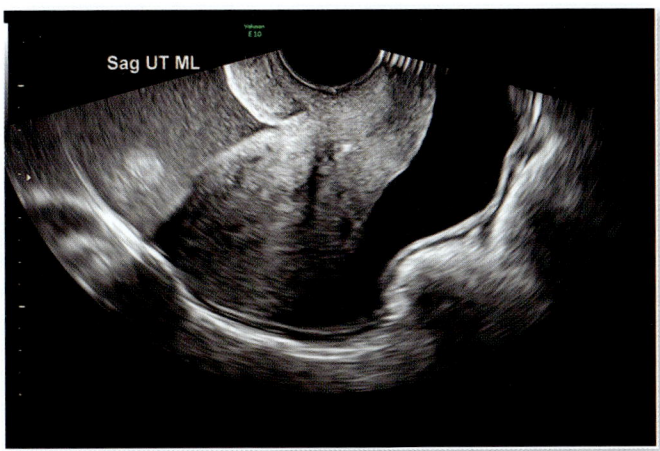

Figure 10.2: Transvaginal scan of free fluid in the cul-de-sac

■ CLINICAL QUESTIONS

1. What is OHSS?
And. OHSS is an exaggerated response to ovulation induction therapy. OHSS is typically a complication of exogenous gonadotropin stimulation and rarely with use of other agents (clomiphene citrate, letrozole and gonadotropin-releasing hormone [GnRH]).[1] It is a self-limiting syndrome, consisting of the broad spectrum of clinical manifestations.

2. What is the pathophysiology of OHSS?
And. Increase in capillary permeability resulting in a fluid shift from intravascular space to the third space. Various factors have been implicated in this process; recent studies have shown that hCG increases VEGF expression in human granulosa cells and raises serum VEGF concentrations.[2] VEGF is an angiogenic cytokine that is a potent stimulator of vascular endothelium. VEGF levels correlate with severity of OHSS.[3] Numerous other factors may be involved directly or indirectly such as angiotensin II, insulin like growth factor 1(IGF-1), epidermal growth factor (EGF), transforming growth factor (TGF), platelet derived growth factor (PDGF) and interleukin-6 and 1beta (IL-6, 1beta).[4]

3. What are the risk factors for development of OHSS?
And. The risk factors for development of OHSS are the following: PCOS, increased estradiol (E2) or rapidly rising levels and higher follicle count, higher dose of exogenous gonadotropins, previous episode of OHSS, lower BMI and younger reproductive age. Pregnancy increases the likelihood, duration and severity of OHSS.[4] Shields et al. created a risk score calculator for development of OHSS based on estradiol level, follicle count and BMI, which can be used to assess patients at high-risk.[5]

4. What are the clinical features of OHSS?

And. OHSS is associated with significant morbidity and mortality. Lower abdominal and pelvic discomfort, nausea, vomiting, diarrhea, and abdominal distension are the most common clinical symptoms. These symptoms typically occur after ovulation induction for oocyte retrieval in an ART cycles, but may be delayed. Hypotension, oliguria, and/or anuria from reduced renal perfusion due to decreased vascular volume, ascites and pulmonary compromise are seen in severe form of OHSS. Life threatening complications from OHSS include renal failure, adult respiratory distress syndrome (ARDS), hemorrhage from ovarian rupture, and thromboembolism.[6] OHSS is classified as mild, moderate or severe OHSS. Early OHSS occurs within 8 days of hCG administration, while late OHSS occurs after 9 days of hCG administration.[4]

5. What is the management of OHSS?

And. Mild disease is managed on an outpatient basis with analgesics, and patient should be informed on sign and symptoms of severe illness. Intercourse should be avoided to decrease a risk of ovarian rupture and hemorrhage. Worsening disease requires antiemetic and closer monitoring, including daily weight assessment, serial laboratory measurements for hematocrit, electrolyte and creatinine.

Pregnant patients with OHSS are at risk of severe and progressive illness, so close observation is required. In ART cycles, cryopreservation and deferring transfer to a subsequent cycle should be considered to avoid development of a severe OHSS. Severe OHSS requires hospitalization and IV fluid to address the acute volume depletion. Strict fluid management is essential and treatment with diuretics may be considered after an adequate intravascular volume has been restored. Thromboembolism is a life threatening complication, so prophylactic intermittent pneumatic compression device and heparin therapy are recommended. Intensive care is required in patients with complications, such as thromboembolism, renal failure or pulmonary compromise.[4]

6. How to prevent a development of OHSS?

And. Recognition of risk factors for OHSS and experience with ovulation induction are keys to prevent OHSS. Be mindful of OHSS risk factors during the course of ovulation induction: rapidly rising serum E2 levels, an E2 level >2,500 pg/mL and multiple number of intermediate sized follicles (10–14 mm).[4]

Withholding further gonadotropin stimulation and delaying hCG administration until E2 levels decreases can reduce a risk of OHSS. Such "coasting" does not adversely affect outcome of IVF cycles unless it is prolonged for more than 3 days. Lower dose of hCG may be prudent for at risk of OHSS patients.[6] Use of exogenous progesterone instead of supplemental dose of hCG for luteal phase support may reduce risk of OHSS.[7]

■ TAKE-HOME MESSAGES

- Knowledge and experience with ovulation induction therapy, familiarity with pathophysiology, risk factors and clinical features of OHSS are very important for its prevention and management.[4]
- Majority of cases are due to controlled ovarian stimulation with ART.[1] Mild OHSS is very common; worsening of OHSS should be monitored closely.

- Moderate to severe forms occur in 3–10% of all ART, but the incidence can reach up to 20% in high-risk patients.[1]
- Precise cause of OHSS is controversial. VEGF plays a key role on pathophysiology of OHSS.[2]
- High response rate with controlled ovarian stimulation (COS) is correlated with the Anti-Müllerian Hormone (AMH) and antral follicle count (AFC) values.[1]
- The risk of OHSS may be predicted by serum estradiol and follicle count. The risk is reduced by the use of cabergoline or other dopamine agonist.[1]
- GnRH agonist for final maturation significantly reduces the risk of OHSS.
- Freezing all oocytes/embryos for later transfer reduces the risk of OHSS significantly, but this conservative approach imposes a financial and emotional burden on the patients.[1]

REFERENCES

1. Nastri CO, Teixeira DM, Moroni RM, LeitHo VMS, Martins WP. Ovarian hyperstimulation syndrome: Pathophysiology, staging, prediction and prevention. Ultrasound Obstet Gynecol. 2015;45(4):377-93. doi:10.1002/uog.14684.
2. Geva E, Jaffe RB. Role of vascular endothelial growth factor in ovarian physiology and pathology. Fertil Steril. 2000;74(3): 429-38. doi:10.1016/S0015-0282(00)00670-1.
3. Levin ER, Rosen GF, Cassidenti DL, et al. Role of vascular endothelial cell growth factor in Ovarian Hyperstimulation Syndrome. J Clin Invest. 1998;102(11):1978-85. doi:10.1172/JCI4814.
4. ASRM. Ovarian hyperstimulation syndrome. Fertil Steril. 2008;90(5 Suppl):S188-93. doi:10.1016/j.fertnstert.2008.08.034.
5. Shields R, Vollenhoven B, Ahuja K TA. Ovarian hyperstimulation syndrome: A case control study investigating risk factors. Aust N Z J Obs Gynaecol. 2016;(Aug 17). doi: 10.1111/ajo.12515. [Epub ahead of print]
6. Whelan JG, Vlahos NF. The ovarian hyperstimulation syndrome. Fertil Steril. 2000;73(5):883-96. doi:10.1016/S0015-0282(00)00491-X.
7. RG Forman, R Frydman, D Egan, C Ross DHB. Severe ovarian hyperstimulation syndrome using agonists of gonadotropin-releasing hormone for in vitro fertilization: a European series and a proposal for prevention. Fertil Steril. 1990;53:502-9.

CHAPTER 11

Preconceptional Ultrasound

Sanja Kupesic Plavsic

■ CLINICAL CASE

SM is a 32-year old G1P1, presenting for preconceptional pelvic ultrasound before an IVF-ICSI/ET attempt. Her first pregnancy three years ago was also conceived through IVF-ICSI/ET. Elective CS was performed at 37 weeks because of breech presentation. Her LMP was seven days ago. Her cycles are regular, every 28 days and periods on average last 4–5 days. Her Pap smear, wet mount, *Chlamydia* and gonorrhea tests, and laboratory findings were performed one month ago and were within normal limits. The patient wants to start her ovulation induction in the next cycle. She is interested whether she may deliver vaginally.

Menarche: Age 14.

Menses: 28/4–5 days.

LMP: 7 days ago.

Obstetric history: One uncomplicated pregnancy, CS performed at 37 weeks (3,500 g/54 cm; Apgar 9/10).

Sexual history: In monogamous relationship with her husband who is diagnosed with severe oligoasthenozoospermia. No history of sexually transmitted disease (STD).

Contraception: None.

Review of Systems

- No chest pain or shortness of breath
- No urinary frequency, hematuria or dysuria
- Past medical history: Non-significant
- Past surgical history: CS and appendectomy.

Vaccines: Up to date (hepatitis B vaccine series, MMR booster and flu shot).

Current medications: None.

Allergies: No known drug allergies.

Social history: CR is a clerk; she does not smoke, social ETOH, no drug abuse.

Family history: Mother: 58 years, with no health issues. Father: 60 years, history of nephrolithiasis.

Physical Examination

Vital signs: T 36.4°C oral; BP 120/70; P 74; BMI 22.

Cardiac examination: No heart murmur was detected.

Chest examination: Clear lungs, breathing sound was clear.

Abdominal examination: Within normal limits.

Bimanual pelvic examination: Unremarkable external genitalia. Normal size uterus, in AVF, mobile, and non-tender. Adnexal masses could not be appreciated. Normal physiologic changes of the ovaries.

Ultrasound findings of the uterus are presented in Figure 11.1.

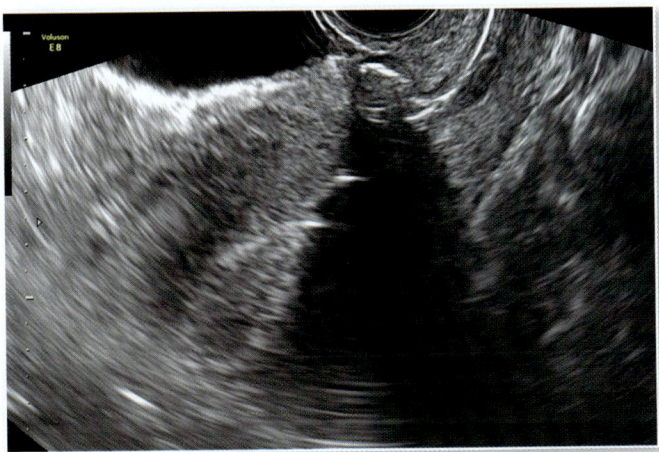

Figure 11.1: Transvaginal sonogram demonstrates normal size uterus in AVF. The endometrium is thin and hyperechogenic. Post C-section scar is visualized in the lower uterine segment

■ CLINICAL QUESTIONS

1. **Native sonogram showed irregular scarring tissue in the lower uterine segment. Can you accurately measure the uterine thickness to assess the risk of defects of scarred uterus?**

And. The quality of the native transvaginal sonogram does not allow precise measurement of the uterine thickness.

2. **What should be done next?**

And. Saline infusion sonography (SIS) should be performed for better assessment of the uterine lower segment thickness (Fig. 11.2).

3. **What is the interpretation of the SIS finding?**

And. High degree of lower uterine segment thinning (2 mm) is a possible indicator of a defective scar (Fig. 11.2). Further assessment of uterine thickness is required in the third trimester of pregnancy (between 35 and 39 weeks gestation). There are no available studies on reliability of preconceptional ultrasound and SIS for evaluating uterine scars among women with a history of cesarean section.

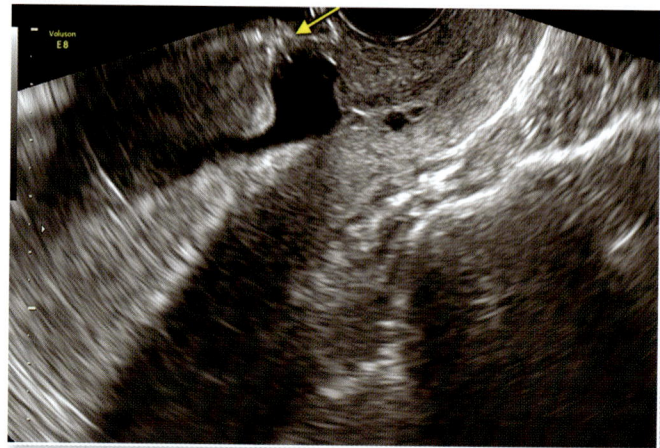

Figure 11.2: Saline infusion sonography (SIS) revealed fluid accumulation at the level of CS scar. Thin myometrial mantle of 2 mm was visualized

4. What is the value of 3D ultrasound in the assessment of lower uterine segment thinning?

And. 3D ultrasound provides a more accurate depiction of the uterine cavity and assessment of the scar shape, thickness, echogenicity, and continuity (Fig. 11.3).

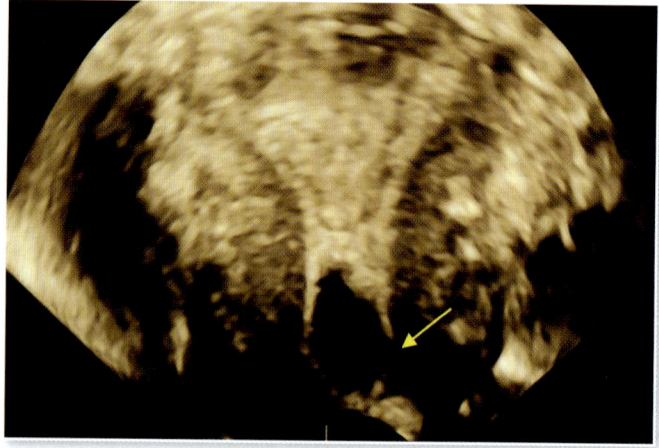

Figure 11.3: 3D ultrasound revealed hyperechogenic balloon shaped C-section scar. Arrow points to the area of discontinuity

■ TAKE-HOME MESSAGES

- Because of the thin muscle layer and poor vascularization lower uterine segment is considered a *locus minoris* resistance to uterine rupture.[1]
- A defective scar is directly related to the degree of thinning of the lower uterine segment on ultrasound at around 37 weeks of pregnancy.[2] There were no defective scars when uterine thickness in the lower uterine segment was greater than 4.5 mm, while 2% of the defective scars appeared with uterine thickness between 3.5 mm and 4.5 mm. With a cutoff value of 3.5 mm, the sensitivity of ultrasonographic measurement was 88.0%, the specificity 73.2%, positive predictive value 11.8%, and negative predictive value 99.3%.[2]

- Other studies confirmed the value of prenatal sonographic examination in the second and third trimesters for diagnosis of a uterine defect to determine the degree of lower uterine segment thinning in patients with previous CS.[3-7] Most of the previous studies measuring the lower uterine segment thickness were conducted between 35 and 39 weeks' gestation. Although they showed high validity, there is still controversy about the optimal threshold that should be used (the actual values ranging from 2.0–3.5 mm). The conclusion is that the measurement of the lower uterine segment can increase the safe use of trial of labor and predict the risk of uterine scar dehiscence.
- The inter- and intraobserver reliability of 3D sonography in the assessment of the lower uterine segment thickness is high, and the interpretation can easily be done offline by an expert.[8]
- The CS scar may be a site of ectopic pregnancy,[9,10] adherent placenta[11] or future dehiscence and uterine rupture.[12,13]

REFERENCES

1. Basic E, Basic Cetkovic V, Kozaric H, Rama A. Ultrasound evaluation of uterine scar after cesarean section. Acta Inform Med 2012;20(3):149-53.
2. Rozenberg P, Goffinet F, Phillippe HJ, Nisand I. Ultrasonographic measurement of lower uterine segment to assess risk of defects of scarred uterus. Lancet. 1996;347(8997):281-4.
3. Gotoh H, Masuzaki H, Yoshida A, et al. Predicting incomplete uterine rupture with vaginal sonography during the late second trimester in women with prior cesarean. Obstet Gynecol. 2000;95(4):596-600.
4. Sen J, Malik S, Salhan S. Ultrasonographic evaluation of lower uterine segment thickness in patients of previous cesarean section. International Journal of Gynecol Obstet. 2004;87:215-9.
5. Rozenberg P, Goffinet F, Philippe HJ, Nisand I. Thickness of the lower uterine segment: its influence in the management of patients with previous cesarean sections. Eur J Obstet Gynecol Reprod Biol. 1999;87(1):39-45.
6. Asakura H, Nakai A, Ishikawa G, et al. Prediction of Uterine Dehiscence by Measuring Lower Uterine Segment Thickness Prior to the Onset of Labor: evaluation by transvaginal ultrasonography. J Nippon Med Sch. 2000;67(5):352-6.
7. Suzuki S, Sawa R, Yoneyama Y, et al. Preoperative diagnosis of dehiscence of the lower uterine segment in patients with a single previous caesarean section. Aust N Z J Obstet Gynaecol. 2000;40(4):402-4.
8. Boutin A, Jastrow N, Roberge S, et al. Reliability of 3-dimensional transvaginal sonographic measurement of lower uterine segment thickness. J Ultrasound Med. 2012;3(6):933-9.
9. Ash A, Smith A, Maxwell D. Caesarean scar pregnancy. BJOG. 2007;114:253-63.
10. Maymon R, Halperin R, Mendlovic S, et al. Ectopic pregnancies in a Caesarean scar: review of the medical approach to an iatrogenic complication. Hum Reprod Update. 2004;10:515-23.
11. Rodgers SK, Kirby CL, Smith RJ, Horrow MM. Imaging after cesarean delivery: acute and chronic complications. Radiographics. 2012;32:1693-712.
12. Rozenberg P, Goffinet F, Phillippe HJ, et al. Ultrasonographic measurement of lower uterine segment to assess risk of defects of scarred uterus. Lancet. 1996;347:281-4.
13. Lydon-Rochelle M, Holt VL, Easterling TR, et al. Risk of uterine rupture during labor among women with a prior cesarean delivery. N Engl J Med. 2001;345:3-8.

CHAPTER 12

Menopause

Sanja Kupesic Plavsic

■ CLINICAL CASE

AF is a 65-year-old G2P2 woman, presenting for her annual pelvic examination. She complains of vaginal dryness and dyspareunia. She has never taken hormonal replacement therapy (HRT) or vaginal estrogen cream. Her history is significant for rheumatoid arthritis for which she was taking steroids. Six years ago she broke her left forearm.

Menarche: Age 15.

LMP: 18 years ago.
Her menstrual cycle used to be regular 28–30/5 days.

OB history: Two uncomplicated pregnancies with vaginal term deliveries.

Sexual history: Three male partners over her lifetime. The patient is sexually active with her husband. Pap smear was performed two years ago and was normal.

Review of Systems

- No headaches, no problems with vision
- No history of blood clots DVT or PE
- No heart palpitations, no shortness of breath
- No abdominal/pelvic pain
- No nausea, vomiting, constipation, and/or diarrhea
- She reports urine leakage with coughing, lifting, and running; no symptoms of UTI.

Past medical history: Six years ago, she broke her left forearm.

Past surgical history: None.

Vaccines : Up to date.

Current medications: None.

Allergies: No known drug allergies.

Social history: AF is a housewife. She used to smoke 1 pack of cigarettes for 30 years; about 10 years ago she quit smoking. Mr AF does not drink alcohol, and reports no history of substance abuse.

Family history: Her mother and sister died of a breast cancer. Mrs AF performed mammography and breast ultrasound 6 months ago, and the results were within normal limits. Her mother had fractured hip.

Physical Examination

- *Vital signs*: T 36.5°C; BP 110/70; P 78; BMI 16
- General physical examination was normal
- Pelvic examination revealed vaginal dryness. The rest of examination was normal. Transvaginal ultrasound was performed and results are presented in Figures 12.1 and 12.2
- Mrs AF was asked to perform bone densitometry (central DXA). The results of DXA scan of her lumbar spine and left hip are shown on Figures 12.3 and 12.4.

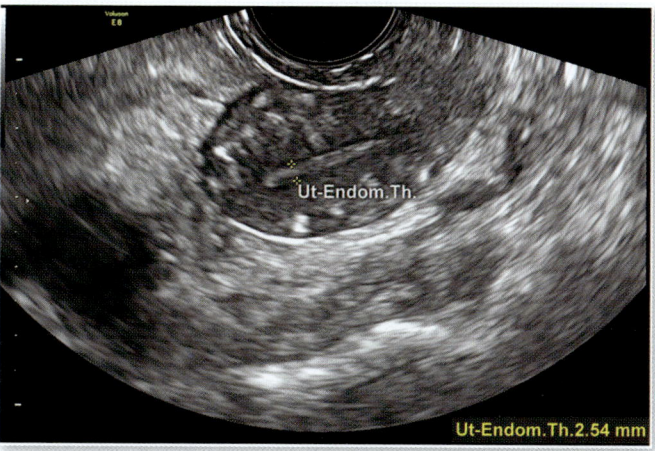

Figure 12.1: Transvaginal ultrasound of the uterus. Note thin endometrium (2.5 mm) and arcuate arterial calcifications in the outer third of myometrium

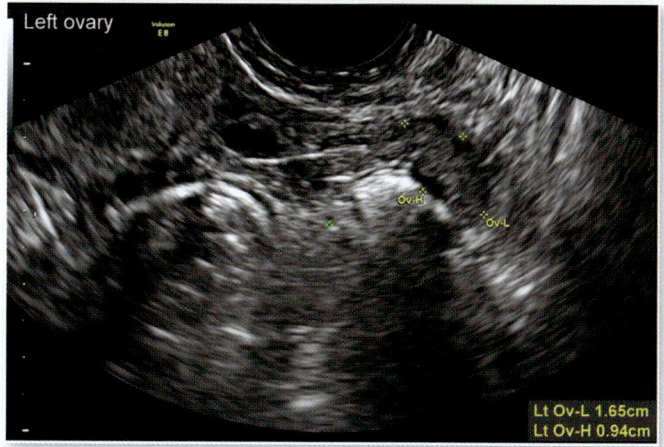

Figure 12.2: Transvaginal ultrasound revealed small ovaries

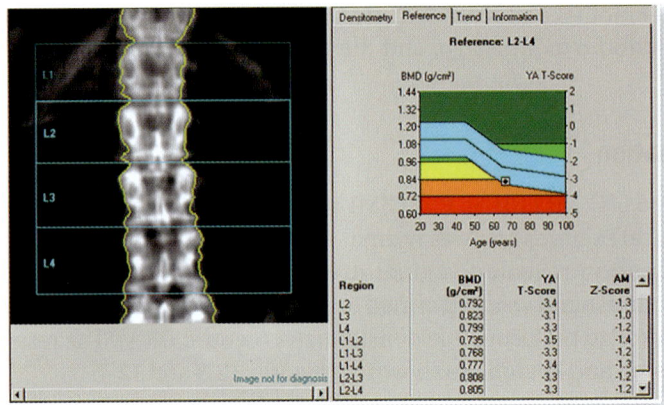

Figure 12.3: DXA scan of the lumbar spine shows osteoporosis (based on the T-score of −3.4 at L1–L4), applying WHO criteria for diagnosis of osteoporosis

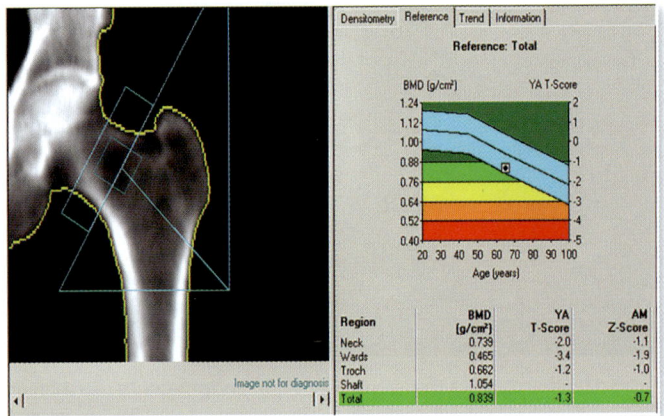

Figure 12.4: DXA scan of the left hip shows low bone mineral density (osteopenia), based on the T-score of −1.3 at total hip (highlighted in green), applying WHO criteria for the diagnosis of osteoporosis

■ CLINICAL QUESTIONS

1. What are the age appropriate screening investigations for this menopausal patient?

Ans. Screening mammography, bone densitometry (central DXA) and colonoscopy.

2. What are the advantages of central DXA?

Ans. Central DXA measures bone mineral density (BMD) in the axial skeleton (spine and the hip). It is cost-effective and keeps radiation exposure to a minimum.[1] Patient's DXA findings are presented in Figures 12.3 and 12.4.

3. List the risk factors for the development of osteoporosis in this patient.

Ans. Nonmodifiable risk factors for osteoporosis in this patient are female gender, menopausal status, late menarche (15 years), an early menopause (47 years), use of steroids, small body size, and history of cigarette smoking.

■ TAKE-HOME MESSAGES

- Osteoporosis is a disease characterized by reduced bone mass, microarchitectural deterioration of bone tissue, normal bone mineralization, and an increased risk of fragility fractures. The disease can be categorized as either being primary or secondary, with the primary form including senile and postmenopausal osteoporosis. Secondary causes of osteoporosis include any medical condition or medication that accelerates bone loss.[1]
- Accelerated bone loss may occur in menopausal women, elderly men and women, and can be secondary to numerous disease states and medications. Postmenopausal osteoporosis is characterized by an estrogen dependent accelerated phase of bone loss that occurs during the decade after a woman's cessation of menses. Estrogen deficiency appears to result in increased synthesis of inflammatory cytokines that augment osteoclastic activity with osteoblasts not being able to compensate for the accelerated loss of bone mass.[1]
- Primary osteoporosis normally lacks any abnormal blood chemistry findings unless a patient has experienced a fracture within the past several months and may exhibit an elevated alkaline phosphatase. The diagnosis of primary osteoporosis is not made by analysis of blood chemistry tests, yet they are important in ruling out secondary causes of osteoporosis. A sound history and physical as well as laboratory work including a comprehensive metabolic profile (CMP), complete blood count (CBC), vitamin D levels, and urinary excretion of calcium is often adequate in excluding secondary causes of decreased bone mass.[1-4]
- Modifiable risk factors for osteoporosis include low estrogen levels, malnutrition, decreased calcium and vitamin D intake, use of certain medications such as glucocorticoids or anticonvulsants, immobility, cigarette smoking and excessive alcohol consumption.[4-7]
- Nonmodifiable risk factors for osteoporosis include female gender, advanced age, small body frame, late menarche/early menopause, Caucasian and Asian race, and family history of osteoporosis.[3-5]
- Patients at risk for osteoporosis should be encouraged to make lifestyle modifications including weight-bearing exercise, smoking cessation, and decreased alcohol consumption.[1]
- In women age 65 and men age 70 an older bone mineral density testing is recommended. Dual-energy X-ray absorptiometry (DXA scan) is the current standard technique for the diagnosis of osteoporosis, due to its ability to measure bone mineral density at a variety of sites. It should normally be measured on two sites, preferably anteroposterior (AP) spine and hip.[1-3] The two sites allow the physician to evaluate both the patient's risk for hip fracture and the risk for vertebral fracture. The spinal measurements are followed to evaluate the effectiveness of interventions.
- Experts recommend that premenopausal women and men consume at least 1,000 mg of calcium per day; this includes calcium in foods and beverages plus calcium supplements. Postmenopausal women should consume 1,200 mg of calcium per day (total of diet plus supplements). It is recommended that men over 70 years and postmenopausal women consume 800 international units of vitamin D each day.[8]
- Drinking alcohol (more than 2 drinks a day) and cigarette smoking increase the risk of fracture.[8]
- Weight-bearing and muscle strengthening exercise (at least 30 minutes three times per week) improve bone mass and helps women to maintain bone density after menopause and reduce the risk of falls and fractures.[8]
- In the United States, the National Osteoporosis Foundation (NOF) recommends use of a medication to treat postmenopausal women (and men ≥50 years) with a history of hip or vertebral fracture or with osteoporosis (T-score ≤−2.5).[9]
- In addition, the NOF recommends drug therapy patients with osteopenia (T-score between −1.0 and −2.5) and an estimated 10-year risk of hip or osteoporosis-related fracture ≥3 or ≥20%, respectively. The absolute risk of fracture can be calculated using the World Health Organization (WHO) Fracture Risk Assessment Tool (FRAX) calculator.[9,10]
- Current FDA-approved pharmacologic options for osteoporosis prevention and/or treatment are bisphosphonates (alendronate, ibandronate, risedronate, and zoledronic acid), calcitonin, estrogens and/or hormone therapy, estrogen agonist/antagonist (raloxifene), and parathyroid hormone, PTH (teriparatide).[9]

- The 1st line medical therapies for osteoporosis are the bisphosphonates (alendronate, risendronate and zolendronic acid are most commonly used bisphosphonates). Because of their extraskeletal side effects, these medications must be taken NPO in the morning with a large glass of water, and the patients must remain upright for at least 30 minutes. The most serious complications of bisphosphonates are osteonecrosis of the jaw, musculoskeletal pain and hypocalcemia. Both daily and weekly forms show increased bone mineral densities and decreased fractures over a 2-year-period.[1]
- Raloxifen is a SERM that has an estrogenic effect on bone but opposes the effects of estrogen in the uterus and breast. It is not a first line agent in the general population because while it does reduce vertebral fractures there is limited evidence that it reduces other higher risk fractures as effectively as the bisphosphonates.[1]
- PTH therapy is reserved for patients with very severe osteoporosis who cannot take bisphosphonates or who have suboptimal results with 1st line therapies.[1]
- BMD testing performed in DXA centers using accepted quality assurance measures is appropriate for monitoring bone loss. For patients on pharmacotherapy, it is typically performed two years after initiating therapy and every two years thereafter; however, more frequent testing may be warranted in certain clinical situations.[9]

REFERENCES

1. Kupesic Plavsic S. Step by Step Case Studies in Obstetrics and Gynecology. New Delhi, London, Philadelphia, Panama: Jaypee Brothers Medical Publisher; 2014. p. 46-60.
2. Siris ES, Miller PD, Barrett-Connor E, et al. Identification and fracture outcomes of undiagnosed low bone mineral density in postmenopausal women: results from the National Osteoporosis Risk Assessment. JAMA 2001;286(22):2815-22.
3. Warriner AH, Patkar NM, Curtis JR, et al. Which fractures are most attributable to osteoporosis? J Clin Epidemiol. 2011;64(1):46-53.
4. Tannenbaum C, Clark J, Schwartzman K, et al. Yield of laboratory testing to identify secondary contributors to osteoporosis in otherwise healthy women. J Clin Endocrinol Metal. 2002;87(10):4431-7.
5. Compston JE, Watts NB, Chapurlat R, et al. Obesity is not protective against fracture in postmenopausal women: GLOW. Am J Med 2011;124(11):1043-50.
6. Herkowitz HN, Garfin SR, Eismont FJ, et al. Metabolic bone disorders of the spine. Rothman-Simeone the spine. 6th ed. Philadelphia: Elsevier; 2011: p 1571-95.
7. Bethel M. Osteoporosis Differential Diagnosis. Medscape 2015. http://emedicine.medscape.com/article/330598-differential. Updated February 26, 2015.
8. Rosen HN. Osteoporosis prevention and treatment. UpToDAte 2015. http://www.uptodate.com/contents/osteoporosis-prevention-and-treatment-beyond-the-basics. Updated September 11, 2014.
9. National Osteoporosis Foundation (NOF).Clinician's Guide to Prevention and Treatment of Osteoporosis. 2010. http://nof.org/files/nof/public/content/file/344/upload/159.pdf. Updated January 2010.
10. FRAX. www.NOF.org and www.shef.ac.uk/FRAX. Accessed December 16, 2015.

CHAPTER

Postmenopausal Bleeding

13

Sanja Kupesic Plavsic, Osvaldo Padilla

■ CLINICAL CASE

UM is a 68-year old Caucasian G2P2 female who presents with complaint of postmenopausal vaginal bleeding. The patient began experiencing the symptoms of vaginal spotting on and off for about two months. She had her LMP at age 51. She had her two children at ages 25 and 28. Her last Pap smear was three years ago, and was within normal limits. She was never using hormonal replacement therapy (HRT).

The patient is currently being treated for breast cancer with tamoxifen for approximately one year. She had a cholecystectomy at age 44 and a CS for her second pregnancy at age 28. She has medically controlled hypertension for the past ten years. She is married to her husband of 44 years, and retired two years ago. The patient is not experiencing other symptoms besides the vaginal bleeding.

On physical examination, the patient is an overweight Caucasian postmenopausal female, with a BMI of 30. She is in no acute apparent distress. Vital signs are unremarkable.

Menarche: Age 14.

Menses: During the reproductive period, her menstrual cycles were regular, 28–30/5 days.

LMP: 17 years ago.

Pregnancies: Two term pregnancies (1 vaginal birth, 1 CS).

Sexual history: She has had two sexual partners in her lifetime, and has never been diagnosed with sexually transmitted infection or other gynecologic pathology. She is currently sexually active with her husband.

Review of Systems

- No chest pain or shortness of breath
- No diarrhea or constipation
- Patient complains of urinary frequency; no hematuria or dysuria.

Section 1: Gynecology

Past medical history: Diagnosed with breast cancer one year ago (treated with surgery and chemotherapy, currently on tamoxifen).

Past surgical history: Cholecystectomy, C-section and lumpectomy.

Vaccines: Up to date (hepatitis B vaccine series, MMR booster and flu shot).

Current medications: Tamoxifen and antihypertensive medications.

Allergies: No known drug allergies.

Social history: UM is retired IT executive; she does not smoke, social ETOH, no drug abuse.

Family history: Non-contributory.

Physical Examination

Vital signs: T 36.4°C oral; BP 140/90; P 78; BMI 30.

Cardiac examination: No heart murmur was detected.

Chest examination: Clear lungs, breathing sound was clear.

Abdominal examination: Within normal limits.

Pelvic examination: Speculum examination reveals blood in the vagina Bimanual examination is unremarkable.

Pelvic ultrasound revealed abnormally thickened endometrium (Fig. 13.1) with increased perfusion (Figs 13.2 and 13.3).

High velocity and low vascular resistance (RI 0.46 and PI 0.59) are suggestive of endometrial neoplasia.

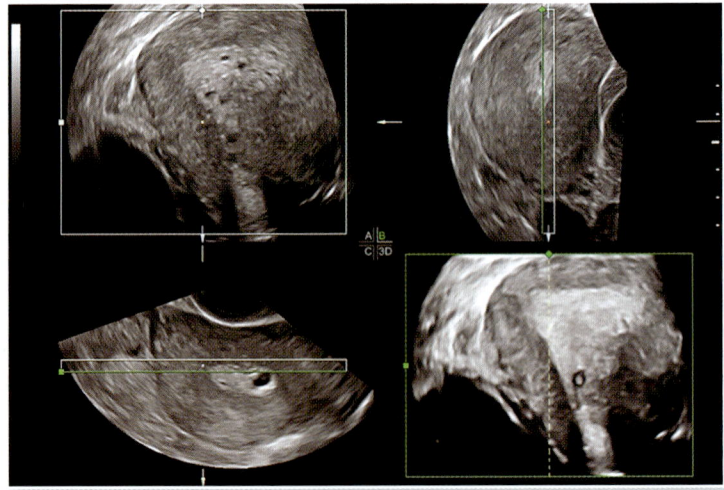

Figure 13.1: Three-dimensional ultrasound demonstrates abnormally thickened endometrium with multiple cystic inclusions

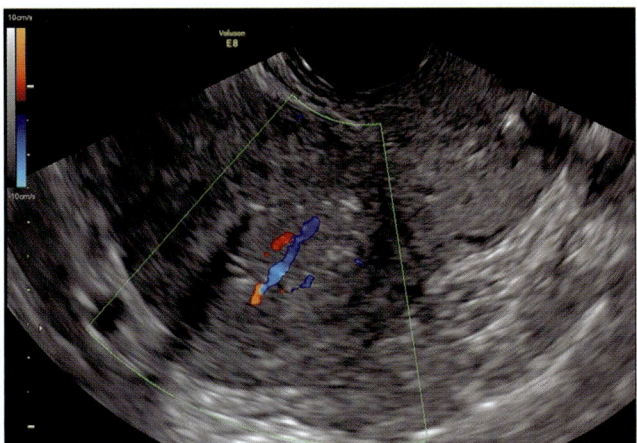

Figure 13.2: Color Doppler demonstrates thickened endometrium with increased perfusion

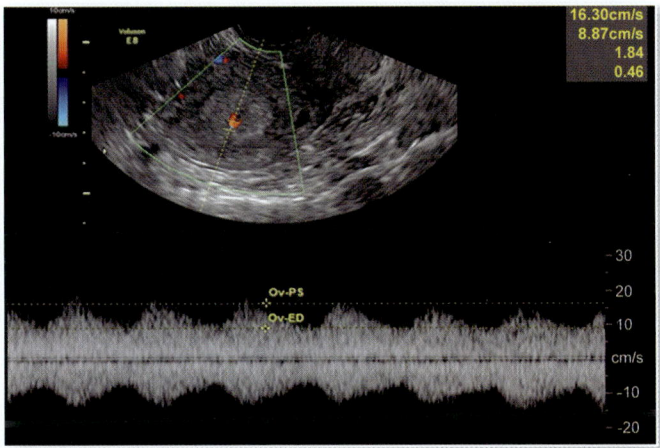

Figure 13.3: Low-to-moderate vascular impedance (RI 0.46) was obtained from intraendometrial vessels

CLINICAL QUESTIONS

1. What is the most appropriate next step in the management of this patient?

Ans. All postmenopausal patients with uncertain endometrial thickness (ill-defined endometrium) should undergo SIS, endometrial biopsy or diagnostic hysteroscopy. SIS, also known as hysterosonography or sonohysterography is a minimally invasive ultrasound technique that involves infusion of a small volume of sterile saline into the uterine cavity. It is performed for better differentiation of intracavitary pathology. Saline acts as a negative contrast medium which clearly delineates the endometrial lining. Contrast enhanced sonographic studies provide high resolution images of the uterine cavity and may reveal solitary or multiple intracavitary lesions. Figure 13.4 illustrates a solitary polyp detected by SIS in our patient, while Figures 13.5 to 13.7 illustrate multiple polyps in another patient using tamoxifen.

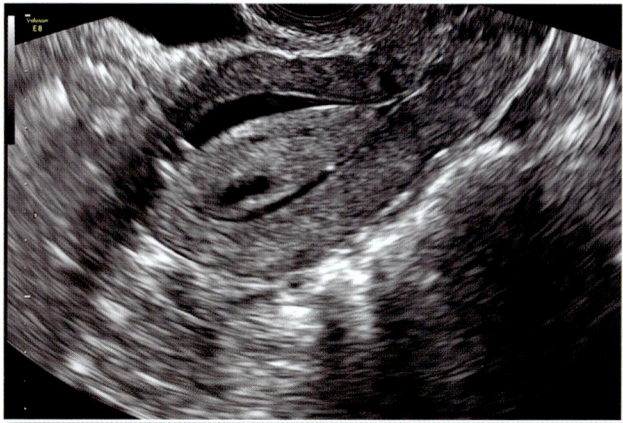

Figure 13.4: Saline infusion sonography demonstrates focal endometrial thickening typical for endometrial polyp. Endometrial polyps are hyperplastic overgrowths of endometrial glands and stroma that form a projection from the surface of the endometrium

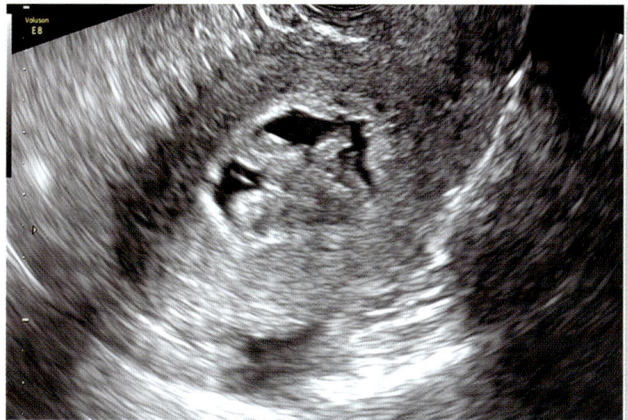

Figure 13.5: SIS reveals multiple irregular polyps in a patient using tamoxifen

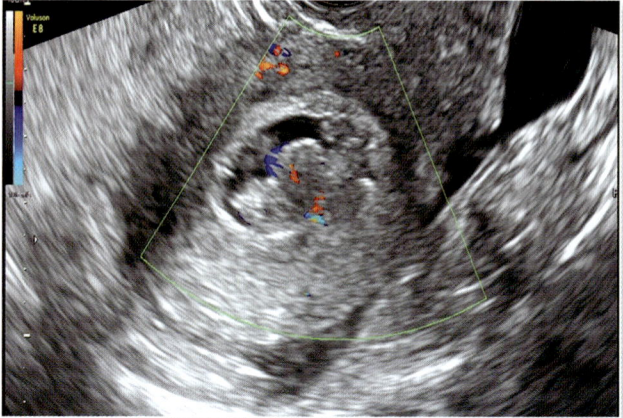

Figure 13.6: Increased vascularity of polypoid lesions is obtained by color Doppler ultrasound

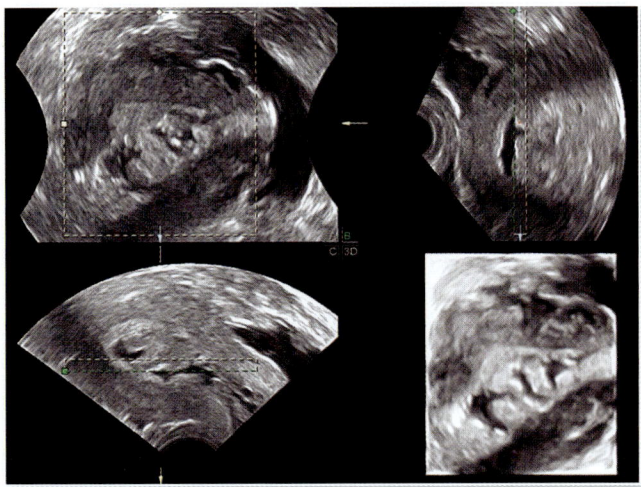

Figure 13.7: Three-dimensional ultrasound of multiple tamoxifen induced polyps

2. List the advantages and limitations of SIS.

Ans. Advantages of SIS:
- Simple and minimally invasive procedure
- Well tolerated by patients
- Enables excellent view of the uterus and endometrial lining and simultaneous visualization of adnexa
- Does not use ionizing radiation
- Few complications.

Limitations of SIS are:
- Cannot be performed in patients with cervical stenosis and uterine adhesions (scarring)
- Absolutely contraindicated in pregnant patients
- Should not be performed in patients with acute pelvic inflammatory disease.

3. What should be performed next?

Ans. The great majority of endometrial polyps are benign, but malignancy may occur in some patients. Therefore, endometrial biopsy should be performed in every postmenopausal patient presenting with vaginal bleeding (Fig. 13.8). It is well documented that tamoxifen may exert a proliferative effect on the endometrium, resulting in focal endometrial thickening. Tamoxifen associated endometrial polyps are often larger than sporadic polyps and are more likely to exhibit epithelial metaplasia and stromal condensation around glands.[1] Histopathology of tamoxifen-induced polyps demonstrates cystic changes, proliferative or inactive glands which are usually peripheral and angulated, fibrous stroma with spindled fibroblast-like cells, and abundant extracellular connective tissue (Fig. 13.9).

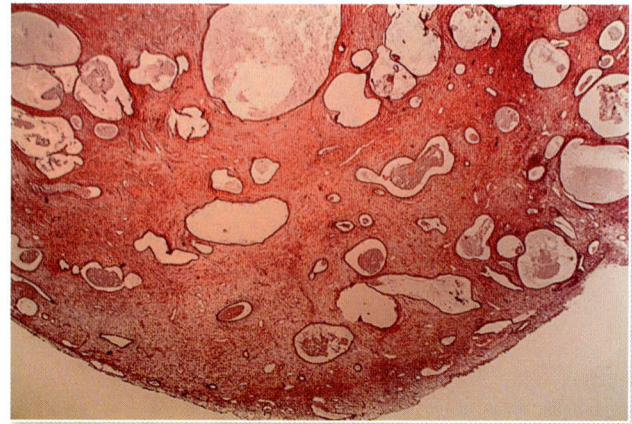

Figure 13.8: A glandulocystic appearance of the polyp, which was also appreciated in sonographic studies

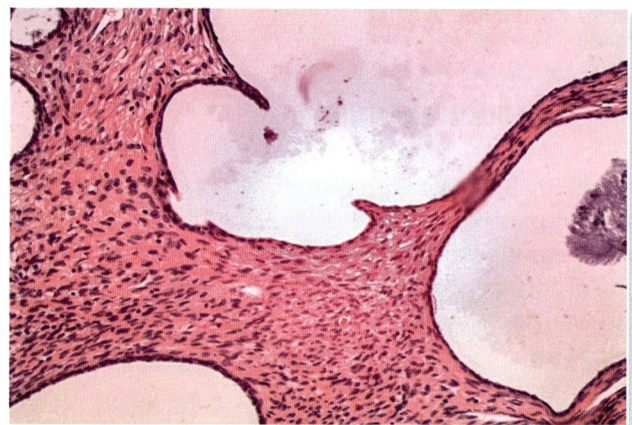

Figure 13.9: Tamoxifen associated endometrial polyp demonstrates stromal fibrosis and dilated, atrophic endometrial glands. No hyperplasia or malignancy was identified in the merging of the polypoid and non-polypoid endometrium

4. List the advantages and limitations of endometrial biopsy.

Ans. Advantages of endometrial biopsy:
- Low cost
- Low complication rate
- High sensitivity
- Easily accessible.

Limitations of endometrial biopsy:
- Requires collaboration with pathology department
- Low sensitivity for detection of structural abnormalities, such as polyps.

5. What is the best treatment option for this patient?

Ans. Polypectomy under hysteroscopy guidance is the treatment of choice for this patient.

6. What is the advantage of 3D ultrasound in the assessment of endometrial lesions?

Ans. The advantage of 3D ultrasound is better visualization of intrauterine lesions, precise volume estimation and assessment of subendometrial halo (Fig. 13.10).

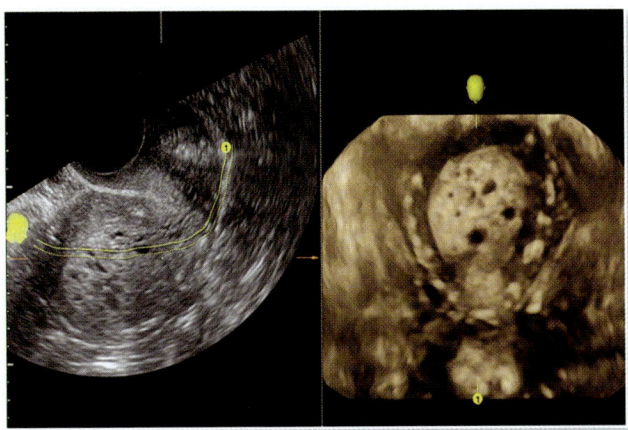

Figure 13.10: Three-dimensional surface reconstruction of the honey-comb appearance of the endometrium in a patient using tamoxifen

■ TAKE-HOME MESSAGES

- Although most patients using tamoxifen have no pathologic endometrial changes, endometrial polyps, hyperplasia and metaplasia are detected in about one third of patients. It is estimated that endometrial polyps develop in 2–36% of postmenopausal women treated with tamoxifen.[2,3] In this group of women polyps may be solitary, multiple and may show molecular alterations.
- Histopathology of tamoxifen induced polyps demonstrates cystic changes, proliferative or inactive glands which are usually peripheral and angulated, fibrous stroma with spindled fibroblast-like cells, and abundant extracellular connective tissue (Figs 13.8 and 13.9).
- It seems that malignant transformation of endometrial polyps occurs more frequently in patients using tamoxifen (up to 11%).[4] Tamoxifen use is associated with an increased risk of endometrial carcinoma.[5] Because women with breast cancer are more likely to develop endometrial carcinoma due to other factors, such as increased socioeconomic status, low parity and hyperestrogenic states, it is difficult to ascertain whether there is a true association between tamoxifen and the development of endometrial cancer.[1] Most epidemiologic studies report that tamoxifen increases the risk of developing an endometrial cancer two to three times compared to the patients with breast cancer who are not using tamoxifen.[1,4]
- Effect of tamoxifen is believed to be due to its estrogenic activity, indicating that most of the endometrial cancers should be of endometrioid type. However, serous carcinoma, carcinosarcomas, and adenosarcomas have also been reported.[1]
- Evidence-based literature is in agreement that all symptomatic polyps should be removed. Polypectomy under hysteroscopy guidance is the treatment of choice.[4-6]
- Color Doppler is useful for distinction between benign and malignant endometrial pathology (Figs 13.2, 13.3 and 13.6).[7]
- Sometimes the patient is sent to be evaluated with SIS because of abnormal endometrial thickening and inconclusive color Doppler findings (Figs 13.4 and 13.5). Data from the literature indicate that SIS does not increase the risk of malignant cell dissemination in patients with endometrial cancer.[8,9]
- Three-dimensional ultrasound enables better visualization of intrauterine lesions, improved estimation of the endometrial volume and superior assessment of subendometrial halo (Figs 13.7 and 13.10).[10]

REFERENCES

1. McCluggage WG. My approach to the interpretation of endometrial biopsies and curettings. J Clin Pathol. 2006;59(8): 801-12.
2. Gul A, Ugur M, Iskender C, et al. Immunohistochemical expression of estrogen and progesterone receptors in endometrial polyps and its relationship to clinical parameters. Arch Gynecol Obstet. 2010;281(3):479-83.
3. Zitao L, Kuokkanen S, Pal L. Steroid hormone receptor profile of premenopausal endometrial polyps. Reprod Sci. 2010; 17(4):377-83.
4. Cohen I. Endometrial pathologies associated with postmenopausal tamoxifen treatment. Gynecol Oncol. 2004;94(2):256-66.
5. Runowicz CD, Costantino JP, Wickerham DL, et al. Gynecologic conditions in participants in the NSABP breast cancer prevention study of tamoxifen and raloxifene (STAR). Am J Obstet Gynecol. 2011;205(6):535.e1-5.
6. Nathani F, Clark TJ. Uterine polypectomy in the management of abnormal uterine bleeding: A systematic review. J Minim Invasive Gynecol. 2006;13(4):260-8.
7. Kupesic S, Shalan H, Kurjak A. Early detection of endometrial cancer by transvaginal color Doppler. Eur J Obstet Gynecol. 1993;49(1-2):46-9.
8. van Hanegem N, Breijer MC, Khan KS, et al. Diagnostic evaluation of the endometrium in postmenopausal bleeding: an evidence-based approach. Maturitas. 2011;68(2):155-64.
9. Takac I. Saline infusion sonohysterography and the risk of malignant extrauterine spread in endometrial cancer. Ultrasound Med Biol. 2008;34(1):7-11.
10. Scofienxa LM, Lacelli F, Caldiera V, et al. Three-dimensional sonohysterography for examination of the uterine cavity in women with abnormal uterine bleeding: Preliminary findings. J Ultrasound. 2010;13(1):16-21.

CHAPTER 14

Endometrial Polyp

Melissa D Mendez, Sireesha Y Reddy, Osvaldo Padilla, Sanja Kupesic Plavsic

■ CLINICAL CASE

GR is a 56-year-old postmenopausal G3P3 who presents to the outpatient gynecology clinic with a chief complaint of low right-sided pelvic pain and irregular vaginal spotting for the past one year. The pain is described as cramping and radiates to the right lower back. She reported a medical history of ovarian cysts. She took naproxen as needed which gave relief for the pain. She denied having an abnormal Pap smear or an abnormal mammogram.

Menarche: Age 10.

Menses: 28/4.

LMP: Six years ago.

Obstetric hisotry: 3 SVDs, all full term, no complications.

Sexual history: Denies ever having any sexually transmitted diseases.

Contraception: Bilateral tubal ligation at age 33.

Review of Systems

- No chest pain or shortness of breath
- No diarrhea or constipation
- Denies any urinary frequency, urgency, hematuria or dysuria.

Past medical history: Ovarian cysts and hypertension, controlled by medication.

Past surgical history: A right ovarian cyst removal at age 19. She is unsure what type of cyst was removed. Bilateral tubal ligation at age 33.

Medications: Lisinopril 10 mg orally daily, calcium daily.

Allergies: None known drug allergies.

Social history: Denies tobacco, drug or alcohol use. Married, is a homemaker, lives with her husband and her youngest child.

Family history: Mother with diabetes, obesity, had a hysterectomy at age 40 for abnormal bleeding.

Physical Examination

Vital signs: T 36.8°C oral; BP 145/92; P 60; BMI 29.

Cardiac examination: Regular rate and rhythm, no murmurs.

Chest examination: Lungs are clear to auscultation bilaterally.

Abdominal examination: Non distended, non-tender, no masses felt.

Pelvic examination: External Genitalia with no abnormalities. No cervical masses. No cervical motion tenderness. Uterus 10-week size, globular, mobile, non-tender. Adnexa within normal limits.

She underwent a transvaginal ultrasound of the pelvis where she was found to have a thickened endometrial stripe of 13.8 mm. Her ovaries were normal. 2D and 3D SIS was performed (Figs 14.1 and 14.2). She subsequently underwent an endometrial biopsy which confirmed

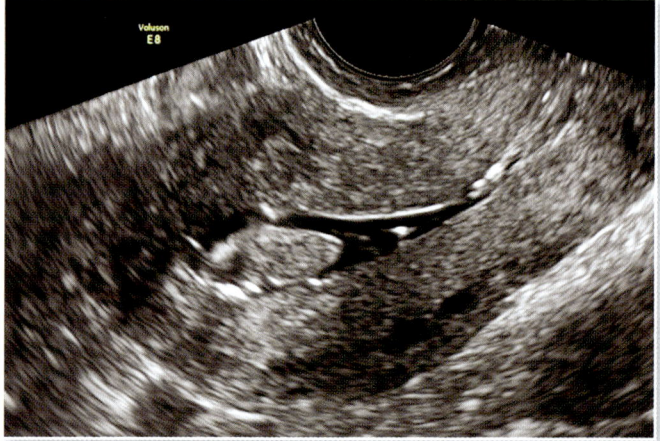

Figure 14.1: Transvaginal saline infusion sonography clearly outlines the focal endometrial lesion, suggestive of an endometrial polyp

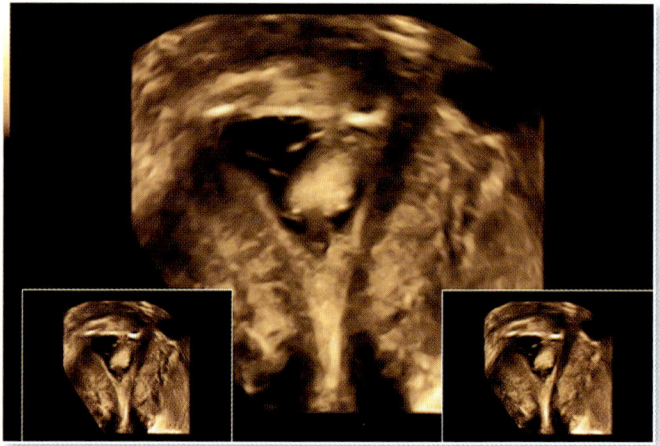

Figure 14.2: Reconstruction on the coronal plane by 3D saline infusion sonography reveals exact location of the endometrial polyp in the left uterine horn

evidence of an endocervical polyp. The patient then underwent hysteroscopic polyp removal as demonstrated in Figures 14.3 and 14.4.

Figures 14.5 and 14.6 illustrate gross anatomy and histopathology images of an endometrial polyp in a postmenopausal patient who underwent hysterectomy.

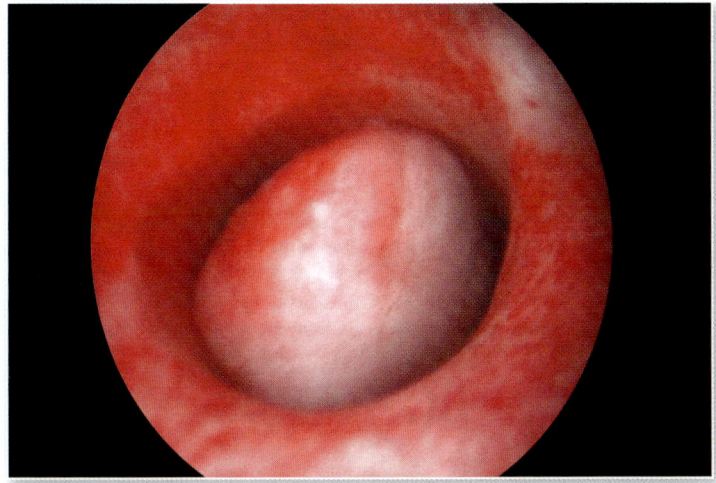

Figure 14.3: Hysteroscopic view demonstrating a large endometrial polyp occupying the endometrial cavity

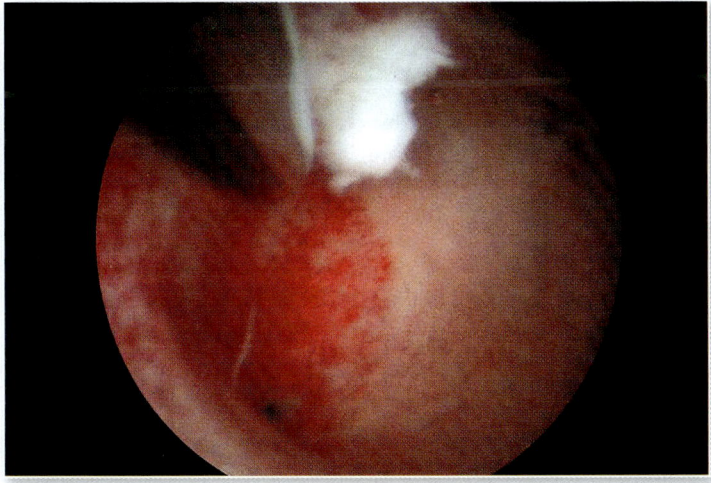

Figure 14.4: Hysteroscopic polyp removal of the polyp in Figure 14.3 using endoshears

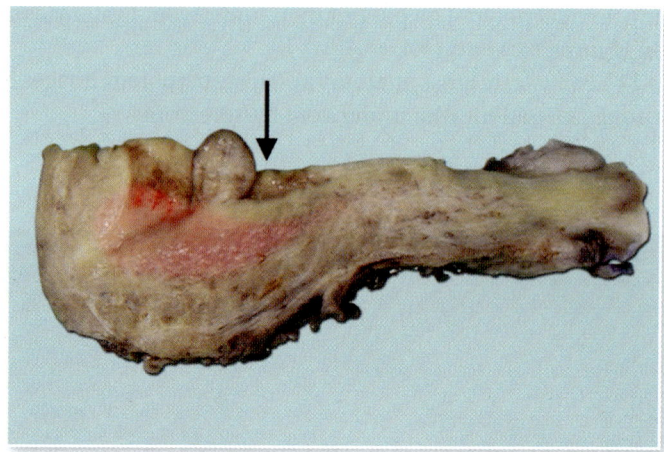

Figure 14.5: Gross specimen of a uterus after a hysterectomy. The arrow points to an endometrial polyp

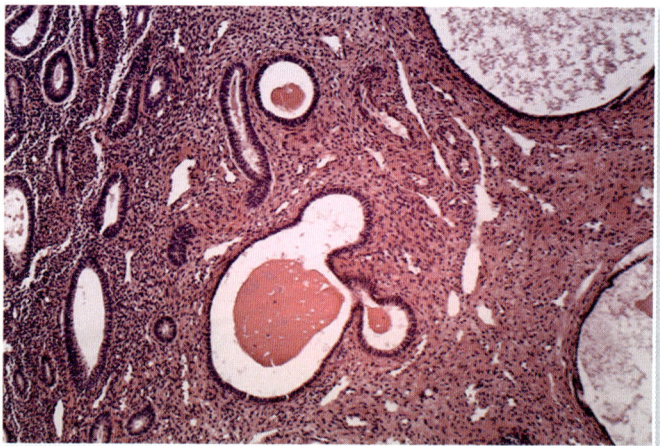

Figure 14.6: The histologic appearance of an endometrial polyp

■ CLINICAL QUESTIONS

1. **What are risk factors for a woman to develop an endometrial polyp?**

Ans. The formation of polyps appears to be linked to excess estrogen. Risk factors include age, late menopause, obesity, and tamoxifen use. Some studies have also linked diabetes and hypertension as risk factors for developing endometrial polyps and some have not.[1]

2. **What is the risk of a postmenopausal woman developing cancer from an endocervical or endometrial polyp?**

Ans. The risk for an endometrial polyp to be malignant appears to be higher for a postmenopausal women with symptomatic vaginal bleeding (4%) than the risk found in a premenopausal woman or postmenopausal woman without vaginal bleeding (1.5%).[1,2]

3. What role does transvaginal sonogram and SIS play in the diagnoses of endocervical and endometrial polyps?

Ans. Endometrial polyps can be diagnosed on transvaginal ultrasound or SIS. SIS has a higher specificity and sensitivity for the diagnosis of endometrial polyps. Operative hysteroscopy is the preferred diagnosis and treatment modality for endometrial polyps.

4. What is the best treatment for endometrial polyps?

Ans. Treatment depends on the menopausal status and presenting symptoms. If the woman is premenopausal and asymptomatic you can observe. If the patient has symptomatic vaginal bleeding or has infertility, the polyp should be removed. If the patient is postmenopausal and has uterine bleeding, the polyp should be removed. Treatment is typically operative hysteroscopy with polyp removal either with polyp forceps, scissors, bipolar energy or morcellation.

■ TAKE-HOME MESSAGES

- Common complaints of women who are found to have endometrial polyps are abnormal menstrual bleeding, intermenstrual bleeding, postmenopausal bleeding and/or vaginal discharge. Many patients are asymptomatic.[1]
- Transvaginal ultrasound (TV US) is the preferred initial diagnostic procedure for evaluating abnormal uterine bleeding.[2] SIS has increased sensitivity and specificity over TV US with and without color Doppler for both endometrial polyps and myomas.[2]
- Diagnostic hysteroscopy seems to have higher diagnostic accuracy compared to TV US and SIS for endometrial polyps and myomas.[2]
- Gel instillation sonography (GIS) may be an alternative for SIS in the evaluation of endometrial polyps and myomas.[3]
- Endometrial polyps are a localized overgrowth of the endometrium. Estrogen stimulation of the endometrium is thought to play an important role in the formation of endometrial polyps, such as late menopause, obesity and tamoxifen use.[4,5] In this group of patients the incidence of endometrial polyps is about 24% with a range of about 7–34%.[4,5]
- Blind dilation and curettage (D and C) or endometrial biopsy is inaccurate for diagnosis.[5,6]
- A polyp is more likely to be malignant in a postmenopausal woman with symptomatic vaginal bleeding, than in a nonsymptomatic postmenopausal woman and therefore the polyp(s) should be removed.[4,5,7]
- Polyps may spontaneously regress in about 25% of patients especially if the polyp is less than 1 cm.[5] This may be considered in women who are premenopausal and asymptomatic.[4,5]
- Polyps in women who are symptomatic or have infertility should be removed to improve symptoms and infertility outcomes.[5,7]
- Some studies have also suggested that risk factors for endometrial polyps include diabetes and hypertension.[8]
- The preferred treatment for endometrial polyps is operative hysteroscopy.[1] Removal of the polyp can be achieved with polypectomy forceps, bipolar systems or hysteroscopic morcellation.[5,9] Polyp removal is associated with a relief or improvement in symptoms.[7,9]

■ REFERENCES

1. Lee SC, Kaunitz AM, Sanchez-Ramos L, Rhatigan RM. The oncogenic potential of endometrial polyps: a systematic review and meta-analysis. Obstet Gynecol. 2010;116(5):1197-205.
2. Grimbizis GF, Tsolakidis D, Mikos T, et al. A prospective comparison of transvaginal ultrasound, saline infusion sonohysterography, and diagnostic hysteroscopy in the evaluation of endometrial pathology. Fertil Steril. 2010; 94(7):2720-5.
3. Werbrouk E, Veldman J, Luts J, et al. Detection of endometrial pathology using saline infusion sonography versus gel instillation sonography: a prospective cohort study. Fertil Steril. 2011;95(1):285-8.

4. Ricciardi E, Vecchione A, Marci R, Schimberni M, et al. Clinical factors and malignancy in endometrial polyps. Analysis of 1027 cases. Eur J Obstet Gynecol Reprod Biol. 2014;183:121-4.
5. American Association of Gynecologic Laparoscopists. AAGLPractice Report: practice guidelines for the diagnosis and management of endometrial polyps. J Minim Invasive Gynecol. 2012;19(1):3-10.
6. Torres ML, Weaver AL, Kumar S, et al. Risk Factors for developing endometrial cancer after benign endometrial sampling. Obstet Gynecol. 2012;120(5):998-1004.
7. Lieng M, Istre O, Qvigstad E. Treatment of endometrial polyps: a systematic review. Acta Obstet Gynecol. 2010;89(8):992-1002.
8. Serhat E, Cogendez E, Selcuk S, et al. Is there a relationship between endometrial polyps and obesity and obesity, diabetes mellitus, hypertension? Arch Gynecol Obstet. 2014;290(5):937-41.
9. AlHilli MM, Nixon KE, Hopkins MR, et al. Long-term outcomes after intrauterine morcellation vs hysteroscopic resection of endometrial polyps. J Minim Invasive Gynecol. 2013;20(2):215-21.

CHAPTER 15

Hematometra in a Postmenopausal Patient

Sushila Arya, Sanja Kupesic Plavsic

■ CLINICAL CASE

SG is a 62-year-old G3P3, who presents to the clinic for complaints of lower abdominal and pelvic pain. Pain is cramping in nature, and started 4–5 weeks ago. She denies any change in bowel or bladder habits, as well as abnormal vaginal discharge, fever, nausea, vomiting, weight or appetite changes. There is no history of postmenopausal bleeding. The patient is not sexually active due to disabled husband. Her history is significant for a cold knife cone biopsy 3 years ago. Follow-up Pap smear one year after the procedure was normal. Patient did not have follow-up or preventive care during the last 2 years.

Menarche: Age 11; Menopause at age 52 years.

Past obstetric history: 3 normal spontaneous vaginal deliveries.

Sexual history: 2 male partners over her lifetime.

Contraception: BTL, menopause.

Past medical history: Prediabetes, no hospitalizations.

Past surgical history: BTL.

Current medications: Multivitamin and fish oil.

Allergies: No known drug allergies.

Social history: SG is a retired schoolteacher. She drinks alcohol occasionally and in moderation. She denies any tobacco or substance abuse.

Family history: Significant for mother with colon cancer at age 68 years. No other family history of hereditary cancers or other chronic medical conditions.

Review of Systems

Positive for abdominal and pelvic pain. All other ROS is negative.

Physical Examination

Vital signs: T 36.7°C oral; BP 131/78; P 71; BMI 29.5.

General: Alert, oriented to time, place and person.

Neck, heart and lungs examination is unremarkable.

Abdominal examination: Soft, lower abdomen is tender, uterus is enlarged ~12 weeks, tender. No guarding or rigidity.

Pelvic Examination

Age appropriate atrophy, but otherwise normal external genitalia. Cervix is atrophic and external os has a small opening. Vagina is smooth with loss of rugoses, otherwise unremarkable. On bimanual examination uterus is enlarged to 12 weeks, tender and in midline. Adnexa were difficult to assess.

Pelvic ultrasound was performed and findings are illustrated in Figures 15.1 and 15.2.

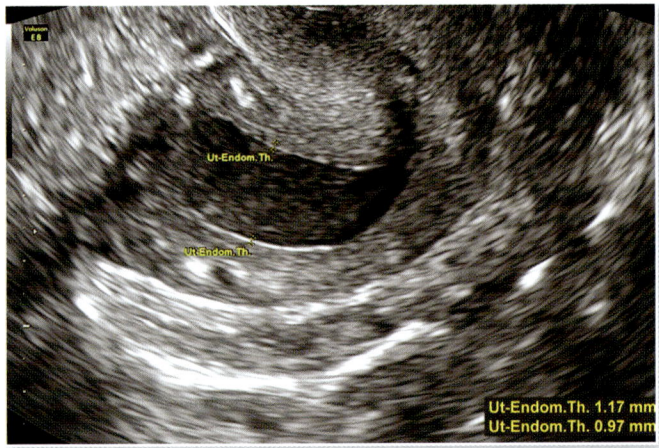

Figure 15.1: Transvaginal scan of a postmenopausal patient with collection of blood in the uterus (hematometra). In the presence of intracavitary fluid, both single endometrial layers should be measured in the sagittal plane

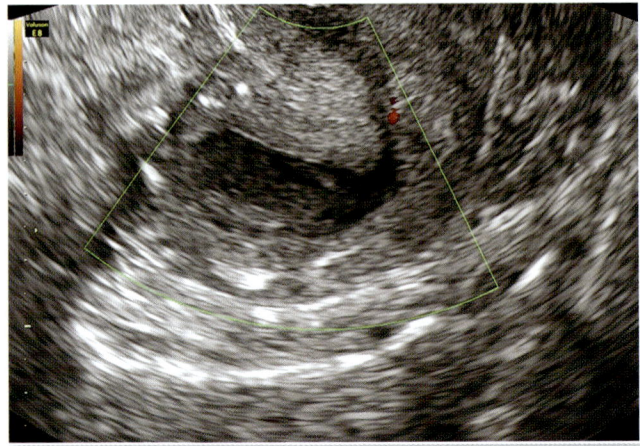

Figure 15.2: Transvaginal color Doppler scan of the same patient. Color Doppler does not reveal endometrial and/or intracavitary vascularity

Patient underwent examination under anesthesia. Following cervical dilatation and drainage of 200 cc chocolate colored blood, hysteroscopy was performed. Hysteroscopy revealed thin atrophic endometrium. Fractional D and C was done and revealed a scant benign and endometrial gland, with no evidence of hyperplasia or malignancy. She was discharged home same day.

CLINICAL QUESTIONS

1. What is clinical presentation of hematometra?

Ans. Presenting symptoms can be different depending upon the cause, duration and severity of distal genital tract obstruction causing hematometra. In a premenopausal female presenting symptoms are usually secondary amenorrhea, or scant irregular periods with cyclic midline lower abdominal pain and lower abdominal mass/distension. In a postmenopausal female typical clinical presentation is lower abdominal pain and/or distension.

2. How is the diagnosis of hematometra established?

Ans. Hematometra (fluid-filled endometrial cavity) allows good sonographic visualization of the endometrial abnormalities. As illustrated in Figures 15.1 and 15.2, the endometrial thickness and contours of the uterine cavity are well visualized since blood accumulation serves as a contrast medium for sonographic assessment.[1] Transperineal sonography can be helpful if endovaginal ultrasound cannot be performed because of severe vaginal stenosis.[2]

3. Which conditions may lead to hematometra?

Ans. Hematometra results from partial or complete obstruction of the lower genital tract, which can be acquired or caused by congenital conditions. In pediatric and adolescent patients common congenital conditions are imperforate hymen, transverse vaginal septum, and noncommunicating Müllerian duct.[3,4] Acquired causes are menopause related atrophy of the endocervical canal or isthmus obliteration from scarring due to surgical procedures related to synechiae, radiotherapy and malignancy.[5]

Various gynecological procedures may be associated with hematometra, such as dilatation and curettage, cervical cone biopsy, electrocautery, cryocoagulation of cervical dysplasia and endometrial ablation. C-section and termination of pregnancy complicated with postprocedural endometritis can also lead to hematometra or pyometra, as well as the use of uterine compression sutures for atonic hemorrhage.[6-8]

4. List the appropriate work up of a patient with hematometra.

Ans. Appropriate work up of hematometra in postmenopausal patients is very important since it can harbor malignancy. Wu et al. reported a case of endometrial adenocarcinoma who presented with hematometra mimicking a large pelvic cyst.[9] The degree of association of uterine fluid collection and malignancy is reported differently by various authors. Breckenridge et al. reported that 94% (16 out of 17) of symptomatic postmenopausal women with pelvic pain, vaginal bleeding, or pelvic masses had active carcinoma involving the uterus or cervix.[10] However, Carlson et al. found only 25% malignancy rate among 20 postmenopausal women with intrauterine fluid collections.[11] Goldstein reported that nodular or thickened endometrium on ultrasound and increasing volumes of fluid seem to correlate with the risk of gynecologic cancer.[12] As in our case, a normal atrophic postmenopausal endometrium in association with cervical stenosis can produce uterine fluid collections in women without malignancy. Endometrial sampling yielded inactive tissues while endometrial thickness was less than 3 mm.

5. What is the treatment of hematometra?

Ans. Examination under anesthesia, cervical dilatation and drainage and endometrial sampling are the major steps in the management of hematometra. In young patients the correction of obstruction (e.g. hysteroscopic adhesiolysis in patients with Asherman syndrome) is necessary. Foley catheter is traditionally used for up to 10 days after hysteroscopic treatment to prevent further formation of adhesions.[13] Intrauterine contraceptive device (IUCD) has been used for the same purpose in the past. Orhue et al. found Foley catheter to be safer and more effective than IUCD in restoring normal menstrual periods and later pregnancies.[13] Overall use of Foley catheter and IUCD resulted in restoration of the normal menstrual cycles in 72.7% patients with adhesiolysis. Estrogen with or without progesterone can be utilized postoperatively to restore the endometrium in premenopausal patients after hysteroscopic lysis of adhesions.[14] Interval ultrasound (preferably SIS) should be performed to confirm the patency of endocervical canal and endometrial cavity.

■ TAKE-HOME MESSAGES

- In postmenopausal women abnormal vaginal serous or bloody discharge, with or without fluid collection within the uterus must prompt immediate assessment of the endometrial mucosa. Uterine malignancy should be suspected until proven otherwise.
- TV US is considered as the first modality for the diagnosis of hematometra. Transperineal ultrasound can be utilized if there is severe vaginal atrophy either due to age related atrophy or radiotherapy.
- Increased endometrial thickness and prominent color Doppler signals with low vascular resistance are good markers of endometrial malignancy.
- Young women with hematometra should be treated timely to prevent retrograde menstruation, hematosalpinx and endometriosis.
- The most common causes of hematometra are congenital conditions (such as imperforate hymen, transverse vaginal septum, and non-communicating Müllerian duct) or acquired causes (such as atrophy of the endocervical canal in postmenopausal patients or isthmus obliteration from scarring due to surgical procedures related to synechiae, radiotherapy, and malignancy).[3-5]
- Various gynecological procedures may be associated with hematometra, such as D and C, cervical cone biopsy, electrocautery, cryocoagulation of cervical dysplasia and endometrial ablation. C-section and termination of pregnancy complicated with postprocedural endometritis can also lead to hematometra or pyometra, as well as the use of uterine compression sutures for atonic hemorrhage.[6-8]
- Correction of obstruction (e.g. incision of imperforate hymen) is treatment of hematometra.

■ REFERENCES

1. Scheerer LJ BL. Transvaginal sonography in the evaluation of hematometra—a report of two cases. J Reprod Med. 1996(41):205.
2. Meyer WR, McCoy R FM. Combined abdominal-perineal sonography to assist in diagnosis of transvaginal septum. Obstet Gynecol. 1995(85):882.
3. Reuter KL, Young SB, Daly B. Hematometra complicating conization with radiologic correlation: A case report. J Reprod Med Obstet Gynecol. 1994;39(5):408-10.

4. Fujimoto VY, Klein NA MP. Late-onset hematometra and hematosalpinx in a woman with a noncommunicating uterine horn-a case report. J Reprod Med. 1998;43:465.
5. Romer T, Grabow D, Muller J. Conservative management of a post-ablation syndrome after transcervical endometrial ablation. Geburtshilfe Frauenheilkd. 1997;57(1):43-5.
6. Kaur G, Jain S, Sharma A VN. Hematometra Formation- A Rare Complication of Cesarean Delivery. J Clin Diagnostic Res. 2014;(8):OD03-OD04.
7. Dadhwal G, Sumana SM. Haematometra following uterine compression sutures. Int J Gynecol Obstet. 2007;99(3):255-6.
8. Louros JM, Danezis GP. Use of intrauterine devices in the treatment of intrauterine adhesions. Fertil Steril. 1968;19:509-28.
9. Wu MP, Wu CC, Chang FM, Yen EYT, Hsieh MF, Chao MH. Endometrial carcinoma presenting as hematometra mimicking a large pelvic cyst. J Clin Ultrasound. 1999;27:541-3.
10. Breckenridge JW, Kurtz AB, Ritchie WE et al. Postmenopausal uterine fluid collection: indicator of carcinoma. Am J Roentgenol. 1982;(139):529.
11. Carlson JA, Arger P, Thompson S, et al. Clinical and pathologic correlation of endometrial cavity fluid detected by ultrasound in the postmenopausal patient. Obs Gynecol. 1991;77:119.
12. Goldstein SR. Postmenopausal endometrial fluid collections revisited: look at the doughnut rather than the hole. Obstet Gynecol. 1994;83(5 Pt 1):738-40.
13. Orhue AAE, Aziken ME, Igbefoh JO. A comparison of two adjunctive treatments for intrauterine adhesions following lysis. Int J Gynecol Obstet. 2003;82(1):49-56.
14. Thomson AJ, Abbott JA, Deans R, Kingston A, Vancaillie TG. The management of intrauterine synechiae. Curr Opin Obs Gynecol. 2009;21(4):335-41.

CHAPTER 16

Endometrial Carcinoma

Sanja Kupesic Plavsic, Osvaldo Padilla

■ CLINICAL CASE

CA is a 68-year-old postmenopausal G0P0, who presents to the gynecology clinic with history of postmenopausal bleeding. The patient started experiencing vaginal bleeding about 3 months ago. She had her LMP at age 53. Her menarche was at age 11. Her last Pap smear was done at age 65, and was normal. The patient has a history of type 2 diabetes mellitus and hypertension. She was diagnosed with breast cancer at age 63, and has since been on tamoxifen. She is currently on medications to treat her hypertension and diabetes, and takes calcium and vitamin D for osteoporosis prevention.

Menarche: Age 11.

Menses: 30–60/5 days, irregular.

LMP: 15 years ago.

OB history: She has never been pregnant.

Sexual history: Sexually inactive. The patient was widowed by her husband at age 68.

Review of Systems

- She complains of shortness of breath and chronic tiredness.
- Denies urinary frequency, hematuria, and dysuria; normal bowel movement.

Past medical history: History of ovulation induction for infertility treatment (3 cycles of clomiphene citrate and 2 cycles of gonadotropin induction).

Past surgical history: Appendectomy, tonsillectomy, and diagnostic laparoscopy for infertility.

Vaccines: Up to date (hepatitis B vaccine series, MMR booster and flu shot).

Current medications: Antihypertensive therapy, insulin, tamoxifen, calcium, and vitamin D supplementation.

Allergies: No known drug allergies.

Social history: CA is a retired high school teacher who lives by herself; does not smoke, social ETOH, no drug abuse.

Family history: Mother: Died of breast cancer at the age of 52; aunt died of colon cancer at the age of 65. Father: Died of myocardial infarction at the age of 76.

Physical Examination

Vital signs: T 36.7°C oral; BP 140/95; P 92; BMI 36.

Physical examination: The patient is an obese female in no acute apparent distress.

Cardiac examination: No heart murmur was detected.
She is short of breath postambulation around the clinic.
Abdominal examination is normal.

Pelvic Examination

External genitalia with no abnormalities. Speculum examination reveals dark blood in the vagina. Bimanual examination is positive for an enlarged uterus. Pap smear and endometrial biopsy were performed.

Laboratory tests (CBC, chemistry profile with liver function tests) and cancer antigen-125 were performed. Pelvic ultrasound findings are presented in Figures 16.1 to 16.4. Endometrial biopsy reveals endometrial malignancy. Chest radiography and MRI are ordered.

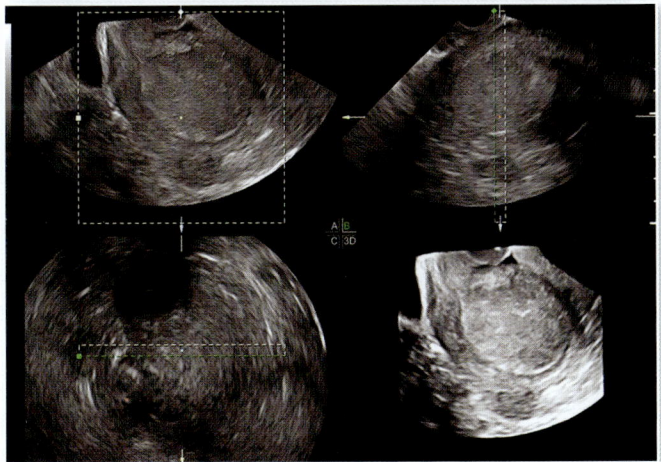

Figure 16.1: Three-dimensional ultrasound of the uterus. The uterus is in RVF. The endometrium is ill defined and maximal endometrial thickness is 39 mm

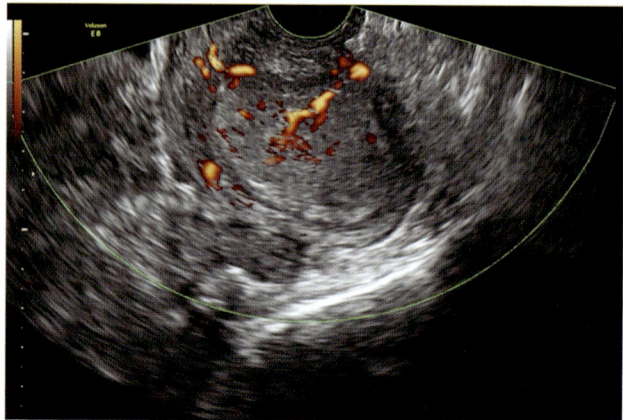

Figure 16.2: Power Doppler ultrasound demonstrates irregularly branching vessels. The subendometrial halo is not clearly visualized

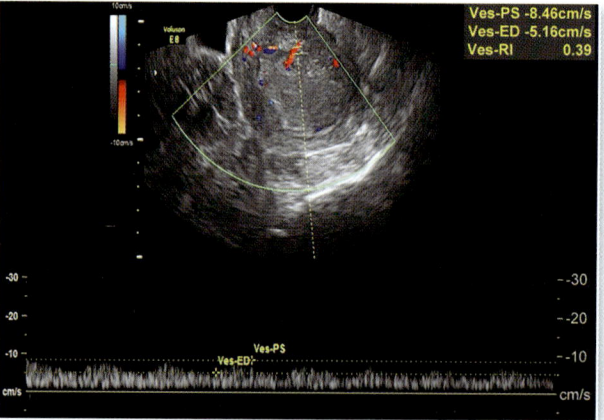

Figure 16.3: Pulsed Doppler waveform analysis reveals low impedance blood flow signals (RI 0.39), suggestive of endometrial neoplasia

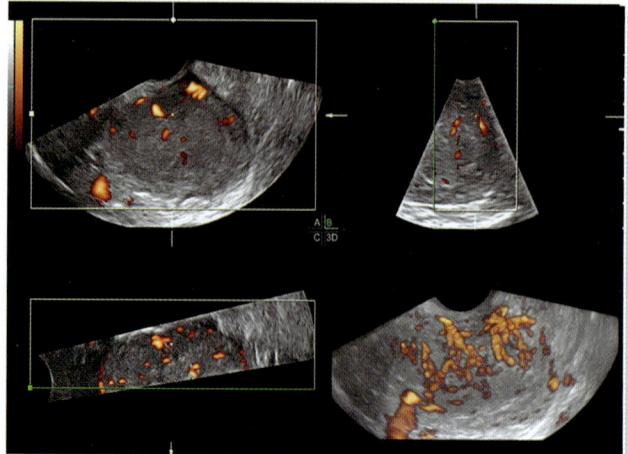

Figure 16.4: Three-dimensional power Doppler image demonstrates randomly dispersed vessels with penetrating pattern toward the anterior myometrium

CLINICAL QUESTIONS

1. What is the most appropriate next step in this patient?

Ans. The most appropriate next step in this patient is to perform pelvic ultrasound, laboratory tests (CBC, chemistry profile with liver function tests), cancer antigen-125, chest radiography and CT scan. Pelvic ultrasound findings are presented in Figures 16.1 to 16.4.

2. What is the indication for endometrial biopsy in postmenopausal patients presenting with uterine bleeding?

Ans. ACOG Committee Opinion from 2009 reviews the use of transvaginal ultrasonography in the evaluation of postmenopausal bleeding.[2] The opinion clarifies that endometrial biopsy or transvaginal ultrasonography may be used in the initial evaluation of postmenopausal bleeding, and both tests may not be necessary. The opinion further concludes that "when an endometrial thickness less than or equal to 4 mm is found, endometrial sampling is not required." When the endometrium cannot be reliably assessed by ultrasonography in women with postmenopausal bleeding because of marked obesity, shadowing caused by uterine fibroids, or other anatomic limitations, an alternative method of evaluation is necessary.

3. What is the role of SIS and hysteroscopy in the assessment of postmenopausal bleeding?

Ans. Saline infusion sonography (SIS) is often used as a second step diagnostic test for the assessment of endometrium in patients with abnormal uterine bleeding. It is particularly useful when ultrasonography suggests a focal lesion (e.g. endometrial polyp). If a focal lesion is noted on SIS, operative hysteroscopy is indicated.[2] Hysteroscopy allows direct endoscopic visualization of the endometrial cavity and is highly accurate in diagnosing endometrial cancer.[3]

4. What would be your focus during evaluation of this patient?

Ans. Initial evaluation of Mrs CA should include physical examination, transvaginal ultrasound, Pap smear, endometrial biopsy, laboratory tests and cancer antigen-125. Because endometrial cancer is found after examining endometrial sample tissues, the following tests should be used in the staging process: chest radiography, CT, and MRI.[4] Preoperative assessment should also focus on detection and optimization of medical comorbidities that could complicate the surgery and postoperative course.

5. What are the prognostic factors in endometrial carcinoma?

Ans. Important prognostic factors in endometrial carcinoma are myometrial invasion, histologic grading of the carcinoma and presence of lymph node metastases. The depth of myometrial invasion is classified as none (stage 1A), superficial (invasion of less than half of the myometrium, stage 1B), or deep (invasion of deep myometrial mantle, stage 1C). The incidence of lymph node involvement is tightly linked to a degree of myometrial invasion. Therefore, estimation of the myometrial invasion depth is crucial in preoperative evaluation of the patients with positive endometrial biopsy.[5] Color Doppler images of the uterus (Figs 16.2 to 16.4) demonstrate irregular branching pattern and low vascular impedance, typical for endometrial cancer, which was confirmed by histology. Penetrating vascular pattern toward the anterior myometrial layer suggests its invasive nature.[6]

6. What are the treatment choices for endometrial cancer?

Ans. In the absence of obvious extrauterine metastases, staging, and initial treatment are accomplished with total hysterectomy, bilateral salpingo-oophorectomy, and peritoneal washings. In patients with myometrial invasion, pelvic and para-aortic lymph node dissection should be performed as a prognostic indicator. Figure 16.5 illustrates endometrial adenocarcinoma with evidence of myometrial invasion. With more advanced stages of disease, tumor debulking is indicated to improve treatment outcomes.[7-10]

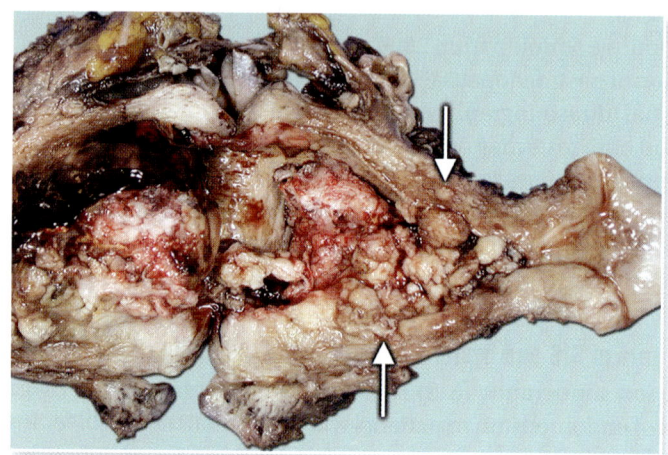

Figure 16.5: This endometrial adenocarcinoma demonstrates a papillary lesion within the uterine cavity with focal areas of myometrial invasion (white arrow)

■ TAKE-HOME MESSAGES

- ACOG Committee Opinion from 2009 reviews the use of transvaginal ultrasonography in the evaluation of postmenopausal bleeding.[2] The opinion clarifies that endometrial biopsy or TV US may be used in the initial evaluation of postmenopausal bleeding, and both tests may not be necessary. The opinion further concludes that "when an endometrial thickness less than or equal to 4 mm is found, endometrial sampling is not required."[2] When the endometrium cannot be reliably assessed by ultrasonography in women with postmenopausal bleeding because of marked obesity, shadowing caused by uterine fibroids, or other anatomic limitations, an alternative method of evaluation is necessary.
- SIS is often used as a second step diagnostic test for the assessment of endometrium in patients with abnormal uterine bleeding. It is particularly useful when ultrasonography suggests a focal lesion (e.g. endometrial polyp). If a focal lesion is noted on SIS, operative hysteroscopy is indicated.[2]
- Hysteroscopy allows direct endoscopic visualization of the endometrial cavity and is highly accurate in diagnosing endometrial lesions.[3]
- Preoperative evaluation should include physical examination, transvaginal ultrasound, Pap smear, endometrial biopsy, laboratory testing, and cancer antigen-125. Chest radiography and MRI are indicated if extrauterine metastases are expected.[4] Preoperative assessment should also focus on detection and optimization of medical comorbidities that could complicate the surgery and postoperative course.[4]
- Important prognostic factors in endometrial carcinoma are myometrial invasion, histologic grading of the carcinoma and presence of lymph node metastases.[5] The depth of myometrial invasion is classified as none (stage 1A), superficial (invasion of less than half of the myometrium, stage 1B), or deep (invasion of deep myometrial mantle, stage 1C). The incidence of lymph node involvement is tightly linked to the degree of myometrial invasion. Therefore, estimation of the myometrial invasion depth is crucial in preoperative evaluation of the patients with positive endometrial biopsy.[5]

- Penetrating vascular pattern of the endometrial vessels towards the myometrial layer assessed by color and/or power Doppler ultrasound, and high velocity - low vascular impedance blood flow signals suggest invasive nature of endometrial carcinoma.[6]
- In the absence of obvious extrauterine metastases, staging and initial treatment are accomplished with total hysterectomy, bilateral salpingo-oophorectomy, and peritoneal washings. In patients with myometrial invasion, pelvic and para-aortic lymph node dissection should be performed as a prognostic indicator. With more advanced stages of disease, tumor debulking is indicated to improve treatment outcome.[7-10]
- Radiation therapy (e.g. external beam radiotherapy or brachytherapy) is an effective treatment for endometrial cancer. In stage I disease, the use of radiation therapy is beneficial for patient subgroups determined by age, tumor grade, depth of myometrial invasion, and lymphovascular space involvement.[8] Radiotherapy is also effective in patients with local recurrence of the disease.
- The use of tamoxifen and progestin have shown increased overall survival rate.[9,10]

REFERENCES

1. Karlsson B, Granberg S, Wikland M, et al. Transvaginal ultrasonography of the endometrium in women with postmenopausal bleeding—a Nordic multicenter study. Am J Obstet Gynecol. 1995;172(5):1488-94.
2. American College of Obstetricians and Gynecologists. ACOG Committee Opinion no. 426: The role of transvaginal ultrasonography in the evaluation of postmenopausal bleeding. Obstet Gynecol. 2009;113(2 pt 1):462-4.
3. Clark TJ, Voit D, Gupta JK, et al. Accuracy of hysteroscopy in the diagnosis of endometrial cancer and hyperplasia: a systematic quantitative review. JAMA. 2002;288(13):1610-21.
4. Hernandez E, American College of Obstetricians and Gynecologists. ACOG Practice Bulletin No. 65: management of endometrial cancer. Obstet Gynecol. 2005;106(2):413-25.
5. Appleton K, Kupesic Plavsic S. Role of ultrasound in the assessment of postmenopausal bleeding. Donald School J Ultrasound Obstet Gynecol. 2012;6(2):197-206.
6. Kupesic S, Kurjak A, Zodan T. Staging of endometrial carcinoma by 3-D power Doppler. Gynaecol Perinatol. 1998;8:1-5.
7. Bristow RE, Zerbe MJ, Rosenshein NB, et al. Stage IVB endometrial carcinoma: the role of cytoreductive surgery and determinants of survival. Gynecol Oncol. 2000;78(2):85-91.
8. HM Keys, JA Roberts, VL Brunetto, et al. A phase III trial of surgery with or without adjunctive external pelvic radiation therapy in intermediate risk endometrial adenocarcinoma: a Gynecologic Oncology Group study. Gynecol Oncol. 2004;92(3):744-51.
9. Sorosky JI. Endometrial cancer. Obstet Gynecol. 2008;111(2 pt 1):436-47.
10. Buchanan EM, Weinstein LC, Hillson C. Endometrial cancer. Am Fam Physician. 2009;80(10):1075-80.

CHAPTER 17

Leiomyosarcoma

Christopher Ortiz, Melissa D Mendez, Osvaldo Padilla, Sanja Kupesic Plavsic

■ CLINICAL CASE

A 59-year-old G4P2 postmenopausal patient complains of a 5–6 month history of lower abdominal pain and right lower quadrant greater than left lower quadrant pain. This lower abdominal pain is associated with vaginal bleeding. The patient went through menopause at 52 years old and her Pap smears have been normal.

Menarche: Age 12.

LMP: Seven years ago, now reports postmenopausal bleeding and pelvic pain.

Last pap: Last year and was normal.

Ob history: Two normal vaginal deliveries with no complications and two miscarriages.

Sexual history: No history of sexually transmitted disease, one lifetime male partner.

Review of Systems

- No chest pain or shortness of breath
- No nausea and vomiting
- Patient complains of postmenopausal bleeding and bloating.
- Patient also complains of dark colored stools and constipation.

Past medical history: Type 2 diabetes, hypertension, high cholesterol, depression, gastritis.

Past surgical history: Colonoscopy with polyp removal three years ago.

Vaccines: Up to date.

Current medications: Celebrex, dicyclomine HCl, omeprazole, vitamin D, metformin, simvastatin, losartan, and zoloft.

Allergies: No known drug allergies.

Social history: Denies drinking, smoking, or drug use; is a homemaker.

Family history: Father: Died of lung cancer at 70 years of age; Mother: 84 years, history of stroke and diabetes type 2.

Physical Examination

Vital signs: T 36.9°C oral; BP 129/80; P 68; BMI 40.02.

General physical examination: Well groomed, in no apparent distress, alert and oriented times three.

Cardiac examination: Regular rate and rhythm, no heart murmur detected.

Chest examination: Clear to auscultation bilaterally.

Abdominal examination: Palpable uterus below the level of the umbilicus. No tenderness to palpation.

Pelvic Examination

Vulva: No lesions, normal hair pattern. Vagina: Smooth, thin walls, atrophic. Cervix: anterior position, scant blood coming from os, no overt lesions. Uterus: 18 week size, mobile, mildly tender to palpation and heterogeneous. Adnexa: Not palpable due to large uterine mass. Rectum: Good sphincter tone, guaiac negative.

Diagnostic imaging results:
1. Transvaginal color Doppler ultrasound revealed asymmetrically enlarged uterus. Myometrial lesion measuring 4.5 cm with randomly dispersed vessels and low vascular resistance (Figs 17.1 and 17.2) is visualized in the anterior uterine wall. The endometrium is ill defined. In the ultrasound images reviewed adnexal masses and free fluid are not detected.
2. CT with contrast shows a low density uterine mass measuring 4.5 cm.
3. MRI of the pelvis showing an enlarged uterus with multiple fibroids (10 × 9 × 8 cm), endometrium could not be identified. No adnexal masses and no free fluid.

Endometrial biopsy revealed malignant spindle cell and epithelioid neoplasm consistent with a high grade sarcoma vs. endometrial stromal sarcoma.

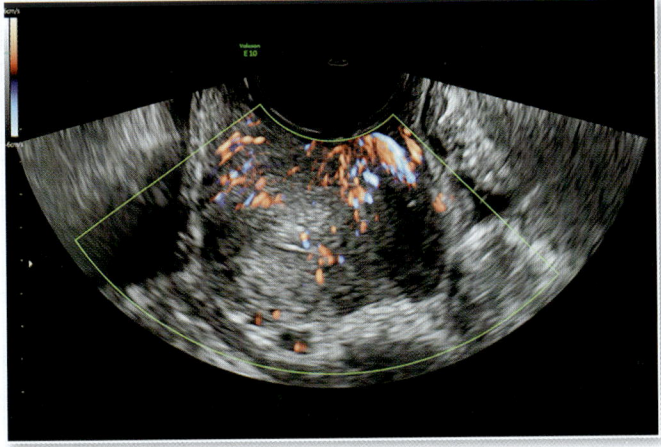

Figure 17.1: Asymmetrically enlarged uterus. Note an anterior myometrial mass with poorly defined margins and randomly dispersed vessels

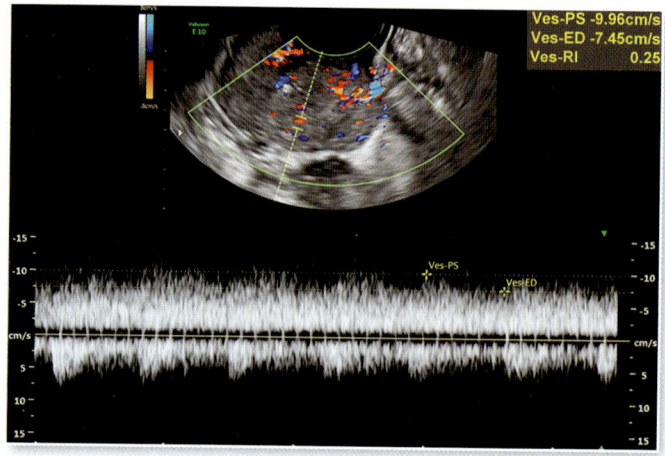

Figure 17.2: Pulsed Doppler waveform signals obtained from the uterine lesion reveal low vascular resistance (RI 0.25)

■ CLINICAL QUESTIONS

1. What is the best next step in the management of this patient?

Ans. Our patient is a postmenopausal woman with abnormal uterine bleeding with confirmed uterine mass on imaging. The patient also has definitive diagnosis of a high-grade sarcoma revealed via endometrial biopsy. For these reasons the most definitive management option for her is a total hysterectomy. A bilateral salpingo-oophorectomy is often performed at the same time particularly for menopausal or perimenopausal women.[1] Lymphadenectomy is usually not indicated for leiomyosarcoma unless there is a suspicious lymph node seen during surgery or imaging. The use of radiation as additional therapy is done on a case by case basis and used primarily to prevent recurrence of disease.[2] Chemotherapy is used primarily to treat recurrent or metastatic leiomyosarcoma. After surgery postoperative surveillance is required. Physical and pelvic examinations every three to four months for two years are recommended, then for the next two years every 6 months.[3]

2. How is a diagnosis of uterine leiomyosarcoma made?

Ans. Diagnosis of uterine leiomyosarcoma is made histologically usually after either a hysterectomy or myomectomy. Uterine sarcomas are rare (3–7 per 100,000) and are associated with poor prognosis. There are three criteria that are important for diagnosis. These are mitotic index (>10 per 10 high power fields), cellular atypia, and geographic areas of coagulative necrosis separated from a viable tumor.[4] Leiomyosarcomas are typically large yellow or tan solitary masses with soft, fleshy cut surfaces with areas of hemorrhage and necrosis. There are two variant forms of leiomyosarcomas:
- Epithelioid—characterized by round to polygonal cells with abundant eosinophilic or clear cytoplasm
- Myxoid—Myxoid appearance may obscure the smooth muscle differentiation, the extent of nuclear pleomorphism and the true number of mitotic figures.[5]

3. How is leiomyosarcoma staged?

Ans. Leiomyosarcomas are staged using the FIGO staging system. This staging system does not predict the prognosis for overall survival for patients with uterine leiomyosarcomas, (Table 17.1).[6]

Chapter 17: Leiomyosarcoma

Table 17.1	FIGO staging system for uterine leiomyosarcoma
I	Tumor limited to the uterus
IA	Tumor 5 cm or less in greatest dimension
IB	Tumor more than 5 cm
II	Tumor extends beyond the uterus, within the pelvis
IIA	Tumor involves adnexa
IIB	Tumor involves other pelvic tissues
III	Tumor infiltrates abdominal tissues
IIIA	One site
IIIB	More than one site
IVA	Tumor invades bladder or rectum
IVB	Distant metastasis (excluding adnexa, pelvic and abdominal tissue)

■ TAKE-HOME MESSAGES

- Leiomyosarcomas represent 1–2% of all uterine cancers.[7]
- Overall 5 year survival rates can be poor, down to 15% but can reach up to 60% for stage I or II leiomyosarcoma.[7]
- Leiomyosarcomas present at a median age of 50–55 years.[7,8]
- Risk factors for endometrial carcinoma are not known to be related to leiomyosarcomas.[7,8]
- Leiomyosarcomas typically spread by local or regional invasion as well as hematogenous dissemination with metastasis most common to the lungs. The prognosis mostly depends on the extent of spread (or tumor stage) with overall 5 year survival rates ranging from 15–25%, but the 5 year survival rate may range from 40–70% in stage I and stage II tumors.[8,9]
- Most recurrences occur within 2 years from the date of diagnosis.[9]
- Rapid increase in uterine size after menopause is suspicious for leiomyosarcomas, although this can also occur in rapidly growing leiomyomas. Patients may also complain of abnormal uterine bleeding and pelvic pain.[10]
- Leiomyosarcoma are characteristically solitary intramural masses with poorly defined margins on imaging studies. Hemorrhage and necrosis are also typically grossly present.[10] Macroscopic examination typically reveals yellow-tan masses with geographic areas of necrosis and hemorrhage (Fig. 17.3).
- Microscopic evaluation typically shows elongated (or spindle-shaped) cells with smooth muscle differentiation and features of malignancy (pleomorphic cells, hyperchromasia, increased mitotic index, and necrosis)[11] (Fig. 17.4).

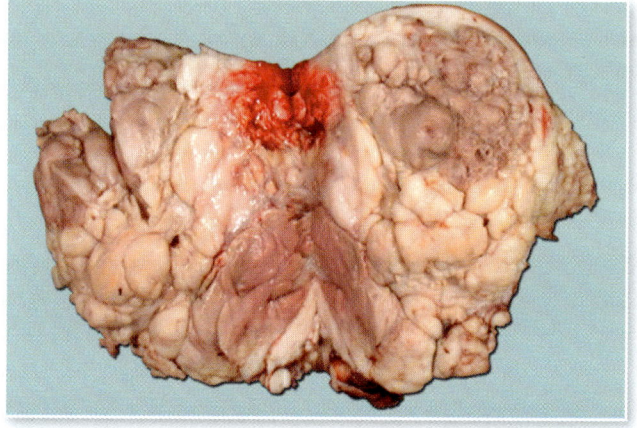

Figure 17.3: Leiomyosarcoma are typically yellow-tan masses with geographic areas of necrosis and hemorrhage

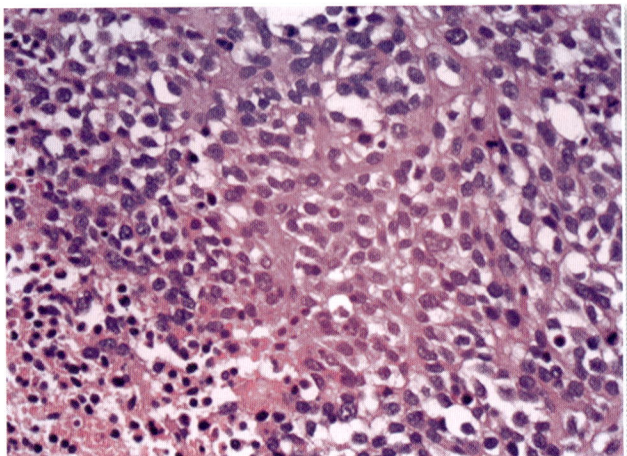

Figure 17.4: This leiomyosarcoma has a round cell sarcoma appearance with pleomorphism, increased mitosis, and focal areas of necrosis

REFERENCES

1. Dinh TA, Oliva EA, Fuller AF Jr, et al. The treatment of uterine leiomyosarcoma. Results from a 10-year experience (1990-1999) at the Massachusetts General Hospital. Gynecol Oncol. 2004;92(2):648-52.
2. Durnali A, Tokluoglu S, Ozdemir N, et al. Prognostic Factors and treatment outcomes in 93 patients with uterine sarcoma from 4 centers in Turkey. Asian Pac J Cancer Prev. 2012;13(5):1935-41.
3. Elit L, Reade CJ. Recommendations for follow-up care for gynecologic cancer survivors. Obstet Gynecol. 2015;126(6):1207-14.
4. Gadducci A, Cosio S, Romanini A, Genazzani AR. The management of patients with uterine sarcoma: a debated clinical challenge. Crit Rev Oncol Hematol. 2008;65(2):129-42.
5. Sandberg AA. Updates on the cytogenetics and molecular genetics of bone and soft tissue tumors: leiomyosarcoma. Cancer Genet Cytogenet. 2005;161(1):1-19.
6. Hensley ML, Barrett BA, Baumann K, et al. Gynecologic Cancer InterGroup (GCIG) Consensus Review: uterine and ovarian leiomyosarcomas. Intl J Gynecol Cancer. 2014;24(S3):S61-6.
7. Pritts EA, Parker WH, Brown J, Olive DL. Outcome of occult uterine leiomyosarcoma after surgery for presumed uterine fibroids: a systematic review. J Minim Invasive Gynecol. 2015;22(1):26-33.
8. Gockley AA, Rauh-Hain A, del Carmen MG. Uterine Leiomyosarcoma: a review article. Intl J Gynecol Cancer. 2014;24(9):1538-42.
9. Rauh-Hain JA, Oduyebo T, Diver EJ, et al. Uterine leiomyosarcoma: an updated series. Intl J Gynecol Cancer. 2013;23(6):1036-43.
10. Bonneau C, Thomassin-Naggara I, Cortez A, et al. Value of ultrasonography and magnetic resonance imaging for the characterization of uterine mesenchymal tumors. Acta Obstet Gynecol Scand. 2014;93(3):261-8.
11. Hewedi IH, Radwan NA, Shash LS. Diagnostic value of progesterone receptor and p53 expression in uterine smooth muscle tumors. Diagn Pathol. 2012; Jan 5;7:1. doi: 10.1186/1746-1596-7-1.

CHAPTER 18

Ovarian Cystadenocarcinoma

Sanja Kupesic Plavsic, Osvaldo Padilla

■ CLINICAL CASE

DP is a 72-year-old postmenopausal patient, G3P0, visiting her gynecologist because of a feeling of persistent abdominal distension, and vague abdominal, pelvic and back pain. During the course of last three months she lost 8 kg "because she feels full after eating a small meal". Her LMP was 20 years ago. During the reproductive years, her cycles were regular, every 26–28 days. Her past medical history is significant for infertility treatment and endometriosis. She had multiple ovulation inductions, six intrauterine inseminations, two IVF/ET cycles, and was diagnosed with three miscarriages at 7, 9, and 10 weeks gestation. She was previously seen by gastroenterologist who ordered upper and lower GI studies, which were both negative. Her last Pap smear was done at age 65, and was normal. She was using hormonal replacement therapy (HRT) for 5 years; currently takes calcium and vitamin D for osteoporosis prevention.

Menarche: Age 11.

Menses: 26–28/5 days, regular.

LMP: 20 years ago.

OB history: Three miscarriages at 7, 9, and 10 weeks.

Sexual history: Sexually inactive.

Review of Systems

- No chest pain; complains of shortness of breath and chronic tiredness.
- Mrs DP complains of abdominal/pelvic fullness, vague abdominal/pelvic pain and bloating, and reports changes in bowel habit (constipation).
- Complains of urinary frequency; denies hematuria and dysuria.

Past medical history: History of ovulation induction for infertility treatment and use of HRT for 5 years.

Past surgical history: Appendectomy and two laparoscopic surgeries.

Vaccines: Up to date (hepatitis B vaccine series, MMR booster and flu shot).

Current medications: Calcium and vitamin D supplementation.

Allergies: No known drug allergies.

Social history: DP is a retired college professor; does not smoke, social ETOH, no drug abuse.

Family history: Mother: Died of breast cancer at the age of 52; aunt died of ovarian cancer at the age of 63. Father: Died of prostate cancer at the age of 74.

Physical Examination

Vital signs: T 36.9°C oral; BP 110/75; P 94; BMI 17.

Cardiac examination: No heart murmur was detected.

Chest examination: Dullness to percussion.

Abdominal examination revealed a pelvic mass. Ascites was detected by inspection, percussion and fluid wave test.

Pelvic examination: External genitalia with no abnormalities. Per-speculum examination was normal. Bimanual pelvic examination revealed a huge pelvic mass.

Laboratory tests (CBC, chemistry profile with liver function tests) and tumor markers (CA-125, CA 19-9, CEA, AFP, beta-hCG, inhibin and LDH) were performed. Pelvic ultrasound and CT scan of the pelvis and abdomen were ordered. Ultrasound and CT findings are illustrated in Figures 18.1 to 18.8. Clinical views are shown in Figures 18.9 and 18.10.

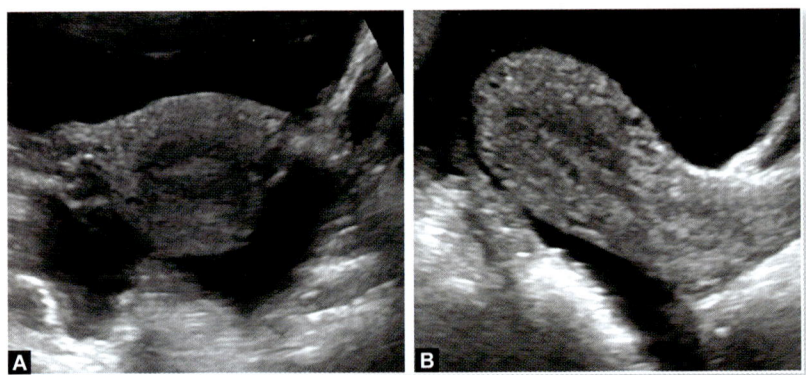

Figures 18.1A and B: Transabdominal ultrasound images of the uterus and free fluid in (A) transverse and (B) longitudinal planes

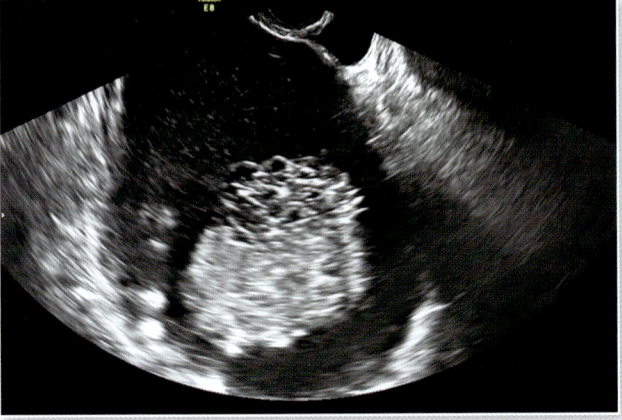

Figure 18.2: Transvaginal ultrasound scan of a complex right adnexal mass

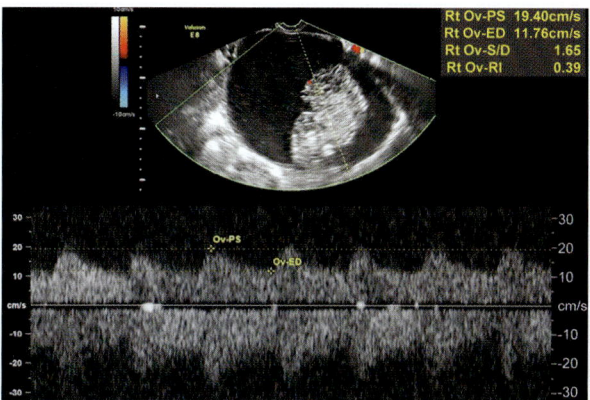

Figure 18.3: Transvaginal color Doppler ultrasound revealed high velocity—low impedance blood flow signals (RI 0.39), typical for tumor neovascularization

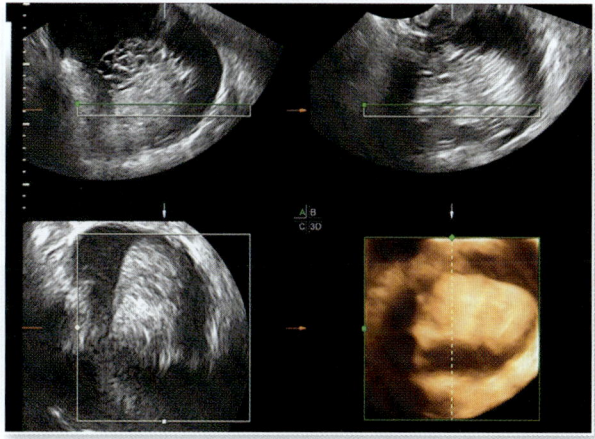

Figure 18.4: Three-dimensional ultrasound (multiplanar and surface rendering) reinforces initial diagnostic impression of conventional 2D sonography. This modality allowed more detailed assessment of internal wall surface irregularities and solid parts

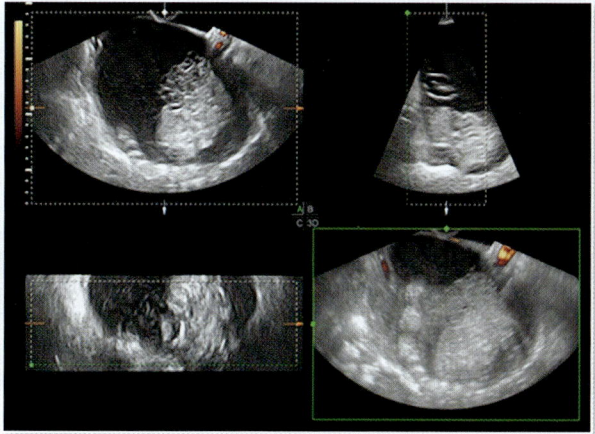

Figure 18.5: Three-dimensional power Doppler ultrasound revealed peripheral flow

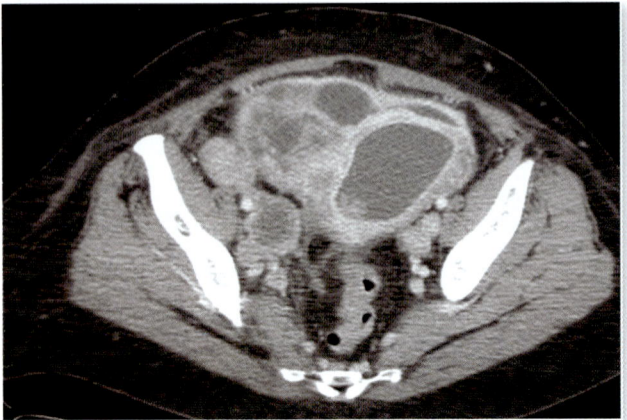

Figure 18.6: CT of complex adnexal mass in the pelvis

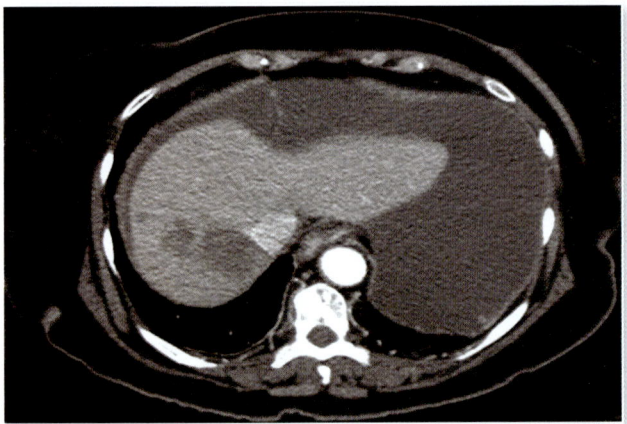

Figure 18.7: Ascites and multiple liver metastases

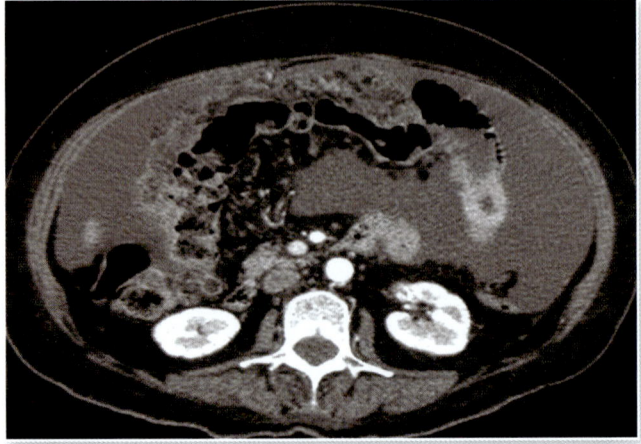

Figure 18.8: Omental caking

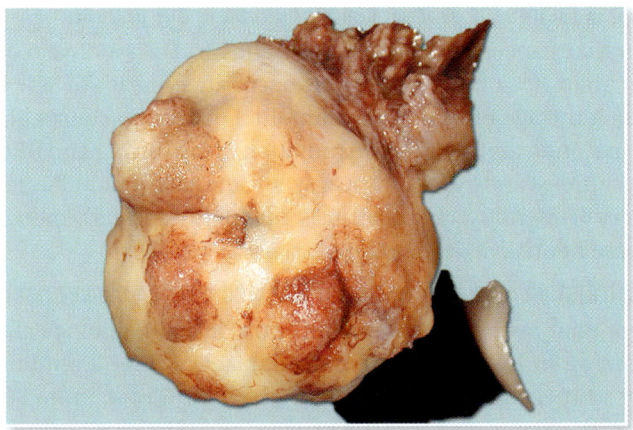

Figure 18.9: In ovarian serous carcinoma, tumor invades the ovarian capsule and may extend to the outer ovarian capsule, as seen in the picture above. These lesions can also be appreciated as malignant omental implants or implants on other pelvic or peritoneal organs

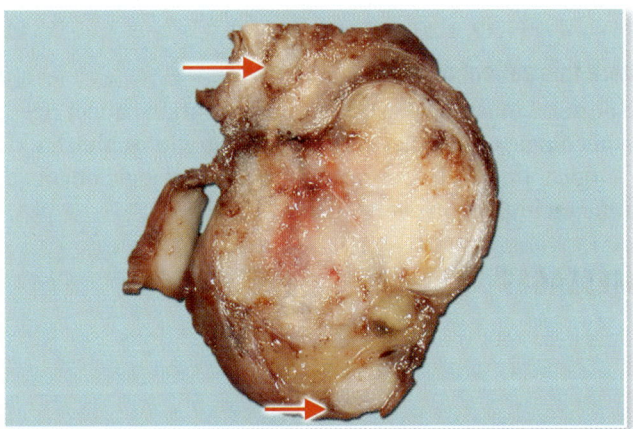

Figure 18.10: Note prominent papillary and solids areas with microscopic and gross evidence of invasion into adjacent structures. In the picture above, one can appreciate tumor nodules (red arrows) extending (or invading) well beyond the ovarian capsule

■ CLINICAL QUESTIONS

1. **Mrs DP presents with a variety of nonspecific symptoms, including abdominal, pelvic and back pain, bloating, pressure effects on the bladder (frequency) and rectum (constipation), shortness of breath, tiredness and weight loss. Her physical findings, sonographic and CT images (Figs 18.1 to 18.8) suggest advanced ovarian cancer. What is the anticipated level of elevation for tumor markers?**

Ans. No tumor marker is completely specific for ovarian carcinoma. In our patient, CA-125 was significantly elevated (140 U/mL; normal 35IU/mL), while other tumor markers were within normal limits.

2. What are the risk factors for ovarian cancer noticed in our patient?

Ans. The risk for ovarian cancer increases with age, and Mrs DP is a 72-year old postmenopausal patient (more than 70% of ovarian cancers occur after the age of 50).[1] Her mother died of breast cancer at the age of 52 and her aunt died of ovarian cancer at the age of 63. This information may indicate an inherited mutation of the BRCA1 and BRCA2 genes. Women with hereditary breast and ovarian cancer syndrome have up to 45% lifetime risk of ovarian cancer.[1] History of infertility, endometriosis, nulliparity and early menarchal age (11 years) further increase her risk of developing ovarian cancer.

3. What is the correlation between the use of HRT and ovarian cancer risk?

Ans. A recent meta-analysis by Collaborative Group on Epidemiological Studies of Ovarian Cancer assessing individual participant datasets from 52 epidemiological studies revealed that women who use hormone therapy for 5 years from 50 years of age have about one extraovarian cancer per 1,000 users and if its prognosis is typical, about one extraovarian cancer death per 1,700 users.[2] Ovarian carcinoma risk was similar in European and American prospective studies and for estrogen-only and estrogen-progestagen preparations, but differed across the four main tumor types, being definitely increased only for the two most common types, serous (RR 1.53, 95% CI 1.40–1.66; $p < 0.0001$) and endometrioid cancer (1.42, 1.20–1.67; $p < 0.0001$).

4. When and where this patient needs to be referred?

Ans. Patients with adnexal mass that is suspicious for ovarian cancer need to be immediately referred to gynecologic oncologist and have surgery to establish a definitive diagnosis. Appropriate surgical treatment performed by a gynecologic oncologist has been shown to have a significant impact on overall survival.[1,3]

■ TAKE-HOME MESSAGES

- Ovarian cancer is the deadliest gynecologic cancer, taking the lives of over 14,000 women annually in the United States.[1,4] Epithelial ovarian cancer is the most common type, accounting for approximately 90% of ovarian cancers. There are six main histologic types of epithelial ovarian cancer: serous, mucinous, endometrioid, clear cell, and transitional (Brenner type).[1,4]
- On physical examination advanced ovarian cancer is palpated as irregular, fixed, sometimes bilateral adnexal mass.[4] The physician should search for other signs of malignant disease, including palpable lymphadenopathy, presence of ascites, abdominal nodules and/or omental cake.
- Transvaginal sonography can recognize sonographic markers of ovarian malignancy, such as complex mass, presence of thick septations, mural nodules, papillary projections and ascites. Evaluation of blood flow by color Doppler and 3D power Doppler studies provides additional information regarding neovascularization characteristics of ovarian malignancy.[5,6]
- Patients with suspicious adnexal masses should undergo the surgical procedure to establish the diagnosis (disease classification), assess the extent of the disease (surgical staging), and remove as much of the visible tumor as possible (cytoreductive or debulking surgery).[1,7] The stage of the disease and the amount of residual tumor at the time of surgery have a significant impact on the prognosis of the patient.[8]
- Complete surgical staging consists of the following steps:[1,7,9]
  - Evaluation of any free fluid for cytology
  - Peritoneal washings from the pelvic cul-de-sac, each paracolic gutter and from beneath each hemidiaphragm

- Removal of the intact adnexal mass to prevent seeding the peritoneal cavity with tumor cells
- If frozen sections indicate presence of ovarian cancer the surgeon should proceed with a complete abdominal exploration, systematic inspection of all intra-abdominal surfaces and biopsy or removal of any suspicious areas or adhesions on the peritoneal surfaces
- If there is no apparent disease, biopsies should be obtained from the peritoneum of the pelvic cul-de-sac, both paracolic gutters, over the bladder and the intestinal mesenteries
- The diaphragm should be sampled by either a biopsy or a scraping for cytologic smear
- Removal of the uterus and the adnexa, bilateral pelvic and para-aortic lymphadenectomy and omentectomy should be performed.

♦ Optimal debulking is defined as tumor resection with residual tumor nodules not exceeding 1 cm in diameter at the close of the procedure.[7,9] Benefits of optimal debulking are optimal response to subsequent chemotherapy, lower rates of platinum resistance and improved survival.[10]

♦ The potential role of laparoscopy in neoadjuvant therapy for ovarian cancer and in surgery for early-stage ovarian carcinoma is currently being assessed.[11]

♦ A number of studies have evaluated the use of serologic markers, such as CA-125, and imaging modalities, such as computed tomography (CT) or positron emission tomography/CT (PET/CT), to determine which patients are ideal candidates for primary cytoreductive surgery vs. neoadjuvant chemotherapy.[12]

REFERENCES

1. ACOG. Ovarian Cancer: Focus on Female Cancers; 2009. http://mail.ny.acog.org/website/OvarianCa.pdf. Published June 2009.
2. Collaborative Group on Epidemiological Studies of Ovarian Cancer, et al. Menopausal hormone use and ovarian cancer risk: individual participant meta-analysis of 52 epidemiologic studies. Lancet, 2015;385(9980):1835-42.
3. Giede KC, Kieser K, Dodge J, Rosen B. Who should operate on patients with ovarian cancer? An evidence-based review. Gynecol Oncol. 2005;99(2):447-61.
4. Berek and Hacker. Practical Gynecologic Oncology. Chapter 11: Epithelial Ovarian Cancer Pennsylvania: Lippincott Williams and Wilkins; 2005.
5. Kupesic S, Kurjak A. Contrast enhanced three-dimensional power Doppler sonography for differentiation of adnexal lesions. Obstet Gynecol. 2000; 96(3): 452-8.
6. Kupesic S, Plavsic BM. Early ovarian cancer: 3-D power Doppler. Abdom Imaging. 2006;31(5):613-9.
7. Chobanian N, Dietrich CS 3rd. Ovarian cancer. Surg Clin North Am. 2008;88(2):285-99.
8. Bristow RE, Tomacruz RS, Armstrong DK, et al. Survival effect of maximal cytoreductive surgery for advanced ovarian carcinoma during the platinum era: A meta-analysis. J Clin Oncol. 2002;20(5):1248-59.
9. Fader AN, Rose PG. Role of surgery in ovarian carcinoma. J Clin Oncol. 2007;25(20):2873-83.
10. Chi DS, Schwartz PE. Cytoreduction vs. neoadjuvant chemotherapy for ovarian cancer. Gynecol Oncol. 2008;111(3):391-9.
11. Gomez Hidalgo NR, Martinez Cannon BA, Nick Am, et al. Predictors of optimal cytoreduction in patients with newly diagnosed advanced-stage epithelial ovarian cancer: Time to incorporate laparoscopic assessment into the standard of care. Gynecol Oncol. 2015;137(3):553-8.
12. Rimbach S, Neis K, Solomayer E, et al. Current and future status of laparoscopy in gynecologic oncology. Geburtshilfe Frauenheilkd. 2014;74(9):852-9.

CHAPTER 19

Borderline Ovarian Tumor

Sanja Kupesic Plavsic, Osvaldo Padilla

■ CLINICAL CASE

SS is a 38-year-old primary infertile patient who comes to your office to discuss ovulation induction protocol prior to her third IVF/ET attempt. Her cycles are regular, every 28–30 days, and menses typically lasts about 5 days. She complains of abdominal discomfort and dyspareunia of 3 months duration. Pap smear, wet mount, *Chlamydia* and gonorrhea tests performed 6 months ago were within normal limits. Sperm analysis reveals oligoasthenozoospermia.

Menarche: Age 13.

Menses: 28-30/5 days, regular.

LMP: 10 days ago.

Sexual history: In monogamous relationship with her husband of 5 years.

Contraception: None.

Review of Systems

- No chest pain or shortness of breath
- Patient complains of abdominal/pelvic fullness and dyspareunia of 3 months duration
- No diarrhea or constipation
- No urinary frequency, hematuria, and dysuria
- *Past medical history*: Noncontributory
- *Past surgical history*: Appendectomy
- *Vaccines*: Up to date (hepatitis B vaccine series, MMR booster and flu shot)
- *Current medications*: None
- *Allergies*: No known drug allergies
- *Social history*: SS is a physical therapist; does not smoke, social ETOH, no drug abuse
- *Family history*: Mother: 64 years, history of diabetes. Father: 66 years, history of prostate cancer.

Physical Examination

- *Vital signs*: T 36.8°C oral; BP 115/70; P 74; BMI 18.
- *Cardiac examination*: No heart murmur is detected.

- *Chest examination*: Clear lungs, breathing sound is clear.
- *Abdominal examination*: Fullness in the right lower abdomen.
- *Pelvic examination*: External genitalia with no abnormalities. Per-speculum examination is normal. Bimanual pelvic examination reveals anteverted, normal size uterus and enlarged right ovary. Left adnexa are normal by palpation.
- Laboratory findings are within normal limits, with exception of tumor markers. CA-125 and CA 19-9 are elevated (75 IU/mL and 85 IU/mL respectively), while CEA is normal.
- Pelvic ultrasound detected a complex right adnexal mass measuring 5 × 4 cm. The cystic lesion had multiple papillary projections, which were vascularized at the base (Figs 19.1 and 19.2). Pulsed Doppler waveform analysis revealed low to moderate impedance blood flow signals (RI 0.52) (Fig. 19.3). Surface rendering was beneficial for depiction of the wall irregularities (Fig. 19.4). Sonographic, Doppler and tumor marker findings were suggestive of neoplastic etiology. CT scan of the abdomen and pelvis confirmed the ultrasound findings.

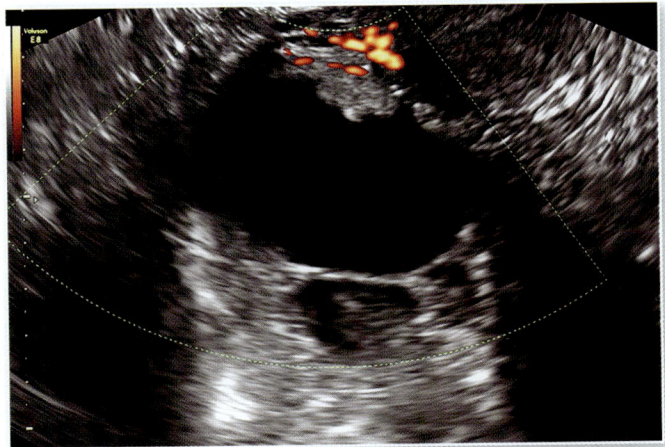

Figure 19.1: Transvaginal power Doppler image of the right ovarian complex cyst. Note blood flow signals spreading from the periphery of the lesion toward the papillary protrusion

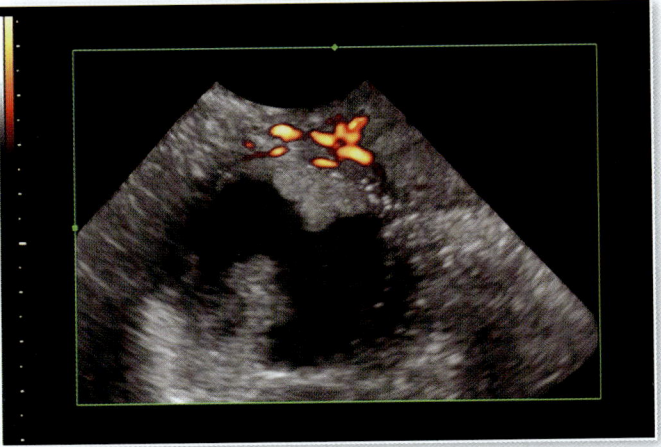

Figure 19.2: Three-dimensional power Doppler scan of the same patient

Section 1: Gynecology

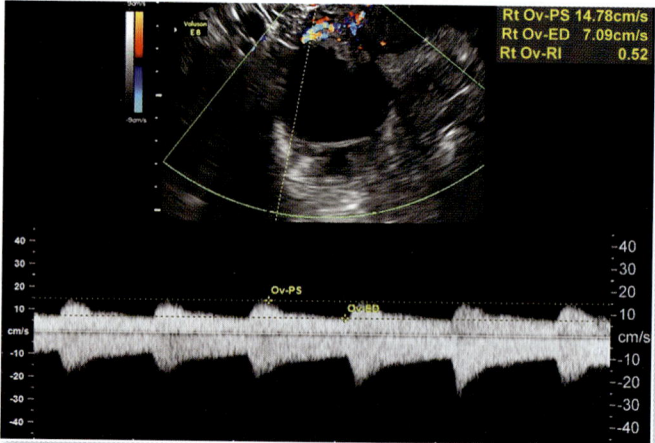

Figure 19.3: Pulsed Doppler waveforms were obtained from the peripheral vessels exhibiting low-to-moderate vascular impedance (RI 0.52)

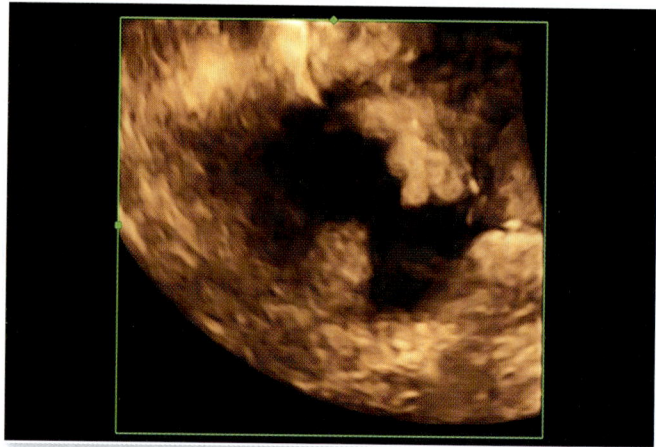

Figure 19.4: Inner cystic wall irregularities were best depicted by three-dimensional ultrasound (surface rendering)

CLINICAL QUESTIONS

1. **How would you counsel this patient who is interested to preserve fertility?**

Ans. Mrs SS should be informed that fertility sparing surgery is an acceptable option in confirmed stage I disease.

2. **The patient insists on laparoscopic surgery. Laparoscopy detects right ovarian tumor with normal left ovary on gross examination. Frozen sections of the right ovary reveal ovarian tumor of a low malignant potential. The tumor is limited to the right ovary and its capsule is intact, without tumor extension on the ovarian surface. There is no ascites and malignant cells are not detected in the peritoneal lavage. What should be done next?**

Ans. There is a need for comprehensive staging. Sampling biopsies from the pelvic peritoneum (cul-de-sac, pelvic wall, bladder peritoneum, abdominal peritoneum (paracolic gutters

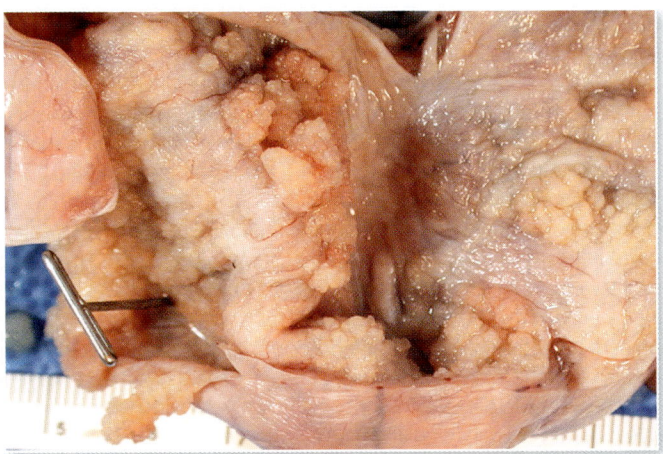

Figure 19.5: Ovarian borderline serous tumors often present as cysts with "patchy" areas of serous epithelial proliferation, resulting in papillary and solid areas of neoplasm attached to a cystic wall. These findings can also be appreciated on imaging studies

and diaphragmatic surfaces), omentum, intestinal serosa, mesentery and retroperitoneal lymph nodes) were negative, and the decision was made regarding the preservation of fertility. Unilateral salpingo-oophorectomy should be performed.

Slides and paraffin blocks were reviewed and the diagnosis of serous borderline ovarian cancer was confirmed (Fig. 19.5).

3. **Patient tolerated surgery well and postoperative period was uneventful. Her CA-125 and CA 19-9 tumor marker values are within normal limits postoperatively and on follow-up at one year. Because of husband's oligoasthenozoospermia, she would like to undergo another IVF/ET attempt. What is her chance to conceive?**

Ans. A systematic review of the literature, searching the relevant electronic databases was performed analyzing conservative surgery of borderline ovarian tumors and pregnancy rates/fertility outcome. Overall, 19 studies met the inclusion criteria for this assessment. From these studies 2,479 patients had borderline ovarian tumors of which 923 (37%) patients were treated by conservative surgery.[1] Nine studies recorded data regarding pregnancy outcome, and the pregnancy rate calculated on these data was 48%. The recurrence rate after conservative treatment was 16% with only five recorded disease-related deaths.[1]

■ TAKE-HOME MESSAGES

- Epithelial tumors of the ovary are divided into the three categories: benign (cystadenomas), malignant (cystadenocarcinomas) and borderline ovarian tumors (BOTs).[2]
- Borderline ovarian tumors (BOTs) usually occur in the 3rd and/or 4th decade of women's life, and majority of them are detected in initial stages.[3]
- Women with more than one delivery have a lower risk of developing BOTs compared with nulliparous patients. Similar to ovarian cancer, breastfeeding was reported as a protective factor. Interestingly, the use of oral contraceptives was not found to be protective against the development of BOTs.[4]

- The histological subtypes of epithelial BOTs are: serous, mucinous, endometrioid, clear and transition cells (Brenner); the first two variants, including 95% of all the BOTs.[5]
- Patients are usually asymptomatic at the time of diagnosis, and are likely to be diagnosed during a routine pelvic examination. Pelvic ultrasound is the first step in the evaluation of these patients. Although there are no typical sonographic features of BOTs, a great proportion of them shows wall irregularities, predominantly papillary protrusions within the cyst (Figs 19.1 to 19.4).[6] Doppler studies revealed no specific color and/or Doppler features for accurate preoperative detection of BOTs.[7] Three-dimensional ultrasound was not shown to be superior to conventional 2D ultrasound.[8] Neither CT nor MRI can reliably discriminate between BOTs and benign or malignant ovarian masses.[9]
- Preoperative serum levels of CA-125, CA-19-9 and CEA may be elevated, but are not specific for BOTs. In many patients, their level is within normal limits, or only minimally elevated.[9,10]
- Surgery consisting of hysterectomy, bilateral salpingo-oophorectomy, omentectomy, multiple biopsies and peritoneal cytology remains the initial treatment for BOTs. For patients who have not met their expectations for reproduction, conservative fertility treatment consisting of removing the entire disease, but preserving the uterus and at least a part of ovary is an alternative option.[1,11]
- Analysis of more than 2,000 published cases, conservative fertility surgery was found to be associated with a major risk of recurrence of the disease but had no impact on the overall survival rate.[12]

REFERENCES

1. Swanton A, Bankhead CR, Kehoe S. Pregnancy rates after conservative treatment for borderline ovarian tumours: a systematic review. Eur J Obstet Gynecol Reprod Biol. 2007;135(1):3-7.
2. Serov SF, Scully RE and Sobin LH. International histological classification of tumors, No 9 Histoloigcal Typing of Ovarian Tumours. Geneva: World Health Organization. 1973.
3. Nikrui N. Survey of clinical behavior of patients with borderline tumors of the ovary. Gynecol Oncol. 1981;12(1):107-19.
4. Riman T, Dickman PW, Nilsson S, et al. Risk factors for epithelial borderline ovarian tumors: results of a Swedish case-control study. Gynecol Oncol. 2001;83(3):575-85.
5. Lalwani N, Shanbhogue AK, Vikram R. Current update on borderline ovarian neoplasms. Am J Roentgenol. 2010;194(2):330-6.
6. Exacoustos C, Romanini ME, Rinaldo D, et al. Preoperative sonographic features of borderline ovarian tumors. Ultrasound Obstet Gynecol. 2005;25(1):50-9.
7. Valentin L. Pattern recognition of pelvic masses by gray-scale ultrasound imaging: the contribution of Doppler ultrasound. Ultrasound Obstet Gynecol. 1999;14(5):338-47.
8. Kurjak A, Kupesic S, Sparac V, Kosuta D. Three-dimensional ultrasonographic and power Doppler characterization of ovarian lesions. Ultrasound Obstet Gynecol. 2000;16(4):365-71.
9. deSouza NM, O'Neill R, McIndoe GA, et al. Borderline tumors of the ovary: CT and MRI features and tumor markers in differentiation from stage I disease. Am J Roentgenol. 2005;184(3):999-1003.
10. Kupesic S, Vujisic S, Kurjak A, et al. Preoperative assessment of ovarian tumors by CA 125 measurement and transvaginal color Doppler ultrasound. Acta Med Croatica. 2002;56(1):3-10.
11. Jones MB. Borderline ovarian tumors: current concepts for prognostic factors and clinical management. Clin Obstet Gynecol. 2006;49(3):517-25.
12. Uzan C, Kane A, Rey A, et al. Outcomes after conservative treatment of advanced-stage serous borderline tumors of the ovary. Ann Oncol. 2010;21(1):55-60.

CHAPTER 20

Ovarian Dermoid

Sireesha Y Reddy, Osvaldo Padilla, Sanja Kupesic Plavsic

■ CLINICAL CASE

About 26-year-old G0 presents for her annual gynecological examination. She has no complaints. Her pregnancy test is negative. During her pelvic examination, her physician palpates a five centimeter non-tender, mobile adnexal mass on the right side. The remainder of her physical examination was normal. A Pap smear is completed and found to be negative for intraepithelial lesion or malignancy. She was told that her cyst was likely a functional cyst related to her reproductive cycle. On a follow-up visit, a repeat pelvic examination detected that the right adnexa was persistently large. Her physician scheduled an ultrasound to better characterize the right adnexa.

Transvaginal ultrasound revealed normal size uterus and left ovary. Figure 20.1 illustrates enlarged right ovary with a complex cyst. A dermoid mesh with hyperechoic lines produced by presence of hair (right) and prominent parietal nodule (left) are typical for dermoid cyst. Morphology and external contours of the cystic lesion are better appreciated by three-dimensional ultrasound (Fig. 20.2). Figure 20.3 illustrates power Doppler imaging features typical for a benign lesion (regularly separated peripheral vessels and absence of penetrating vascularity).

The physician reviewed findings with the patient. She counsels the patient that the cyst will continue to be persistent and is likely benign. She recommends a follow-up ultrasound in 2 months. In case lesion will persist, surgical removal of the dermoid cyst contained within the right ovary will be recommended (Figure 20.4).

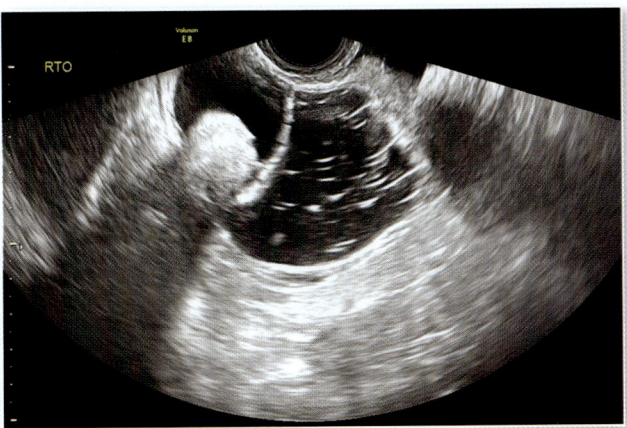

Figure 20.1: Transvaginal ultrasound of a complex cyst with a large hyperechoic area (left) demonstrating the Rokitansky nodule (dermoid plug). Hyperechoic band like echoes on the right are produced by hair

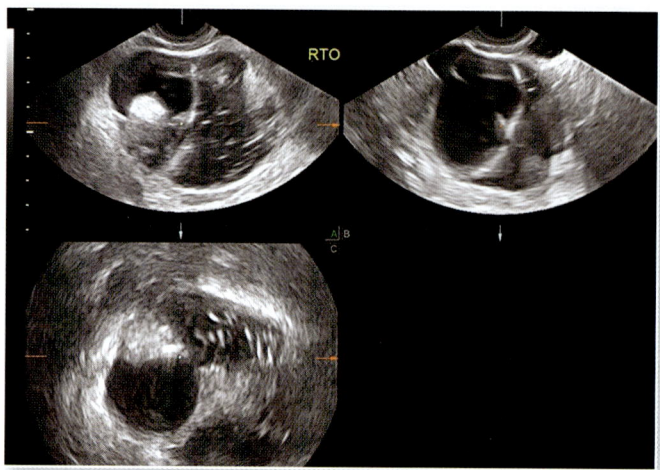

Figure 20.2: Three-dimensional ultrasound of the same lesion

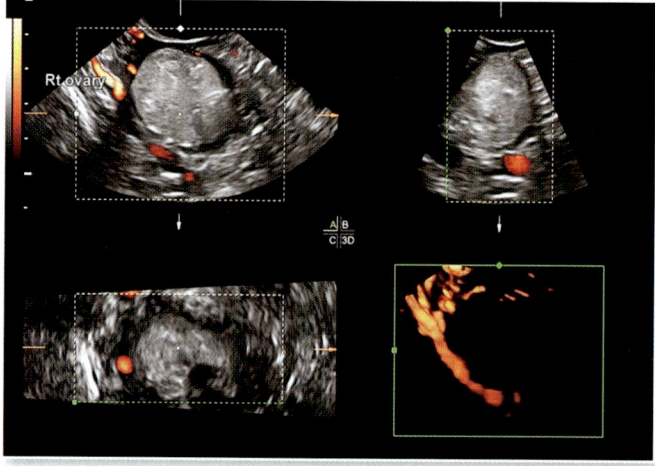

Figure 20.3: Three-dimensional power Doppler ultrasound demonstrates regularly separated peripheral vessels and absence of penetrating vascularity

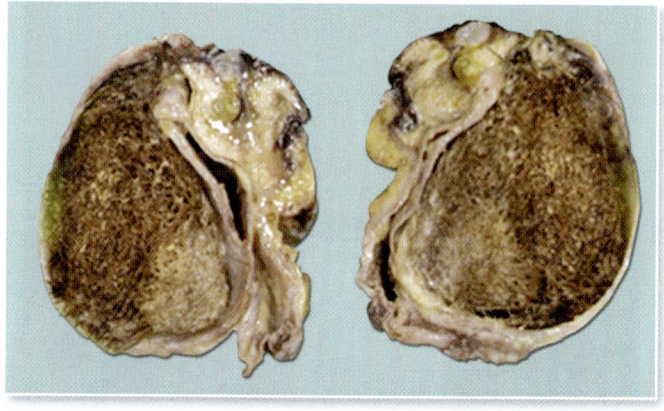

Figure 20.4: Macroscopic image of a dermoid cyst

CLINICAL QUESTIONS

1. What is the clinical approach to asymptomatic masses in young reproductive age women?

Ans. The approach taken in this patient is a reasonable one. Initially, the provider may choose to observe the mass. A vast majority in this age group will be benign and associated with their menstrual cycle or reproduction (follicular cyst, corpus luteum or hemorrhagic cyst).[1] A follow-up visit to ensure the resolution of the cyst indicates thoroughness in the diagnostic evaluation.

2. What is the imaging modality generally used in adnexal masses in young reproductive age women?

Ans. A pelvic transvaginal ultrasound is the imaging modality of choice to characterize pelvic organs and associated pathologies.[2] In comparison to CT or MRI, ultrasound provides a similar diagnostic accuracy and less expense. The other images can be used to better characterize pelvic lesions, if it is unclear from the ultrasound.

3. What are the sonographic features that help define the benign nature of this mass?

Ans. Dermoids have typical polymorph appearance: hyperechoic regions or foci that may show acoustic shadowing (Rokitansky protuberance), hypoechoic areas with band-like hyperechoic echoes (dermoid mash), and less frequently, echogenic fluid, calcifications and floating globules.[3] Sometimes, bone or teeth are visualized as calcification with posterior shadowing.

4. What are the most common pitfalls in the ultrasound diagnosis of ovarian dermoid cysts?

Ans. Hemorrhagic cysts with blood clot which may imitate Rokitansky protuberance, and ovarian endometrioma which may appear echogenic, similar to the sebaceous fluid of a mature teratoma. Sometimes echogenic bowel can also be mistaken for echogenic teratoma.

5. What are the complications associated with dermoid cysts?

- Ovarian torsion
- Cyst rupture which can lead to acute peritonitis
- Malignant degeneration (< 2%)[5]

6. What is malignant degeneration of an ovarian dermoid?

Ans. Malignant degeneration of an ovarian dermoid is a malignancy arising *de novo* in a preexisting benign mature cystic teratoma. This is a rare complication, reported to occur in less than 2% of the cases.[5] In contrast, immature teratomas do not arise from mature cystic teratomas.

7. How are teratomas pathologically classified?

Ans. Pathologically, teratomas are classified into three groups:
- Mature cystic teratoma—a benign tumor that contains mature forms of three germ-cell layers (endoderm, mesoderm, ectoderm), also known as mature cystic teratoma, benign cystic teratoma, and dermoid cyst;
- Monodermal teratoma—a benign tumor, composed only or predominantly of one highly specialized tissue type (i.e. struma ovarii—predominantly composed of thyroid tissue);
- Immature (malignant) teratoma—a malignant neoplasm, consisting of immature tissues from one, two, or all three germ-cell layers; can coexist with mature elements.

■ TAKE-HOME MESSAGES

- Mature teratomas, or dermoid cysts, are the most common germ-cell tumor of the ovary, accounting for more than 95% of all ovarian teratomas.[1,2,6]
- Cystic teratomas can present at any age; however, they are diagnosed most frequently in the reproductive years.[3]
- Mature teratomas are bilateral in 8–14% of cases.[2,3]
- There is a 2% chance of mature teratomas developing into a malignant tumor. If malignancy develops, the most common type of malignancy to develop from a mature teratoma is a squamous cell carcinoma.[4,5]
- Most women with mature cystic teratoma are asymptomatic. Clinical manifestations depend on the size of the lesion. Complications include torsion and rupture, which is associated with the spillage of the sebaceous material into the abdominal cavity, leading to formation of dense adhesions secondary to chemical peritonitis.[7]
- Ultrasound is a method of choice for diagnosis of cystic teratoma, with high specificity between 98% and 100%.[8,9]
- The addition of the three-dimensional ultrasound allows better visualization of the inner wall irregularities, visualization of the solid areas, measurement of the wall and septation thickness, evaluation of the echogenicity of the lesion and analysis of the distal shadowing.[10]
- Evaluating the presence or absence of intratumoral blood flow, together with assessment of blood flow resistance in tumor vessels using transvaginal color Doppler imaging may be useful to differentiate malignant from benign cystic teratomas.[11]
- Ovarian cystectomy is suggested to avoid complication such as torsion, rupture, and malignant transformation (rare).

■ REFERENCES

1. Borgfeldt C, Andolf E. Transvaginal sonographic ovarian findings in a random sample of women 25-40 years old. Ultrasound Obstet Gynecol. 1999;13(5):345-50.
2. American College of Obstetricians and Gynecologists. ACOG Practice Bulletin. Management of adnexal masses. Obstet Gynecol. 2007;110:201-14.
3. Patel MD, Feldstein VA, Lipson SD, et al. Cystic teratomas of the ovary: diagnostic value of sonography. AJR Am J Roentgenol. 1998;171(4):1061-5.
4. Brown DL, Doubilet PM, Miller FH, et al. Benign and malignant ovarian masses: selection of the most discriminating gray-scale and Doppler sonographic features. Radiology. 1998;208(1):103-10.
5. Talerman A. Germ cell tumors of the ovary. In: Kurman RJ, eds. Blaustein's pathology of the female genital tract. 4th ed. New York, NY: Springer-Verlag. 1994;849-914.
6. Ayhan A, Bukulmez O, Genc C, Karamursel BS, Ayhan A. Mature cystic teratomas of the ovary: case series from one institution over 34 years. Eur J Obstet Gynecol Reprod Biol. 2000;88(2):153.
7. DiSaia PJ, Creasman WT. Germ cell, stromal and other ovarian tumors. In: Clinical Gynecologic Oncology, 7th, Mosby-Elsevier, 2007; p.381.
8. Patel MD, Feldstein VA, Lipson SD, et al. Cystic teratomas of the ovary: diagnostic value of sonography. AJR Am J Roentgenol 1998;171:1061.
9. Tongsong T, Luewan S, Phadungkiatwattana P, et al. Pattern recognition using transabdominal ultrasound to diagnose ovarian mature cystic teratoma. Int J Gynaecol Obstet. 2008;103:99.
10. Kurjak A, Kupesic S, Babic MM, Goldenberg M, Ilijas M, Kosuta D. Preoperative evaluation of cystic teratoma: What does color Doppler add? J Clin Ultrasound 1997;25:309-15.
11. Emoto M, Obama H, Horiuchi S, Miyakawa T, Kawarabayashi T. Transvaginal color Doppler ultrasonic characterization of bening and malignant ovarian cystic teratomas and comparsion with serum squamous cell carcinoma antigen. Cancer 2000;15(88):2298-304.

CHAPTER 21

Hemorrhagic Cyst

Sanja Kupesic Plavsic, Osvaldo Padilla

■ CLINICAL CASE

JE is a 19-year-old G0 who presents to your office with history of RLQ pain. Two days ago, she was evaluated in ER. Her urine pregnancy test was negative and laboratory tests were within normal limits. Abdominal and pelvic CT showed a normal appendix and a complex 5 × 4 cm right adnexal mass.

Menarche: Age 12.

Menses: 28/5, regular.

LMP: Three weeks ago.

OB history: The patient was never pregnant.

Sexual history: Sexually active with her long-term boyfriend who is currently in military service.

Contraception: None.

Review of Systems

- No headaches, no problems with vision
- No history of blood clots, DVT or PE
- No heart palpitations, no shortness of breath
- Positive for RLQ colicky abdominal/pelvic pain; Intensity: 4–6/10
- No constipation, no diarrhea; no nausea and vomiting
- *Past medical history*: None; no hospitalizations
- Vaccines are up to date
- *Past surgical history*: None
- *Current medications*: None
- *Allergies*: None known drug allergies
- *Social history*: College student; denies tobacco, drug, and alcohol use
- *Past family history*: Nonsignificant.

Physical Examination

- *Vital signs*: T 36.7°C oral; BP 125/80; P 82; BMI 19
- Normal heart, lungs, thyroid, and neck examination
- *Abdominal examination*: RLQ with tenderness to palpation without rebound tenderness
- *Pelvic examination*: External genitalia and cervix with no abnormalities. The uterus and left adnexa are normal size. There is tenderness and enlargement of the right adnexa
- *Laboratory tests*: *Urinalysis*: normal; *CBC*: normal; *beta-hCG*: negative
- Pelvic ultrasound with color Doppler imaging was performed. Figures 21.1 and 21.2 illustrate patient's imaging findings. Complex ovarian cyst 5 × 4 cm with reticular pattern and discrete peripheral flow was visualized. Spectral Doppler analysis revealed low impedance blood flow signals, typical for luteal conversion (Fig. 21.2).

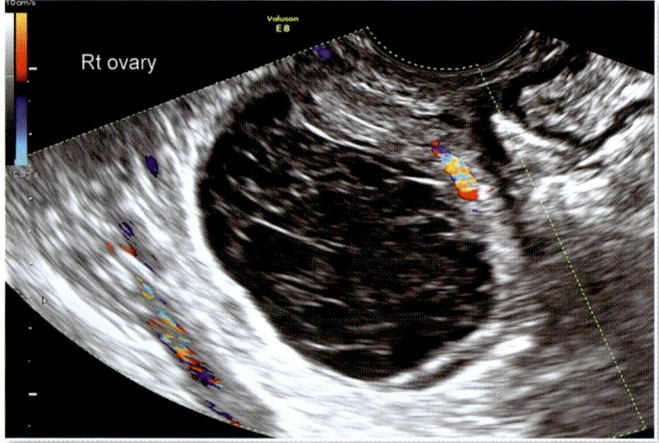

Figure 21.1: Transvaginal color Doppler imaging revealed a complex ovarian cyst with discrete peripheral blood flow

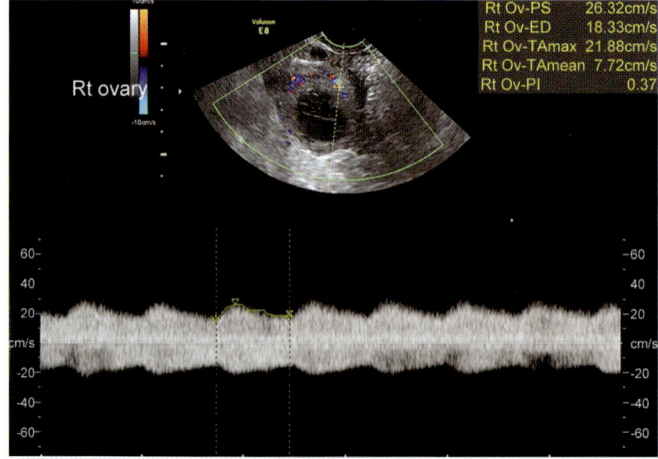

Figure 21.2: Pulsed Doppler waveform analysis of the same patient demonstrated low vascular impedance blood flow signals (RI 0.37) obtained from peripheral vessels

CLINICAL QUESTIONS

1. What is the most likely diagnosis of this patient?
Ans. Patient's symptoms, clinical and sonographic findings are suggestive of a hemorrhagic cyst.

2. What is the mechanism of formation of a hemorrhagic cyst?
Ans. When follicle ruptures to release an oocyte at the time of ovulation, it is transformed into a corpus luteum. Thin walled vessels invade the blood filled cavity of a follicle, and form the corpus luteum.[1] This may cause bleeding into the corpus luteum, resulting in the formation of a hemorrhagic ovarian cyst.

3. What is the typical sonographic appearance of hemorrhagic ovarian cysts?
Ans. The appearance of hemorrhagic ovarian cysts varies and depends on the stage of formation and duration of the cystic lesion.[2] There are four typical appearances:
- Fishnet reticular pattern, consisting of multiple fine strands of fibrin giving a net-like appearance (Figs 21.1 and 21.2). The septations are thin and avascularized on color Doppler
- Retracting clot appearance, consisting of an organized blood clot and sonolucent fluid occupying the remainder of the cyst (Fig. 21.3)
- Rupture of hemorrhagic cyst can mimic an ectopic pregnancy, and is seen as accumulation of sonolucent or echogenic free fluid surrounding the cyst (Fig. 21.4)
- Hemorrhagic cyst with diffuse low level internal echoes mimicking an ovarian endometrioma (Fig. 21.5)
- Complex hemorrhagic cyst, with a clot mimicking a solid part of an ovarian neoplasm (Fig. 21.6).

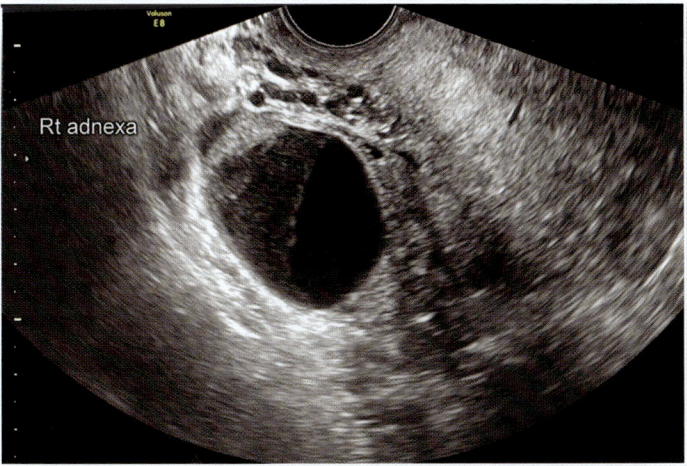

Figure 21.3: Transvaginal scan of a patient with retracting clot appearance of hemorrhagic cyst

Section 1: Gynecology

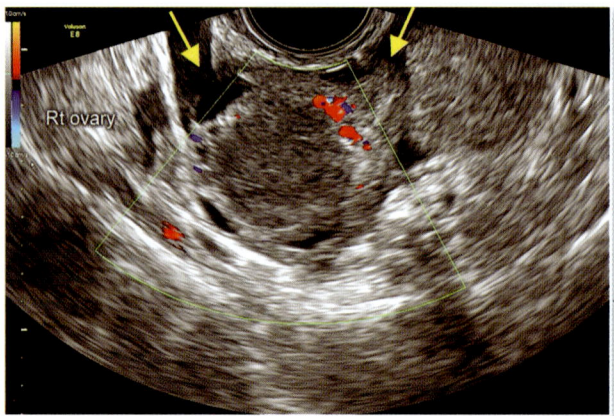

Figure 21.4: Ruptured hemorrhagic cyst is seen as accumulation of free fluid surrounding the cyst (marked by arrows). The fluid is either sonolucent or echogenic. This appearance can be confused with an ectopic pregnancy. Make sure to evaluate hemoglobin level before discharging the patient

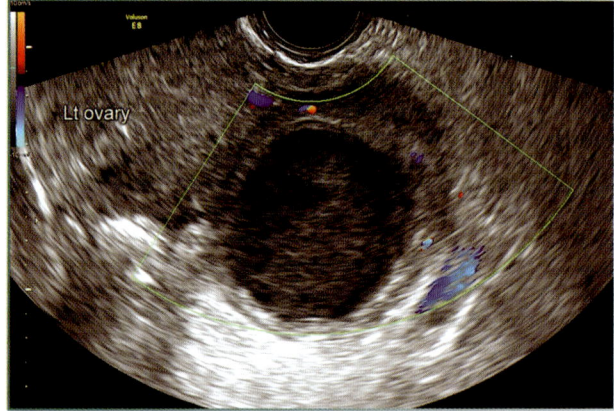

Figure 21.5: Transvaginal color Doppler scan of a hemorrhagic cyst with diffuse low level internal echoes mimicking ovarian endometrioma

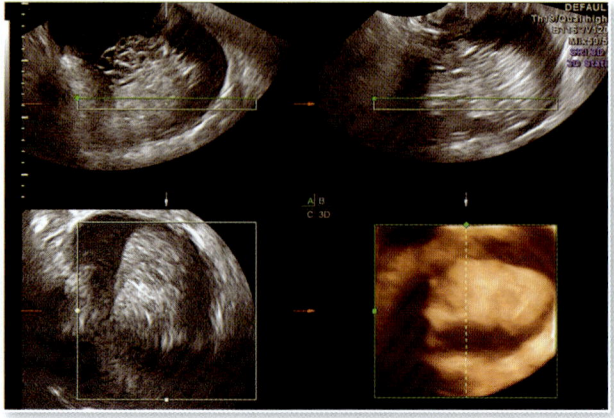

Figure 21.6: Three-dimensional ultrasound image of a complex hemorrhagic cyst. Clot formation within the cyst can mimic a solid part of an ovarian neoplasm

4. What is the role of color Doppler in differentiation of hemorrhagic cyst from other ovarian pathologies?

Ans. Absence of color flow signals within the clot (solid part) and fibrin strands (thin septations) caused by clot retraction is typical for hemorrhagic cyst.[3] Low impedance blood flow signals can be extracted from the peripheral vessels (referred as "ring of fire").

5. What is the best time for follow-up of this patient?

Ans. Follow-up sonogram should be scheduled in 6–8 weeks.[1,2]

■ TAKE-HOME MESSAGES

- Acute onset of abdominal and/or pelvic pain in the second phase of the menstrual cycle is suggestive of a hemorrhagic cyst. Patients typically present with mid-cycle pelvic pain, negative pregnancy test and absence of fever and leukocytosis.[2]
- The definitive diagnosis is usually made by transvaginal sonography. Fibrin strands and a retracting clot are paramount observations in allowing high confidence in the diagnosis of hemorrhagic ovarian cysts. Approximately, 90% of hemorrhagic ovarian cysts will exhibit at least one of these two sonographic features.[3]
- Follow-up ultrasound examination in 6 weeks usually reveals spontaneous resolution of the cystic mass.[4] In patients with positive findings on serial sonography, oral contraception may be prescribed.[5]
- Differential diagnosis includes: ectopic pregnancy, ovarian torsion, pelvic inflammatory disease, ovarian neoplasm and GI pathology (such as appendicitis, Crohn's disease, etc.)[6]
- Patients with presumed rupture of hemorrhagic cyst should be managed conservatively. In stable patients, conservative medical care consists of outpatient treatment with oral analgesics, while unstable patients require admission and anticipatory management with serial sonographic examinations and laboratory testing and pain relief.[7,8]
- Patients with continued intra-abdominal bleeding and/or ovarian torsion should be treated surgically. Warning signs include: nausea, vomiting, syncope, shoulder tenderness and circulatory collapse. Depending on clinical presentation, patient stability, amount of intra-abdominal bleeding and operator skills, laparotomy or laparoscopy should be performed.[9,10] Figure 21.7 illustrates a hemorrhagic cyst with clot formation within the cyst mimicking a solid part.

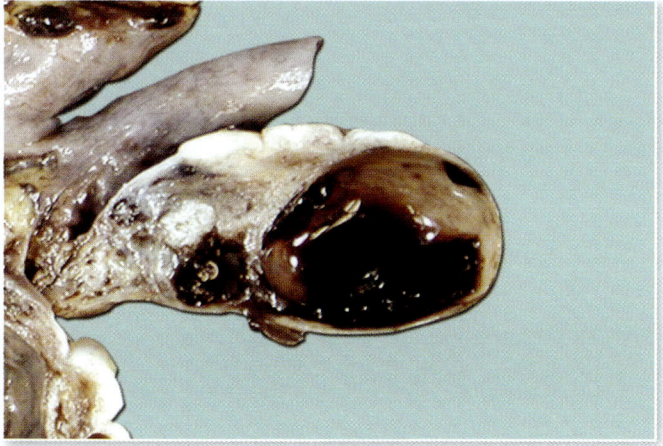

Figure 21.7: Gross anatomy image of hemorrhagic cyst with clot formation

REFERENCES

1. Kupesic S, Hafner T, Bjelos D. Events from ovulation to implantation studied by three-dimensional ultrasound. J Perinat Med. 2002;30(1):84-98.
2. Jain KA. Sonographic spectrum of hemorrhagic cyst. J Ultrasound Med. 2002;21(8):879-86.
3. Kupesic S, Aksamija A. Sonographic evaluation of gynecological and obstetric causes of acute pelvic pain. Ultrasound Rev Obstet Gynecol. 2003;5:192-202.
4. Patel MD, Feldstein VA, Filly RA. The likelihood ratio of sonographic finding for the diagnosis of hemorrhagic ovarian cysts. J Ultrasound Med. 2005;24(5):607-14.
5. Christensen JT, Boldsen JL, Westergaard JG. Functional ovarian cysts in premenopausal and gynecologically healthy women. Contraception. 2002;66(3):153-7.
6. Swire MN, Castro-Aragon I, Levine D. Various sonographic appearance of the hemorrhagic corpus luteum cyst. Ultrasound Q. 2004;20(2):45-58.
7. Raziel A, Ron-El R, Pansky M, et al. Current management of ruptured corpus luteum. Eur J Obstet Gynecol Reprod Biol. 1993;50(1):77-81.
8. Teng SW, Tseng JY, Chang CK, et al. Comparison of laparoscopy and laparotomy in managing hemodynamically stable patients with ruptured corpus luteum with hemoperitoneum. J Am Assoc Gynecol Laparosc. 2003;10(4):474-7.
9. Odejinmi F, Sangrithi M, Olowu O. Operative laparoscopy as the mainstay method in management of hemodynamically unstable patients with ectopic pregnancy. J Minim Invasive Gynecol. 2011;18(2):179-83.
10. Okaro E, Condous G, Khalid A, Timmerman D, Ameye L, Huffel SV, Bourne T. The use of ultrasound-based 'soft markers' for the prediction of pelvic pathology in women with chronic pelvic pain: can we reduce the need for laparoscopy? BJOG. 2006;113(3):251-6.

CHAPTER 22

Ectopic Pregnancy

Sushila Arya, Sireesha Y Reddy, Sanja Kupesic Plavsic

■ CLINICAL CASE

MD is a 28-year-old G3P1, who presents to ER with abdominal pain and vaginal spotting which started a few hours ago. She reports sudden left lower quadrant pain (LLQ) radiating to her upper abdomen. Patient also reports feeling low-grade fever and chills since last 2 hours. Her LMP was 5 weeks ago.

She has not been using any contraceptive, and desires pregnancy. Her history is significant for left ectopic pregnancy 2 years ago, which was treated with methotrexate (MTX). Her pregnancy test is positive; beta-HCG is 2,300 mIU/mL, Hb/Hct is 11.5/34, chemistry panel, and urine analyses are all within normal limits.

Results of her transvaginal ultrasound examination are presented on Figures 22.1 to 22.3.

Menarche: Age 11; Menstrual periods: 28–20 days/5–7 days; LMP: 5 weeks ago.

Obstetric history: One normal spontaneous vaginal delivery; 1 ectopic pregnancy, medically treated.

Sexual and GYN history: 5 male partners over her lifetime. History of *Chlamydia* at age of 19 years. Recent STD testing and Pap smear were performed 4 months ago, and were normal.

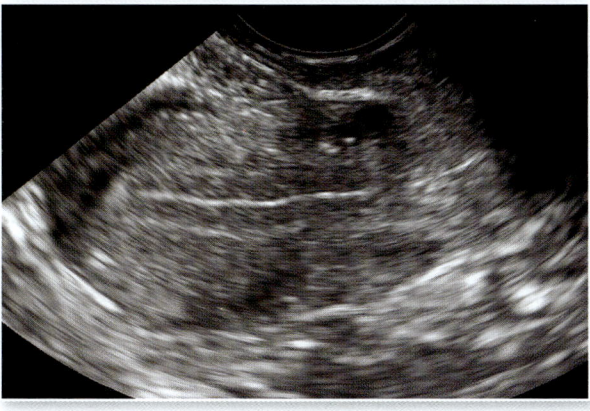

Figure 22.1: Transvaginal ultrasound demonstrates a triple line endometrium. An ectopic pregnancy should be suspected if transvaginal sonography does not show intrauterine gestation when the beta-hCG is higher than 1,500 mIU/mL

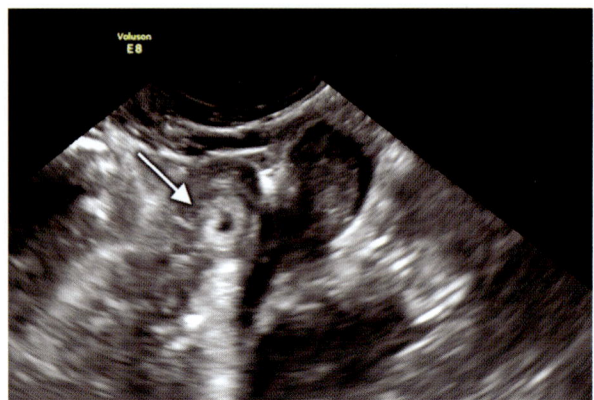

Figure 22.2: B-mode transvaginal ultrasound of the left adnexa. Tubal ring measuring 1 x 2 cm, consisting of echogenic tissue surrounding a hypoechogenic center is visualized adjacent to the left ovary ("bagel sign")

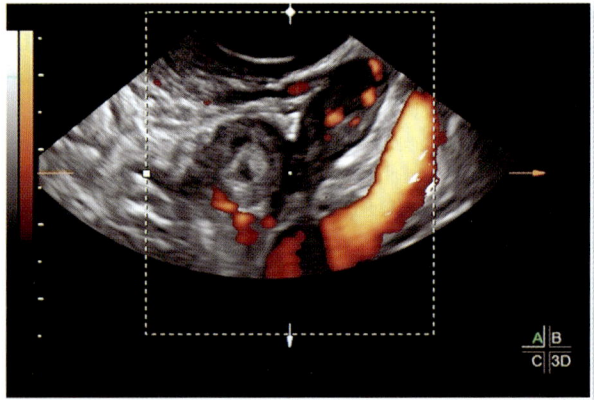

Figure 22.3: Power Doppler image of the same patient, showing dilated tubal vessels next to ectopic pregnancy and corpus luteum

Contraception: None, desires pregnancy.

Past medical history: None, no hospitalizations.

Past surgical history: None.

Current medications: None.

Allergies: No known drug allergies.

Social history: MD is a house maker. She drinks alcohol occasionally and in moderation. She reports 2–3 cigarettes daily for last 10 years, and reports no history of substance abuse.

Family history: Significant for mother who had breast cancer at age of 61 years. No other family history of hereditary cancers or other chronic medical conditions.

Review of Systems

Positive for abdominal/pelvic pain, low-grade fever with chills and dizziness. All other ROS is negative.

Physical Examination

- *Vital signs:* T 37.0°C oral; BP 104/61; P 71; BMI 30.2.
- *General:* Alert, oriented to time, place and person. In mild distress related to pain
- Neck, heart, and lungs examination is unremarkable
- *Abdomen:* Soft, lower abdomen is tender, guarding +, no mass palpable
- *Pelvic examination:* Normal external genitalia, minimal old blood on speculum examination, cervix and vagina unremarkable. On bimanual examination, uterus and adnexa were difficult to assess secondary to guarding and patient discomfort. Left adnexal tenderness noticed. Evidence of fullness in the cul-de-sac.

■ CLINICAL QUESTIONS

1. What is the most likely diagnosis?

Ans. The clinical, laboratory, and imaging results are suggestive of the left tubal ectopic pregnancy. This patient had acute onset sharp abdominal pain, vaginal bleeding, and missed period.[1-3] Her serum beta-hCG was 2,300 mIU/mL. Transvaginal ultrasound revealed an empty uterine cavity and left adnexal mass consistent with ectopic pregnancy.

2. What risk factors you do you see in this patient for ectopic pregnancy?

Ans. History of *Chlamydia* and left ectopic pregnancy.[4,5]

3. Besides ultrasound and beta-hCG what are other helpful laboratory test to diagnose ectopic pregnancy?

Ans. Beta-hCG discriminatory zone 1,500 mIU/mL for transvaginal sonogram of empty uterus.[6] At early gestation (4–5 weeks), there is good sensitivity and specificity of serum progesterone, for example at 4 weeks gestation progesterone level 5 ng/mL has 100% sensitivity and 97% specificity in diagnosing ectopic pregnancy.[7]

4. What is the most appropriate treatment for this patient?

Ans. Left salpingectomy, which should be done laparoscopically since the patient is hemodynamically stable (Fig. 22.4). She is not a candidate for medical management or salpingostomy due to recurrent ectopic pregnancy.

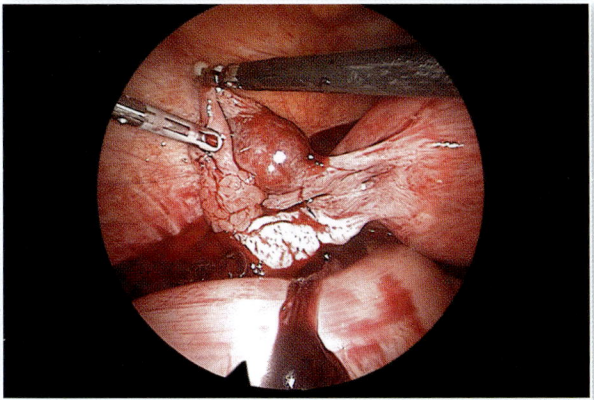

Figure 22.4: Laparoscopic evaluation showing hemoperitoneum and erythematous, dilated ampullary part of the fallopian tube

5. Patient desires future fertility and inquires about tube sparing surgery. What is the most appropriate answer to this request?

Ans. Salpingostomy is appropriate for unruptured ectopic pregnancies, but there is a concern of persistent trophoblastic tissue.[5] Single-dose of MTX after tube sparing procedure has reduced risk of persistent ectopic pregnancy (PEP).[8] Due to prior history of ectopic pregnancy, she is not an appropriate candidate for tube sparing surgery.

6. If she was asymptomatic and had no prior history of ectopic pregnancy how would you have treated her?

Ans. Single or multidose regimens of MTX are two main protocols used to treat asymptomatic patients who qualify for medical treatment. Multidose regimen has higher toxicity so it considered appropriate for patients presenting with beta-hCG higher than 5,000 mIU/mL.

7. Describe follow up after medical treatment of ectopic pregnancy.

Ans. After medical treatment, beta-hCG is measured on day 1, 4 and, 7. At least 15% decrease in beta-hCG on day 7 compared to day 4 is expected. A second dose is given on day 7 if beta-hCG does not decrease for at least 15% between days 4 and 7. If less than 15% decrease, MTX should be considered for maximum 3 doses. After salpingostomy beta-hCG should be measured initially on day 6 and with 3-day interval thereafter to detect persistent ectopic pregnancy. Typically, mean time to undetectable beta-hCG values is 3 weeks after salpingostomy, and 27 days after initiation of MTX.[10]

■ TAKE-HOME MESSAGES

- Ectopic pregnancy occurs at a rate of 1–2% of all pregnancies.[1] There is increase in its incidence, stable since 1992, mainly due to: (1). Improved diagnostic tools, and (2). Increase in sexually transmitted diseases such as *Chlamydia trachomatis*.[1]
- Most common symptoms of ectopic pregnancy are abdominal pain, irregular vaginal bleeding, amenorrhea and syncope. Before rupture pain is vague, colicky, and becomes intense with rupture.[1]
- Important risk factors are salpingitis, tubal surgeries, smoking, older age, IUD, infertility and abdominal/pelvic surgeries.[2,3] With salpingitis, there is agglutination of plicae of endosalpinx, which prevents normal transfer of blastocyst.
- Medical management is increasingly used for ectopic pregnancies due to early diagnosis with smaller size and lower beta-hCG.[9] There is evidence of increased intrauterine pregnancy (IUP) rates after conservative surgical treatment.
- Salpingostomy should be considered for patients who desire future fertility and have unruptured ectopic pregnancy.[5] Salpingostomy is done by performing a tubal incision on antimesenteric border to evacuate the ectopic pregnancy, followed by flushing out the products of conception by suction-irrigator. The incision is not sutured, but instead left to close on its own (closure by secondary intention).
- Persistent ectopic pregnancy (PEP) is getting more common due to conservative management of ectopic pregnancies. After salpingostomy, serum beta-hCG or progesterone must be measured on day 6 and at 3-day interval thereafter. Beta-hCG >1,000 mIU/mL or more than 15% of baseline value are indicative of PEP.[6]
- In asymptomatic patients, PEP should be treated by medical management, otherwise salpingectomy should be considered.[6]
- The crude IUP rates up to 24 months after surgery were 55.5% for salpingectomy, 50.9% for salpingostomy and 40.3% for tubal anastomosis treatments.[11]
- There is 25% risk of repeat ectopic pregnancy even in those who were treated with unilateral salpingectomy. Rate of ectopic pregnancy after salpingostomy or salpingoplasty is 15–25%.[9-11]

REFERENCES

1. Roger A. Lobo Chapter 17. Ectopic pregnancy. Comprehensive Gynecology, 6th edition, Atlanta, GA: Elsevier Mosby 2012.
2. Fernandez H, Gervaise A. Ectopic pregnancies after infertility treatment: Modern diagnosis and therapeutic strategy. Hum Reprod Update. 2004;10:503.
3. Corson SL, Batzer FR. Ectopic pregnancy. A review of the etiologic factors. J Reprod Med. 1986;31:78.
4. Breen JL. A 21 year survey of 654 ectopic pregnancies. Am J Obstet Gynecol. 1970;106:1004.
5. Tulandi T, Guralnick M. Treatment of tubal ectopic pregnancy by salpingotomy with or without tubal suturing and salpingectomy. Fertil Steril. 1991;55:53.
6. Vermesh M, Silva PD, Rosen GF, et al. Persistent tubal ectopic gestation: Patterns of circulation β-human chorionic gonadotropin and progesterone and management options. Fertil Steril. 1988;50:584.
7. McCord ML, Arheart KL, Muram D, et al. Single serum progesterone as a screen fro ectopic pregnancy: exchanging specificity and sensitivity to obtain optimal test performance. Fertil Steril. 1996;66:513.
8. Graczykowski W, Mishell DR. Jr. Methotrexate prophylaxis for persistent ectopic pregnancy after conservative treatment by salpingostomy. Obstet Gynecol. 1997;89:118.
9. Medical treatment of ectopic pregnancy: A committee opinion. Practice Committee of American Society for Reproductive Medicine. Fertil Steril. 2013;100(3):638-44. doi: 10.1016/j.
10. Saraj AJ, Wilcox JG, Najmabadi S, et al. Resolution of hormonal markers of ectopic gestation: a randomized trial comparing single-dose intramuscular methotrexate with salpingostomy. Obstet Gynecol. 1998;92:989.
11. Jingwel L, Kallel J, Fujle Z. Fertility outcome analysis after surgical management of tubal ectopic pregnancy: a retrospective cohort study. BMJ Open. 2015;5:e007339 doi:10.1136/bmjopen-2014-007339.

CHAPTER 23

Ovarian Torsion

Sanja Kupesic Plavsic, Sireesha Y Reddy

■ CLINICAL CASE

NV is a 15-year-old G0 who presents to ER with her mother for a colicky RLQ pain. She feels nauseous with two bouts of vomiting before coming to the hospital. She denies vaginal bleeding. The ER doctor initially suspected, she had appendicitis and ordered a CT scan after obtaining a negative beta-hCG. The CT showed a normal appendix and a right adnexal mass. A pelvic ultrasound was then ordered.

Menarche: Age 11.

Menses: Regular, bleeds every 26 days for 7 days.

LMP: 10 days ago.

Pregnancies: None.

Sexual history: She adamantly denies any sexual activity. (This was asked while she was alone).

Review of Systems

- No headaches, no problems with vision
- No history of blood clots DVT or PE
- No heart palpitations, no shortness of breath
- Positive for right lower abdominal/pelvic pain
- No constipation, no diarrhea. Complains of nausea and vomiting
- *Past medical history*: None, no hospitalizations
- *Past surgical history*: None
- *Vaccines*: Uptodate per mother
- *Current medications*: Tylenol for pain
- *Allergies*: None known drug allergies
- *Social history*: Sophomore in high school—attends a magnet school and is on the honor roll. Denies tobacco, drug, and alcohol use
- *Past family history*: Maternal grandmother age 70, had breast cancer age 65, status post mastectomy and chemotherapy; No other gynecologic cancers in the family.

Physical Examination

- *Vital signs*: T 100.1°F (37.8°C) oral; BP 125/85; P 112; BMI 19
- Normal heart, lungs, thyroid and neck examination
- *Abdominal examination*: RLQ with tenderness to palpation with rebound tenderness
- *Pelvic Examination*: Deferred
- *Laboratory tests*: Urinalysis: normal; CBC: normal; Beta-hCG: negative
- Transabdominal ultrasound with color/power Doppler imaging was performed. Figures 23.1 and 23.2 illustrate patient's imaging findings. Patient underwent laparoscopic procedure. The diagnosis of right ovarian torsion was confirmed by direct visualization of the rotated ovary containing a simple ovarian cyst. Detorsion, followed with ovarian cystectomy and ovarian conservation are demonstrated in Figures 23.3 to 23.6.

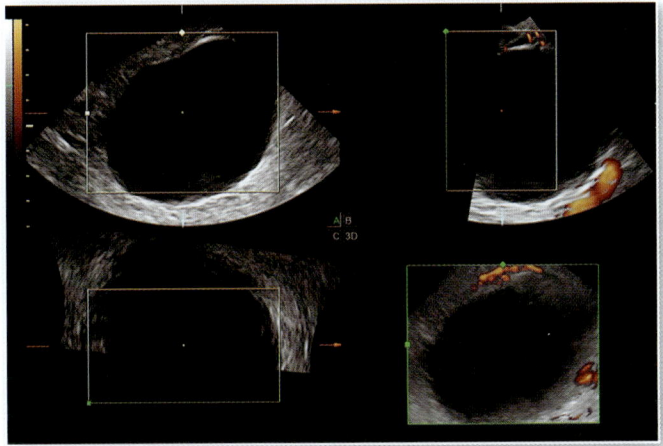

Figure 23.1: Three-dimensional transabdominal power Doppler US of the right ovary demonstrates enlarged right ovary with a simple ovarian cyst. Right lower image demonstrates heterogeneous appearance of the cystic lesion due to edema and hemorrhage with peripheral vessels

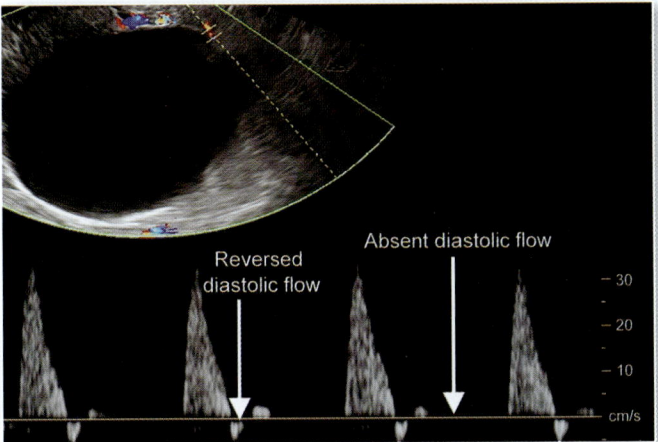

Figure 23.2: Pulsed Doppler waveform analysis of the same patient reveals absent and reversed diastolic flow in the ovarian artery, suggesting an inflow obstruction. Sonographic and Doppler findings are typical for complete ovarian torsion

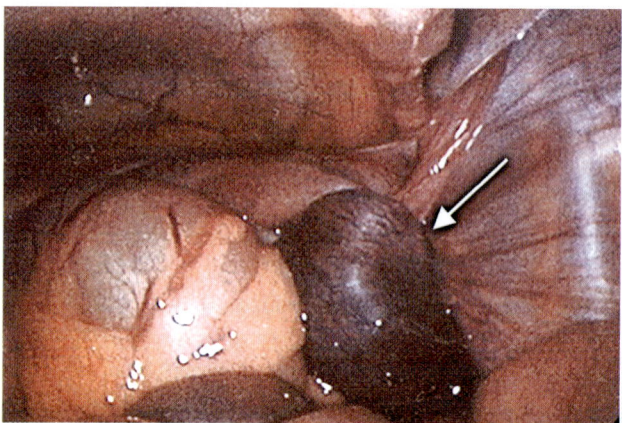

Figure 23.3: Torsion of the right fallopian tube and ovary is seen with a purplish-blue hue showing signs of marked edema suggesting decreased perfusion. Arrow points to torsion

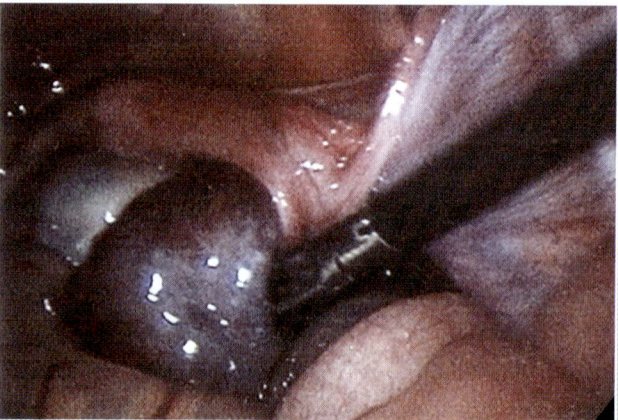

Figure 23.4: Surgeon attempts to detorse the ovary and fallopian tube to return perfusion

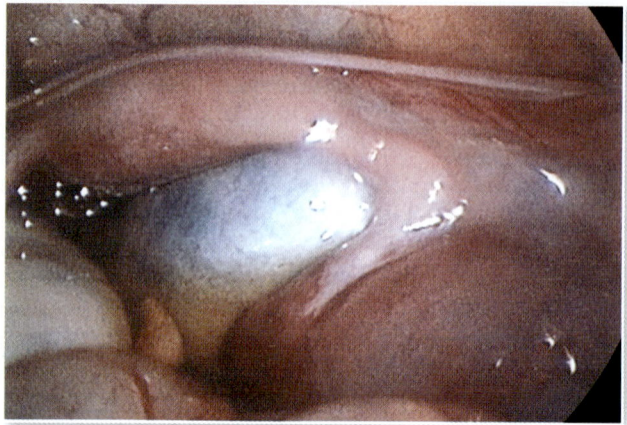

Figure 23.5: Ovary and fallopian tube are detorsed. Immediate reperfusion is seen. There is still marked edema that will likely resolve

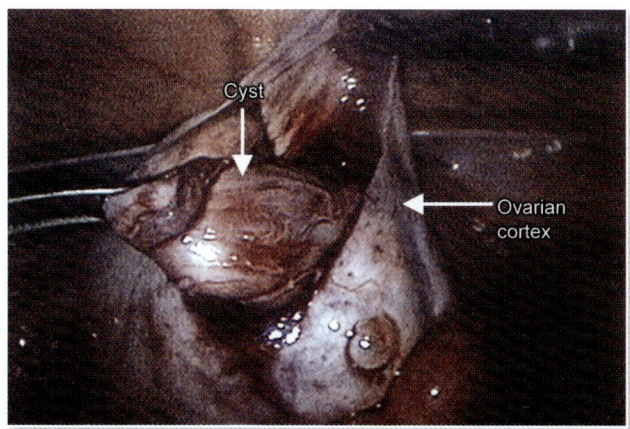

Figure 23.6: An ovarian cyst within the ovary is the cause of the torsion. The cyst wall is apparent and is separated from the ovarian cortex. Ovarian cortex is well perfused and ovary is conserved. Arrows point to the ovarian cyst and ovarian cortex

■ CLINICAL QUESTIONS

1. **What is the mechanism of ovarian torsion? What is the difference between ovarian and adnexal torsion?**

   Ans. Ovarian torsion is defined as rotation of the ovary on its ligamentous support: the infundibulopelvic and the utero-ovarian ligaments. When fallopian tube twists along with the ovary, this is referred as adnexal torsion.

2. **What are the risk factors for ovarian torsion?**

   Ans. The presence of an ovarian mass (functional cysts, dermoid cysts, hyperstimulated ovary, PCOS, etc. usually bigger than 5 cm in diameter) increases the risk of torsion. Benign ovarian lesions (such as functional and dermoid cysts) are more likely to torque than malignant neoplasms, possibly because malignant adnexal masses are fixed to the nearby pelvic structures. Similarly, ovarian endometrioma and tubo-ovarian abscess are at lower risk for torsion because they are fixed in place due to adhesions. Ovarian torsion may occur with normal size ovaries, particularly in pediatric population. Because of the risk for normal sonograms, the diagnosis of ovarian torsion is largely a clinical diagnosis. Possible explanation for this event is the elongated utero-ovarian ligament, which allows excessive ovarian movement. The majority of cases of ovarian/adnexal torsion occur in reproductive age. Pregnancy and ovulation induction are also associated with an increased risk of torsion.

3. **What is the mechanism of the ovarian injury described in Doppler ultrasound image (Fig. 23.2)?**

   Ans. Rotation of the infundibulopelvic ligament first impedes venous and lymphatic outflow. In the first stage of ovarian/adnexal torsion the arterial supply is not interrupted, because the arterial muscular layer is less compressible than the thin venous walls. Blocked outflow and continued arterial inflow lead to ovarian edema and enlargement. In later stages of ovarian/adnexal torsion, the ovarian artery shows absent and/or reversed diastolic flow. If untreated, the final results of compromised ovarian vascularization are ovarian necrosis and infarction.

■ TAKE-HOME MESSAGES

- The most common presenting symptom of ovarian/adnexal torsion is abdominal pain, nausea and vomiting.[1]
- The most common physical examination findings are tenderness, adnexal mass and low grade fever.[2,3]
- Laboratory tests (beta-hCG, urinalysis and CBC) are useful to rule out other causes of acute pelvic pain.[3,4]
- Pelvic ultrasound is the primary imaging modality in patients with suspected ovarian torsion.[5]
- Adolescents and children cannot undergo endovaginal US examination, so it is important that they are scanned with a full bladder.[5,6]
- The addition of color and pulsed Doppler imaging improves diagnostic accuracy of ovarian/adnexal torsion.[7]
- Absence of diastolic flow in the ovarian artery and/or complete absence of ovarian perfusion are suggestive of ovarian/adnexal torsion.[7]
- If ultrasound findings are inconclusive, MRI and CT are recommended as adjunctive diagnostic modalities.[5-7] Urgent surgical evaluation (preferably laparoscopy) to confirm the presence of torsion and evaluate the viability of the ovary is recommended.[8]
- Gross visual inspection is the standard approach to determine the ovarian viability. However, multiple studies confirmed that a "bluish-black" appearance of the ovary at surgery is not an indication of a nonviable ovary.[8-10]
- Detorsion consists of untwisting the torsed ovary and any other torsed lesion or structure by an atraumatic grasper (during laparoscopy), or manually (during laparotomy).[9]
- The key factor for ovarian conservation is to perform detorsion as quickly as possible.[10] A study in rats found that ovarian necrosis occurs 36 hours after occlusion of the ovarian arterial supply.[11]
- Ovarian conservation is the preferred approach for children, adolescents and reproductive age patients.[8,9]
- Ovarian cystectomy is usually performed, if a benign ovarian lesion is visualized.[9]
- Patients with evidence of ovarian necrosis or suspicious malignant ovarian lesion require salpingo-oophorectomy.[12] Salpingo-oophorectomy is also recommended for postmenopausal patients.[12]

■ REFERENCES

1. McWilliams GD, Hill MJ, Dietrich CS 3rd. Gynecologic emergencies. Surg Clin North Am. 2008;88(2):265-83.
2. Huchon C, Fauconnier A. Adnexal torsion: a literature review. Eur J Obstet Gynecol Reprod Biol. 2010;150(1):8-12.
3. Liu YP, Shih SL, Yang FS. Sudden onset of right lower quadrant pain after heavy exercise. Am Fam Physician. 2008;78:379.
4. Kirkham YA, Lacy JA, Kives S, Allen L. Characteristics and management of adnexal masses in a Canadian pediatric and adolescent population. J Obstet Gynaecol Can. 2011;33(9):935-43.
5. Albayram F, Hamper UM. Ovarian and adnexal torsion: spectrum of sonographic findings with pathologic correlation. J Ultrasound Med. 2001;20(10):1083-9.
6. Servaes S, Zurakowski D, Laufer MR, et al. Sonographic findings of ovarian torsion in children. Pediatr Radiol. 2007;37(5):446-51.
7. Kupesic S, Plavsic B. Adnexal torsion: color Doppler and three-dimensional ultrasound. Abdom Imaging. 2009;31(5):602-6.
8. Oelsner G, Cohen SB, Soriano D, et al. Minimal surgery for the twisted ischaemic adnexa can preserve ovarian function. Hum Reprod. 2003;18(12):2599-602.
9. Bristow RE, Nugent AC, Zahurak ML, et al. Impact of surgeon specialty on ovarian-conserving surgery in young females with an adnexal mass. J Adolesc Health. 2006;39(3):411-6.
10. Harkins G. Ovarian torsion treated with untwisting: second look 36 hours after untwisting. J Minim Invasive Gynecol. 2007; 14(3):270.
11. Taskin O, Birincioglu M, Aydin A, et al. The effects of twisted ischaemic adnexa managed by detorsion on ovarian viability and histology: an ischaemia-reperfusion rodent model. Hum Reprod. 1998;13(10):2823-7.
12. Growdon WB, Laufer MR. Ovarian and fallopian tube torsion. UpToDAte. http://www.uptodate.com/contents/ovarian-and-fallopian-tube-torsion. Accessed, 2015.

Pelvic Congestion Syndrome

CHAPTER 24

Sanja Kupesic Plavsic

■ CLINICAL CASE

AS is a 40-year-old G2P2 who was referred to the clinic with chronic pelvic pain for last four years. Her pain typically worsens after sitting and standing, at the end of the day and just before the onset of menstrual bleeding. She also complains of dysmenorrhea and dyspareunia.

Laboratory studies were performed: hemoglobin was 12.1 g/dL and hematocrit was at 35% (normal). No abnormalities were detected in WBC and platelet counts, and blood coagulation. Liver and renal function tests were also normal. Hepatitis antibody tests (HBsAg, HBcAB) and syphilis test were negative. Pap smear, wet mount, *Chlamydia* and gonorrhea tests performed three months ago were within normal limits. Pelvic ultrasound and color Doppler imaging was performed (results presented in Figs 24.1 to 24.4).

Menarche: Age 15.

Menses: 28/6–7 days, regular.

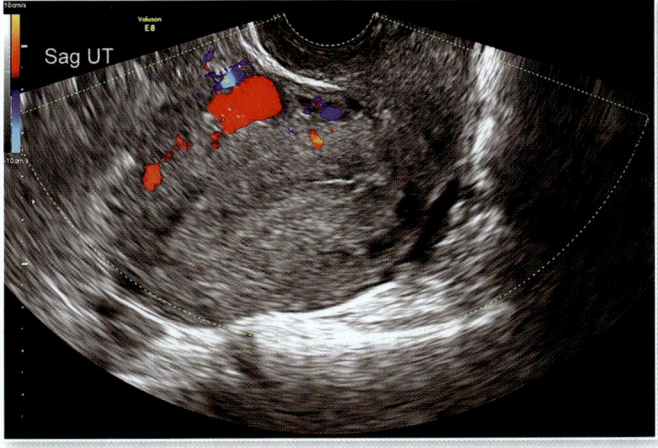

Figure 24.1: Color Doppler ultrasound demonstrates dilated arcuate veins (intraparenchymal venous congestion)

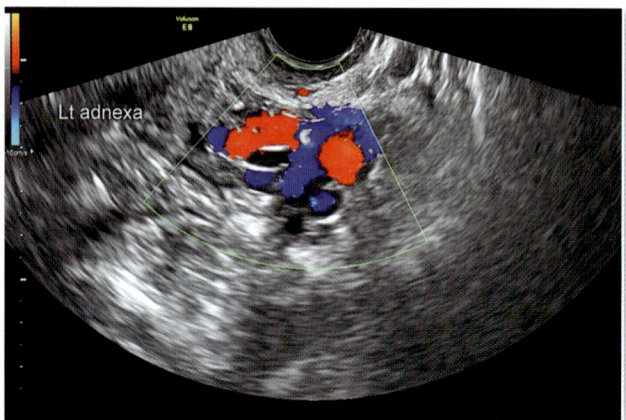

Figure 24.2: The same patient. Note markedly dilated venous plexus in the left adnexal region (extraparenchymal venous congestion)

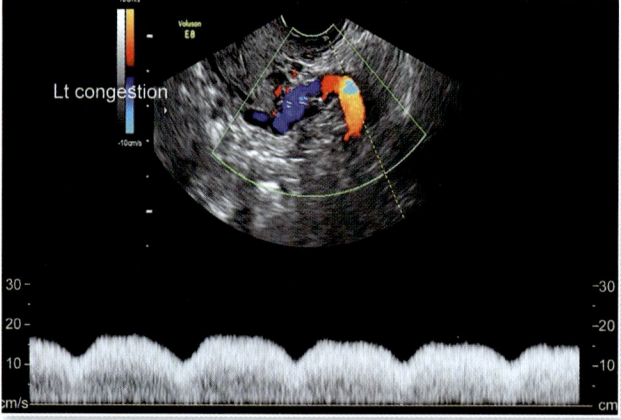

Figure 24.3: Venous blood flow signals are obtained from markedly dilated veins

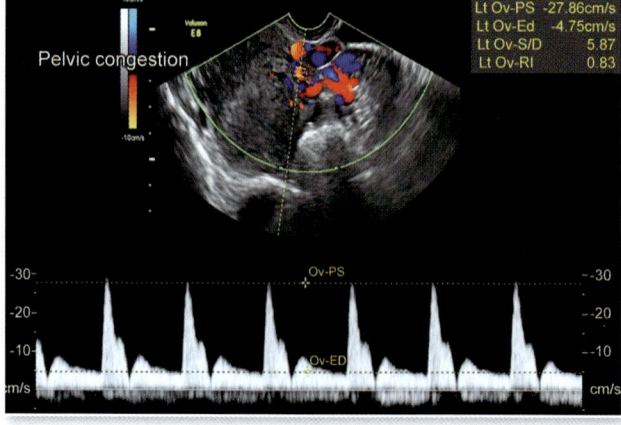

Figure 24.4: Arterial blood flow signals are obtained from the dilated uterine vessels

LMP: Three weeks ago.

OB history: Two uncomplicated pregnancies eight and five years ago. Two normal spontaneous vaginal term deliveries.

Sexual history: In monogamous relationship with her husband of 10 years.

Contraception: Bilateral tubal ligation four years ago.

Review of Systems

- No chest pain or shortness of breath
- No headache, no fever
- The patient complains of chronic pelvic pain, dysmenorrhea, and dyspareunia
- No diarrhea or constipation
- No hematuria or dysuria
- *Past medical history*: Noncontributory
- *Past surgical history*: Tonsillectomy and appendectomy
- *Vaccines*: Up to date (hepatitis B vaccine series, MMR booster and flu shot)
- *Current medications*: Pain medications over the counter
- *Allergies*: No known drug allergies
- *Social history*: She is a designer; does not smoke, social ETOH, no drug abuse
- *Family history*: Mother: 68 years, with no health issues. Father: 70 years, history of type 2 diabetes mellitus.

Physical Examination

- *Vital signs*: T 36.7°C oral; BP 130/80; P 72; BMI 26
- *Cardiac examination*: No heart murmur was detected
- *Chest examination*: Clear lungs, breathing sound was clear
- *Abdominal examination*: Soft, with tenderness in suprapubic area
- *Pelvic examination*: External genitalia with no abnormalities. Cervical motion tenderness is noted. The uterus and adnexa are normal size. There is tenderness in the left adnexa and suprapubic area.
- *Extremities*: Varicose veins of lower extremities noted.

■ CLINICAL QUESTIONS

1. What is the frequency and differential diagnosis of chronic pelvic pain?

Ans. Chronic pelvic pain accounts for 10–15% of outpatient visits in the US.[1] Differential diagnosis of chronic pelvic pain includes:
- Endometriosis
- Fibroids
- Pelvic inflammatory disease
- Fibromyalgia
- GI causes

- Urologic causes
- Pelvic adhesions, and
- Pelvic congestion syndrome.

2. **Clinical presentation of our patient (chronic pelvic pain, worsened by sitting, standing, at the end of the day, dyspareunia and dysmenorrhea), pelvic examination findings (normal size uterus and ovaries, cervical, suprapubic and left adnexa point tenderness) and varicose veins of the lower extremities are suggestive of pelvic congestion syndrome. What is the first imaging modality for evaluation of this patient?**

Ans. Pelvic US with color Doppler imaging is the first imaging modality for evaluation of this patient.

3. **What are the criteria for sonographic diagnosis of pelvic varices?**

Ans. Criteria for sonographic diagnosis of pelvic varices include:
- Dilated tortuous arcuate veins in the myometrium that communicate with bilateral pelvic varicose veins (intraparenchymal type of pelvic congestion) (Fig. 24.1)
- Visualization of dilated ovarian veins greater than 4 mm in diameter (extraparenchymal type of pelvic congestion) (Fig. 24.2)
- Slow blood flow (less than 3 cm/s), and reversed caudal or retrograde venous blood flow particularly in the left ovarian vein[2,3] (Fig. 24.3).
- The venous plexuses are thick and in most cases observable by endovaginal ultrasound. The arteries are much thinner and have a tendency to show their dilatation in intraparenchymal locations, and are typically demonstrated by color flow and pulsed Doppler imaging[4] (Fig. 24.4).

■ TAKE-HOME MESSAGES

- Data from the literature indicate that pelvic varicosities with concomitant vascular stasis and congestion are consistently found in women with chronic pelvic pain syndrome.[2,4]
- Varicose veins are more frequently present with increasing parity.[5] Multiparous women seem to be predisposed to develop pelvic congestion syndrome (PCS). At each term gestation, vein capacity increases by approximately 60%. Over time, venous distension can lead to defective and incompetent valves.[6] Weight gain and exposure to estrogen are additional factors that contribute to the pathogenesis of PCS.
- Many methods have been employed to detect PCS, such as color Doppler ultrasound, angiography, contrast enhanced CT, MRI/MRI venogram (MRV), and laparoscopy.[5,6]
- Treatment options for PCS include medical management with analgesics or hormone analogs, and surgical therapy. Medical treatment includes progestins (such as medroxyprogesterone acetate—MPA), danazol, GnRH agonists, dihydroergotamine and NSAIDs. MPA is given orally 30 mg/day for 6 months, while goserelin acetate is given as an injection of 3.6 mg monthly over 6-month period.[6]
- Surgical management consists of transcatheter embolization of the affected veins, ligation of ovarian veins, and hysterectomy with or without salpingoophorectomy.[7-9]
- Interventional radiology is most promising for offering definitive diagnosis and symptomatic relief to patients suffering from PCS. Transcatheter embolization (TCE) is usually performed at diagnostic venography. During the TCE, sclerosant and coil are used to form an embolus within vein for angio-infarction. About 73–78% of patients were cured or relieved of pain after the procedure.[10]

REFERENCES

1. Robinson JC. Chronic pelvic pain. Curr Opin Obstet Gynecol. 1993;5(6):740-3.
2. Beard RW, Highman JH, Pearce S, et al. Diagnosis of pelvic varicosities in women with chronic pelvic pain. Lancet. 1984; 2(8409):946-9.
3. Park SJ, Lim JW, Ko YT, et al. Diagnosis of pelvic congestion syndrome using transabdominal and transvaginal sonography. AJR Am J Roentgenol. 2004;182(3):683-8.
4. Kupesic S, Kurjak A. Color Doppler assessment of patients with pelvic pain. In: Kurjak A, Kupesic S (Eds.) An Atlas of Transvginal Color Doppler, 2nd edition. London: Parthenon Publishing. 2000, pp 241-4.
5. Hughes RR, Curtis DD. Uterine plebography: correlation of clinical diagnoses with dye retention. Am J Obstet Gynecol. 1962;83:156-64.
6. Ignacio EA, Dua R, Sarin S, et al. Pelvic Congestion Syndrome: diagnosis and treatment. Semin Intervet Radiol. 2008; 25(4):361-8.
7. Ganeshan A, Upponi S, Hon L, et al. Chronic pelvic pain due to pelvic congestion syndrome: the role of diagnostic and interventional radiology. Cardiovasc Intervent Radiol. 2007;30(6):1105-11.
8. Garguilo T, Mais V, Brokaj L, et al. Bilateral laparoscopic transperitoneal ligation of ovarian veins for treatment of pelvic congestion syndrome. J Am Assoc Gynecol Laparosc. 2003;10(4):501-4.
9. Malux G, Stockx L, Wilms G, et al. Ovarian vein embolization for the treatment of pelvic congestion syndrome: long term technical and clinical results. J Vasc Interv Radiol. 2000;11(7):859-64.
10. Edwards RD, Robertson IR, Mac Lean AB, Hemingway AP. Case report: pelvic pain syndrome—successful treatment of a case by ovarian vein embolization. Clin Radiol. 1993;47(6):429-31.

Incisional Endometriosis

CHAPTER 25

Sireesha Y Reddy, Sanja Kupesic Plavsic

■ CLINICAL CASE

MS is a 46-year-old woman G1P1 whose LMP was two months ago. She reports worsening pain in the LLQ since her cesarean section (CS) which took place over 10 years ago. She reports irregular menstrual cycles. She has tried medical management with oral contraceptive pills and an intrauterine device. She reports that the left lower quadrant pain is cyclical. She notices a painful swelling in the left lower edge of her incision. This area is sensitive and painful to the touch. She started menses at age 12 with 28-day intervals lasting 5–6 days. Recently, menstrual flow has increased to 10–14 days; intervals are now 20–45 days. Pap smear: all normal. Denies any history if sexually transmitted diseases.

Chief complaint: Left lower quadrant incisional pain.

OB history: Primary low transverse cesarean section for failure to progress in labor.

Past medical history: Hypertension.

Past surgical history: CS 10 years ago.

Allergies: Penicillin.

Current medications: Hydrochlorothiazide 25 mg daily.

Social history: She works as a nurse and lives with her daughter. She smokes tobacco (2–3 cigarettes per day). She denies any alcohol or drug abuse.

Family history: Mother with diabetes; father with heart disease; sister with hypothyroidism.

Review of Systems

- Head, eyes, ears, nose, and throat (HEENT): Denies
- Respiratory: Denies shortness of breath (SOB), wheezing, and cough
- Cardiovascular: Denies chest pain, dizziness
- Gastrointestinal: Denies nausea, vomiting
- Psych: Denies feeling sad, suicidal ideation, anxiety
- Neurological: Denies headache
- Musculoskeletal: Denies pain and edema.

Physical Examination

- Well appearing, well-dressed female
- *Vital signs*: T 36.2°C oral; P 74; RR 16; BP 100/60
- *Heent*: Normocephalic, atraumatic; EOMI; hearing grossly normal
- *Neck*: No thyromegaly
- *Respiratory*: Clear to auscultation bilaterally
- *Cardiovascular*: Regular rate rhythm; no murmurs, rubs, gallops
- *Abdomen*: Bowel sounds present and normal; no rebound, guarding; tender at the incisional site–prior Pfannenstiel incision; firm, nodular area 3 × 4 cm at the superior edge of incision; tender to palpation, mobile; just below the skin
- *Genitourinary*: Normal external genitalia: normal clitoris, urethra, vulva, vagina, and rectum
- *Speculum examination*: Normal vaginal mucosa, normal cervix; uterus mobile, 7-week size, anteverted, non-tender
- *Pelvic ultrasound*: Transvaginal ultrasound revealed 7 week size uterus. The endometrium was diffusely thickened (15.1 mm). There was a cystic lesion with echogenic content in CS scar measuring 2.1 × 1.7 cm (Fig. 25.1). Three-dimensional ultrasound revealed echogenic cystic lesion extruded beneath the fascia (Fig. 25.2). Sonographic findings are suggestive of endometriotic cyst in a CS scar (Fig. 25.2). There were no adnexal masses and/or free fluid in the cul-de-sac
- *Endometrial biopsy*: Proliferative endometrium
- *Laboratory tests*: Hct 32, TSH 2.5, prolactin 12.1
- *Preventative screening tests*: Normal Pap smear
- Patient decided that she wanted definitive therapy because bleeding was affecting her daily activities. She underwent an uncomplicated hysterectomy. During examination under anesthesia and skin incision, a firm 3 × 4 cm nodule was palpable at the superior left edge of her Pfannenstiel scar, confirming the physical examination in the office and on ultrasound imaging (Figs 25.3 A to C).

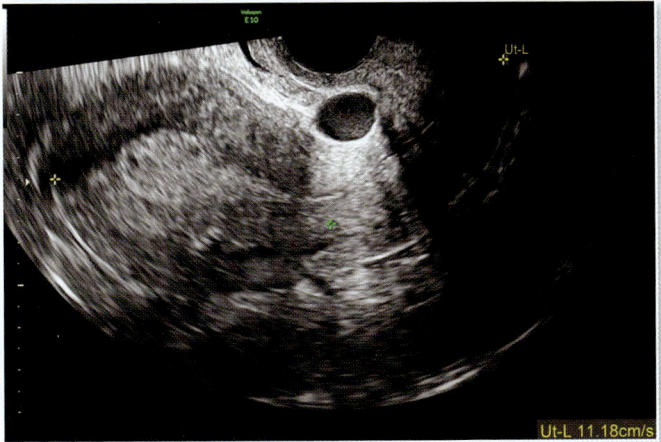

Figure 25.1: Transvaginal ultrasound of the 7-week size uterus with diffusely thickened endometrium. Cystic lesion in the isthmic region 2.1 x 1.7 cm is suggestive of an incisional or scar endometriosis

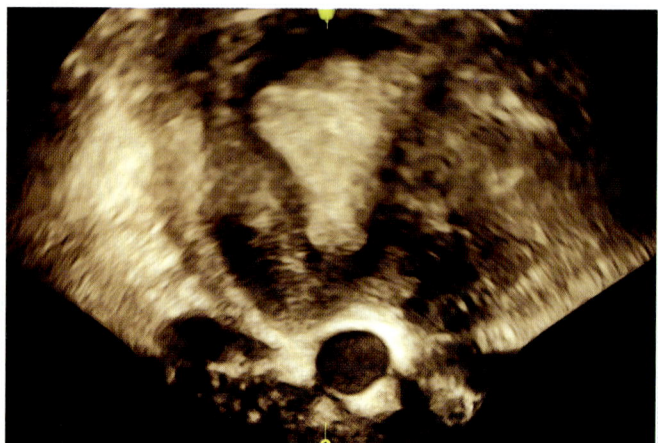

Figure 25.2: Three-dimensional ultrasound of the same patient

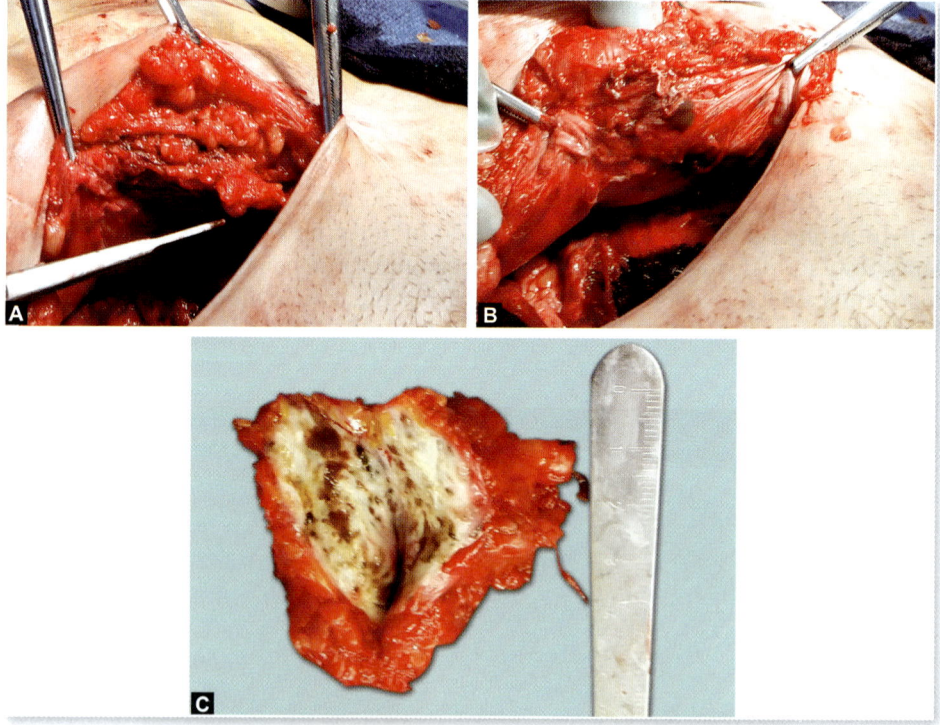

Figures 25.3A to C: (A) The 3 × 4 cm nodular, indurated area in the subcutaneous fat can be visualized. There is a dark hue that suggests that there may be the presence of an endometrioma; (B) As the area is manipulated and resected, there is an area of endometriotic fluid that extruded just beneath the fascia and above the rectus; (C) Bivalving the fibrotic area shows areas of endometriotic cysts

CLINICAL QUESTIONS

1. What is the classical symptom of this patient with incisional or scar endometriosis?

Ans. The classic symptom for a majority of patients with incisional endometriosis is catamenial or cyclical pain. However, it is not universal. Other symptoms can be complaints of a mass or simply pain.[1]

2. What diagnostic tests could have aided the diagnosis of scar endometriosis prior to the surgery?

Ans. Sonogram is the first step as a diagnostic imaging modality to aid in the diagnosis of incisional endometriosis. CT and MRI can be useful in patients with large scar endometriosis especially if fascial implants are suspected for surgical planning.[2] However, these tests cannot provide a definitive diagnosis.

3. What is the treatment of choice?

Ans. Patients may be initially treated with OCPs, progestins, medroxy-progesterone acetate and a hormonal IUD. Although these may help with symptoms of endometriosis of pain and irregular bleeding, if an incisional endometrioma is suspected, wide local excision of the lesion with negative margins is the optimal treatment. The definitive management is surgical excision in the operating room.[3] Recurrence rate is about 4%.

TAKE-HOME MESSAGES

- Majority of the patients with incisional endometriosis present with a history of prior CS.
- The incidence of incisional endometriosis is from 0.3 to 1%.[4]
- The classic symptom is cyclical painful mass at the site of a prior surgical scar.
- Typically there is delayed onset of symptoms, generally 4 years after the initial surgery.[5]
- Diagnostic tests are not definitive but can aid in surgical planning for large fascial defects.
- The pathogenesis for incisional endometriosis is direct inoculation of the endometrial cells during surgical intervention on the fascia and abdomen.[6]
- Treatment of incisional endometriosis is wide local excision.
- Malignant transformation of incisional endometriosis is rare. It is estimated that 21.3% of cases of malignant changes of endometriosis occur at extragonadal sites, and 4% of cases in scars after laparotomy.[7]

REFERENCES

1. Chatterjee SK. Scar endometriosis: a clinicopathologic study of 17 cases. Obstet Gynecol. 1980;56:81-4.
2. Nirula R, Greaney GC. Incisional endometriosis: an underappreciated diagnosis in general surgery. J Am Coll Surg. 2000; 190:404-7.
3. Seydel AS, Sickel JZ, Warner ED, et al. Extrapelvic endometriosis: diagnosis and treatment. Am J Surg. 1996;171:239.
4. Singh KK, Lessells AM, Adam DJ, et al. Presentation of endometriosis to general surgeons: a 10-year experience. Br J Surg. 1995;82:188-90.
5. Horton JD, DeZee KJ, Ahnfeldt EP, et al. Abdominal wall endometriosis: a surgeon's perspective and review of 445 cases. Am J Surg. 2008;196 (2):207-12.
6. Hensen JH, Ven Breda Vriesman AC, Puylaert JB. Abdominal wall endometriosis: clinical presentation and imaging features with emphasis on sonography. Am J Roentgenol. 2006;186:616-20.
7. Sergent F, Baron M, Le Cornec JB, Scotté M, Mace P, Marpeau L. Malignant transformation of abdominal wall endometriosis: a new case report. J Gynecol Obstet Biol Reprod. 2006;35(2):186-90.

CHAPTER 26

Secondary Dysmenorrhea

Sushila Arya, Luis S Noble, Sanja Kupesic Plavsic

■ CLINICAL CASE

EB is a 29-year-old G3P1 who presented to the clinic with complaints of lower abdominal and pelvic pain. Pain started 8 years ago, and is moderate to severe. It is aggravated during menstrual periods and intercourse, and has affected her lifestyle significantly since last 2 years. Pain is partially relieved with Ibuprofen and Percocet. Menarche at age 10 years. Menstrual periods are regular and painful, occurring every 28–30 days, last for 5–7 days with average flow. She has been using OCPs for contraception, with minimal relief in her symptoms.

Obstetric history: C-section for breech presentation at term; history of ectopic pregnancy, treated by laparoscopic right partial salpingectomy and one spontaneous abortion at 9 weeks gestational age.

Patient denies history of STD and pelvic inflammatory disease. She has two lifetime sexual partners.

Past medical history: Significant for chronic pelvic pain.

Past surgical history: C-section, appendectomy, and laparoscopic right salpingectomy.

Allergies: None.

Current medications: Oral contraceptive pills, Ibuprofen, and percocet.

Social history: House maker, lives with child and husband; nonsmoker, occasional alcohol, and history of marijuana use.

Family history: Mother had history of endometriosis and dysmenorrhea.

Review of Systems

Positive for abdominal and pelvic pain, dyspareunia and painful periods. Rest review of systems is negative.

Physical Examination

- *General*: Well nourished, well appearing female
- *Vital signs*: T 36.8°C oral; P 84; RR 18; BP 120/78
- *HEENT*: Atraumatic, normocephalic; EOMI: Grossly normal

- *Neck*: Supple, no lymphadenopathy, no neck masses
- *Respiratory*: Clear to auscultation
- *Cardiovascular*: Regular in rate and rhythm, no added sounds
- *Abdomen*: Soft, non-distended, RLQ tenderness, no guarding or rigidity
- *Genitourinary and pelvic examination*: Normal external genitalia; speculum examination: normal vaginal mucosa and cervix, uterus is anteverted, 8 weeks in size, nontender, mobile. Left adnexal tenderness. No nodularity in fornices
- Transvaginal ultrasound revealed anteverted uterus measuring 8 × 4 × 4.2 cm. Normal endometrium and myometrium. Left adnexa with 5.2 × 4 × 4.5 cm complex mass, suggestive of endometrioma (Figs 26.1 and 26.2). Minimal free fluid in cul-de- sac
- *Laboratory tests*: Hb/Hct 12/36; CA-125: 58
- *Preventive screening tests*: Normal Pap smear.

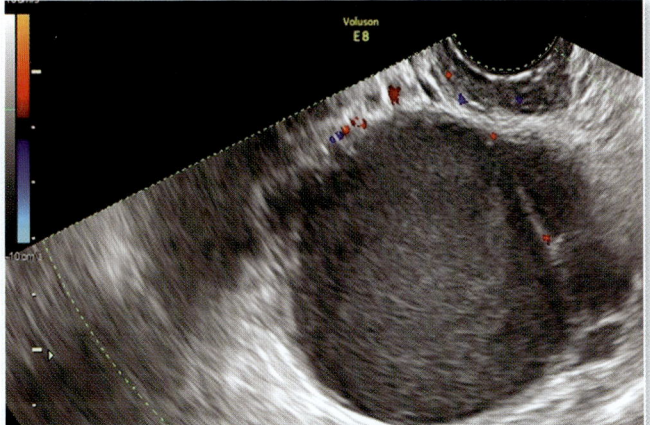

Figure 26.1: Transvaginal color Doppler image of the left adnexa with classic "chocolate cyst" diffuse low-level internal echoes. Color Doppler displays discrete peripheral and septal blood flow signals

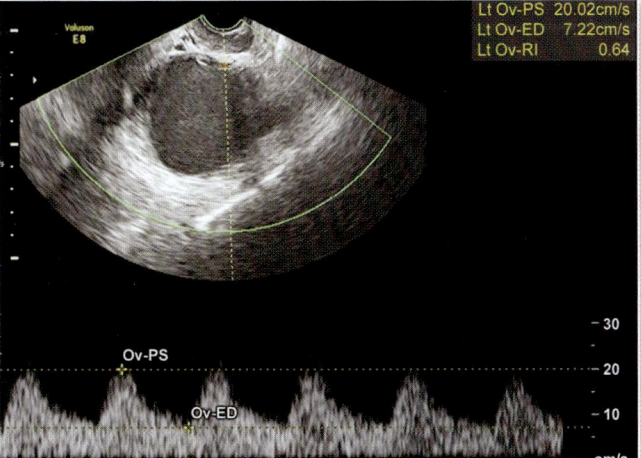

Figure 26.2: Pulsed Doppler signals show moderate to high blood flow impedance (RI of 0.64), indicating benign nature of the lesion

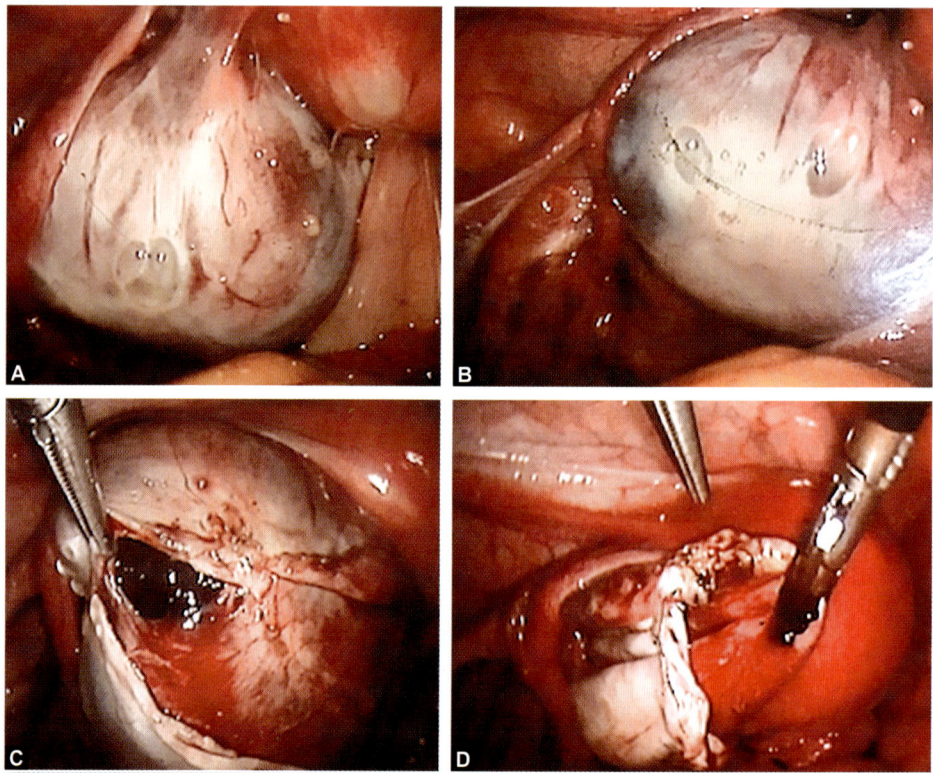

Figures 26.3A to D: 5 × 4 cm chocolate cyst from the left ovary was removed by laparoscopy

Our patient received combined OCPs, followed by norethindrone acetate and then 3 months of Leuprolide acetate with add-back estrogen therapy. Further use of GnRH was not considered due to concern of deleterious effect on bone mineral density (BMD). Despite medical therapy she continued to have significant pain. Patient was offered laparoscopy. Removal of endometrioma and endometriosis implants was performed. Figures 26.3A to D illustrates intraoperative findings. Symptoms were improved after surgery.

■ CLINICAL QUESTIONS

1. **What is dysmenorrhea?**
Ans. Primary dysmenorrhea is a crampy lower abdominal pain which begins with onset of periods. Secondary dysmenorrhea starts after many years of painless periods. Pain is secondary to a pathological condition like cervical stenosis, endometriosis, adenomyoisis, fibroid, pelvic inflammatory disease, and pelvic congestion syndrome.[1]

2. **What are the optimal tests to diagnose dysmenorrhea?**
Ans. The diagnosis of primary dysmenorrhea is usually based on history. Ultrasound, STD testing, hysteroscopy and laparoscopy are helpful to identify different causes of secondary

dysmenorrhea. Most commonly performed test is ultrasound; rarely MRI is required. If the cause is unidentified, diagnostic laparoscopy may be helpful to diagnose endometriosis, adhesions and pelvic congestion syndrome.

3. **What are ultrasonographic features of an endometrioma?**

Ans. Ultrasound is preferred initial imaging to diagnose endometriosis. The characteristic appearance of an endometrioma on ultrasound is hypoechoic mass containing diffuse low-level internal echoes (Fig. 26.1). Diffuse low-level internal echoes are sonographic characteristics in 95% of endometriomas. The appearance may vary due to degradation of blood in the cyst.[2]

4. **What is the treatment of endometriosis related dysmenorrhea?**

Ans. Treatment for secondary dysmenorrhea should be tailored to the pathological condition causing dysmenorrhea. For endometriosis OCPs and progesterone therapy are considered the 1st line treatment. Norethindrone acetate is the most commonly used adjunctive therapy in treating endometriosis.[3] GnRH is used when 1st line treatment fails. Long-term GnRH use has deleterious effect on BMD. There can be 5–10% loss of BMD in adults with 3–6 months of GnRH treatment.[4] Combination of oral norethindrone acetate plus conjugated equine estrogen is safe and effective for increasing BMD and content in young women with endometriosis during 1st year of GnRH agonist treatment and is superior to norethindrone acetate add back only.[5]

■ TAKE-HOME MESSAGES

- Dysmenorrhea is a debilitating disease affecting 45–95% women.[1]
- Greater sensitivity to pain was observed in nonmenstrual days of the cycle in women with dysmenorrhea.[1] Enhanced pain sensitivity may increase pain susceptibility to other painful conditions in later life. This further emphasizes the importance of treating dysmenorrhea.
- Dysmenorrhea affects quality of life, sleep and mood during menstruation, and is commonly disregarded by physicians and patients.[6]
- Increased levels of prostaglandin F2α in secretory endometrium are closely related with the symptoms of dysmenorrhea.[7]
- NSAIDs are usually effective in relieving the symptoms. If one NSAID is not effective, switching to a different class of NSAIDs may be helpful.[7]
- OCPs relieve symptoms of primary dysmenorrhea in 90% of patients.[3]
- Ultrasound is preferred initial test to diagnose pelvic pathology.
- Sensitivity of CA-125 is low for detection of endometriosis, because it can be can be elevated in other conditions. CA-125 is more sensitive to diagnose moderate or severe endometriosis compared with minimal disease.[8]
- In women with secondary dysmenorrhea due to endometriosis suppression of ovulation with combined contraceptives, GnRH and LNG-IUD are beneficial.[7]
- Laparoscopic treatment of endometriosis should be reserved to those who had failed medical therapy.[9,10]
- Persistent pain and concern of malignant transformation in endometriomas lead to surgery.[9]
- Performing a radical surgery is a difficult decision to make; however, it can provide optimal results in terms of improvement of quality of life and, therefore, should be considered when conservative therapy fails.[11]

REFERENCES

1. Lentz G. Primary and secondary dysmenorrhea, Premenstrual syndrome, and premenstrual dysphoric disorder. (Chapter 36). In: Lentz GM, Lobo RA, Gershenson DM, Katz VL, eds. Comprehensive Gynecology; 6th ed. Philadelphia, PA: Elsevier Mosby 2012.
2. Moore J, Copley S, Morris J, Lindsell D, Golding S, Kennedy S. A systematic review of the accuracy of ultrasound in the diagnosis of endometriosis. Ultrasound Obstet Gynecol. 2002;20:630-4.
3. Surrey ES. Gonadotropin-releasing hormone agonist and add- back therapy: what do the data show? Curr Opin Obstet Gynecol. 2010;22:283-8.
4. Matsuo H. Prediction of the change in bone mineral density induced by gonadotropin-releasing hormone agonist treatment for endometriosis. Fertil Steril. 2004;81:149-53.
5. DiVasta AD, Feldman HA, Sadler Gallagher J, Stokes NA, Laufer MR, Hornstein MD, Gordon CM. Hormonal Add-Back Therapy for Females Treated With Gonadotropin-Releasing Hormone Agonist for Endometriosis: A Randomized Controlled Trial. Obstet Gynecol. 2015;126(3):617-27.
6. Lacovides S, Avidon I, Baker FC. What we know about primary dysmenorrhea today: a critical review. Hum Reprod Update. 2015;21(6):762-78.
7. Dawood MY. Nonsteroidal anti-inflammatory drugs and reproduction. Am J Obstet Gynecol. 1993;169:5.
8. Hirsch M, Duffy J, Davis CJ, Nieves Plana M, Khan KS. Diagnostic accuracy of cancer antigen 125 for endometriosis: a systematic review and meta-analysis; International Collaboration to Harmonise Outcomes and Measures for Endometriosis. BJOG. 2016; doi: 10.1111/1471-0528.14055.
9. Heaps JM, Nieberg RK, Berek JS. Malignant neoplasms arising in endometriosis. Obstet Gynecol. 1990;75:1023-8.
10. Patel MD, Feldstein VA, Chen DC, Lipson SD, Filly RA. Endometriomas: diagnostic performance of US. Radiology. 1999;210:739-45.
11. De la Hera-Lazaro CM, Muñoz-González JL, Perez RO, Vellido-Cotelo R, Díez-Álvarez A, Muñoz-Hernando L, Alvarez-Conejo C, Jiménez-López JS. Radical surgery for endometriosis: Analysis of quality of life and surgical procedure. Clin Med Insights Womens Health 2016; 9:7-12.

CHAPTER 27

Uterine Fibroid

Sanja Kupesic Plavsic, Osvaldo Padilla

■ CLINICAL CASE

EL is a 42-year-old G3P3, presenting with heavy menstrual flow, abdominal discomfort, and pelvic and back pain that is not relieved with NSAIDs. Her last menstrual period started two weeks ago and she is still bleeding in clots. Her cycles are regular, every 28–30 days. During her periods she has 7–8 days of flow, usually in clots. She also complains of dysmenorrhea of one year duration.

Laboratory studies are typical for iron-deficiency anemia. No abnormalities are detected in WBC and platelet counts, and blood coagulation. Liver and renal function tests are normal. Pap smear, wet mount, *Chlamydia*, and gonorrhea tests performed six months ago were within normal limits.

Menarche: Age 14.

Menses: 28–30/7–8 days, regular.

LMP: 2 weeks ago.

OB history: Three uncomplicated pregnancies 8, 6, and 5 years ago; three normal spontaneous vaginal term deliveries.

Sexual history: In monogamous relationship with her husband of 10 years.

Contraception: Bilateral tubal ligation (BTL) five years ago.

Review of Systems

- No chest pain or shortness of breath
- Patient complains of premenstrual headache, abdominal/pelvic fullness and dysmenorrhea
- Patient also complains of urinary frequency; no hematuria or dysuria
- No diarrhea or constipation
- *Past medical history*: Noncontributory
- *Past surgical history*: Appendectomy
- *Vaccines*: Up to date (hepatitis B vaccine series, MMR booster and flu shot)
- *Current medications*: Ibuprofen over the counter.

Section 1: Gynecology

- *Allergies*: No known drug allergies
- *Social history*: EL is a housewife; does not smoke, social ETOH, no drug abuse
- *Family history*: Mother: 62 years, with no health issues. Father: 65 years, history of hypertension.

Physical Examination

- *Vital signs*: T 36.5°C oral; BP 135/80; P 76; BMI 28
- *Cardiac examination*: No heart murmur was detected
- *Chest examination*: Clear lungs, breathing sound was clear
- *Abdominal examination*: Midline lower abdominal mass
- *Pelvic examination*: External genitalia with no abnormalities. The cervix is anteriorly located. An irregular, midline mass of approximately 15 weeks' gestational size is palpable and moves in conjunction with the cervix. No adnexal masses are appreciated.

■ CLINICAL QUESTIONS

1. What is the most likely diagnosis of this patient?

Ans. Complaints of progressively heavier and longer menstrual periods with clots, iron deficiency anemia and an enlarged uterus on pelvic examination are typical for uterine fibroids. Uterine fibroids are the most common solid pelvic tumor in women.[1,2]

2. What is the best next step?

Ans. Pelvic ultrasound is the most appropriate imaging modality for further evaluation of this patient. Transabdominal and transvaginal ultrasound was performed and Figures 27.1 to 27.3 present the uterine findings.

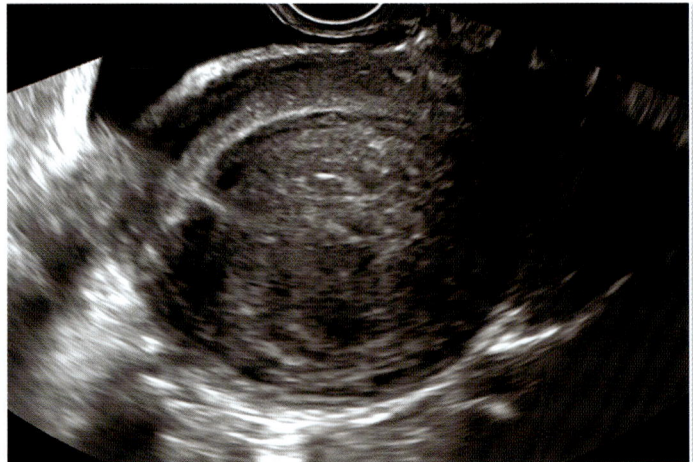

Figure 27.1: Transvaginal ultrasound demonstrates enlarged uterus with well-delineated intramural fibroid measuring 7 × 6 cm

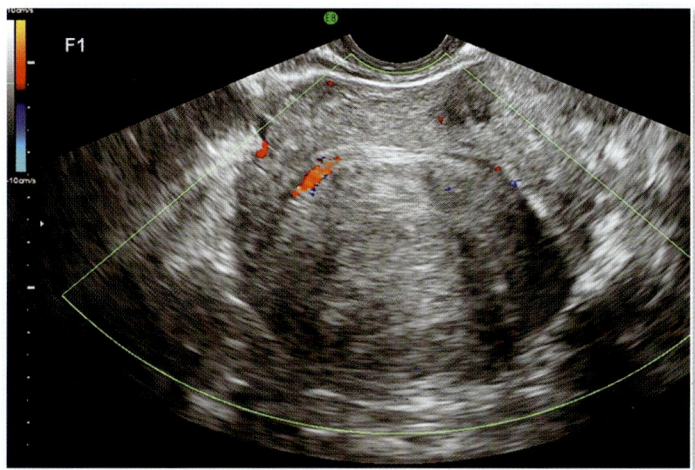

Figure 27.2: Color Doppler ultrasound depicts peripheral vessels

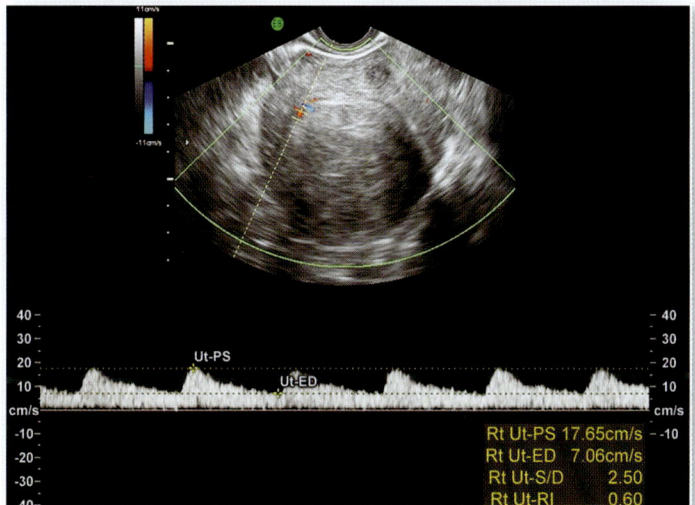

Figure 27.3: Pulsed Doppler waveform analysis demonstrates moderate to high vascular impedance in the fibroid's vessels (RI 0.60)

3. Which therapeutic options are most appropriate for this patient?

Ans. The patient has BTL and is not interested in future pregnancy. Conservative management of abnormal uterine bleeding during the course of last year was unsuccessful. The patient should be informed about non-surgical (e.g. uterine artery embolization, UAE), and surgical treatment options. After appropriate counseling the patient decided to do hysterectomy. Pathology and histology results are presented in Figures 27.4 and 27.5.

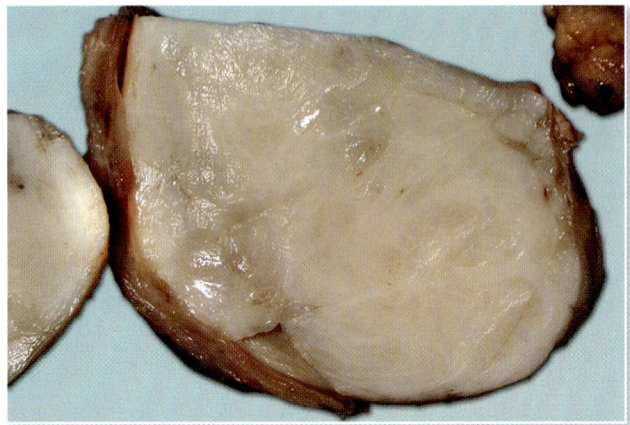

Figure 27.4: Pathology revealed solid, white homogenous uterine mass with a "swirl"-like cut surface, typical for uterine fibroid

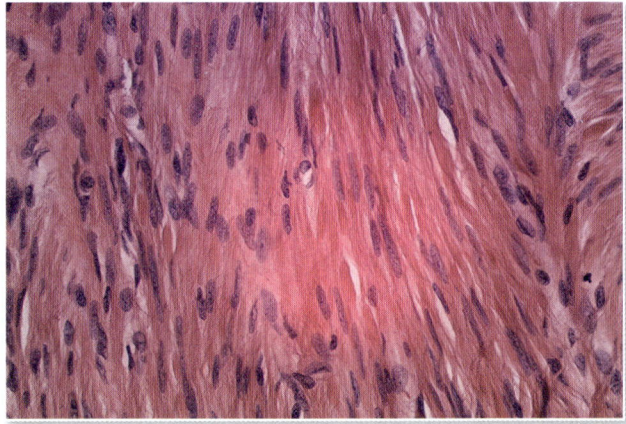

Figure 27.5: Elongated cells (or spindle cells) with "cigar"-shaped nuclei are identified, which are consistent with smooth muscle cells. These cells also demonstrated a typical smooth muscle profile by immunohistochemical stains

■ TAKE-HOME MESSAGES

- Uterine fibroids (leiomyomas) are the most common benign tumors of female pelvis, arising from the smooth muscle cells.[1,2] Typically, they arise in reproductive age and present with symptoms of heavy and prolonged menstrual bleeding, iron deficiency anemia, dysmenorrhea, pelvic pressure, lower back pain and frequent urination. Uterine fibroids decrease in size after menopause.
- Uterine fibroids are diagnosed by pelvic examination and by ultrasound. Intervention depends on the type and severity of symptoms, location and size of fibroid(s).[3] Uterine fibroids can undergo degenerative changes with necrosis resulting in cystic degeneration (Figs 27.6 to 27.8).
- Asymptomatic fibroids require no treatment. Possible exceptions from expectative treatment of asymptomatic fibroids are significant submucosal or intracavitary fibroids in patients who wish to conceive, and women with significantly enlarged uterus with ureteral compression and hydronephrosis.[4,5]
- Conservative management includes iron and vitamins, NSAID (ibuprofen and naproxen), hormonal birth control (e.g. progestin releasing intrauterine device) and medroxyprogesterone acetate (Depo Provera) leading to reduced bleeding and pain during menstrual period and watchful waiting.[6,7] Medications that block the production of estrogen and progesterone such as gonadotropin releasing hormone (GnRH) agonists

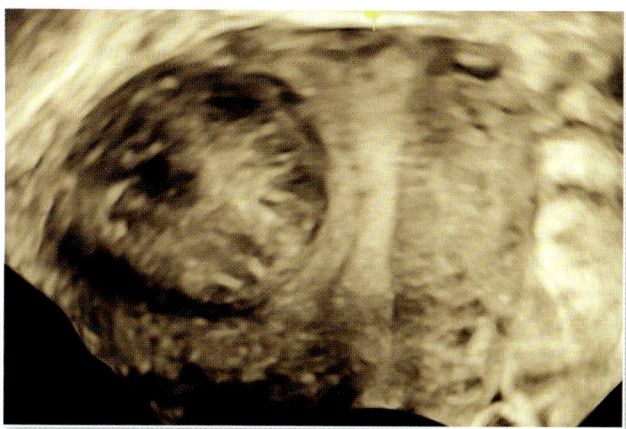

Figure 27.6: Three-dimensional scan (surface rendering) of an intramural fibroid with cystic degeneration in a patient presenting with acute pain

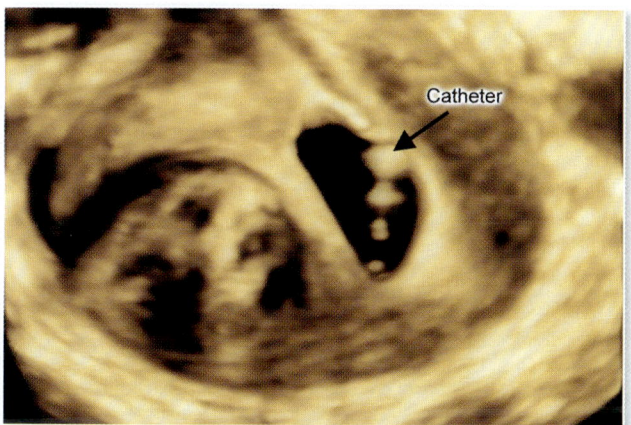

Figure 27.7: The same patient was assessed by SIS, which was performed to rule out intracavitary pathology

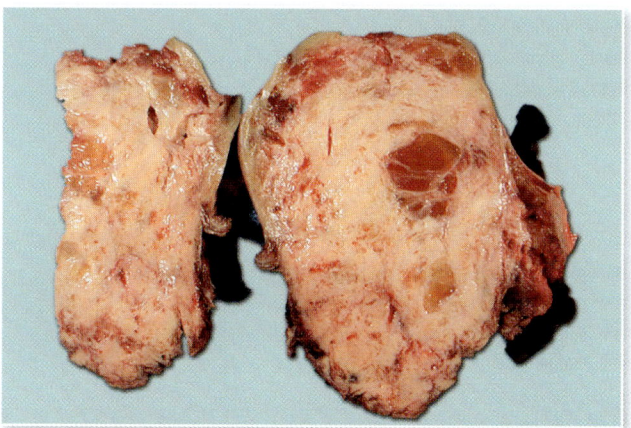

Figure 27.8: A leiomyoma with myxoid degeneration, which appears as cystic-like structures filled with mucinous material, which were visualized in the imaging study

(Lupron, Synarel, etc.) are beneficial for treating symptoms and shrinking the size of the fibroids before a planned surgery. After cessation of treatment, menses usually returns in 4–10 weeks, and fibroids begin to re-grow at their previous rate. GnRH agonists can also be used prior to hysterectomy in premenopausal or perimenopausal women to induce a menopausal state, which results in decreased uterine size facilitating surgical removal. Long-term use of GnRH agonists causes bone density loss which can lead to osteoporosis.[8]

- UAE is a treatment that blocks the blood supply to uterine fibroids, leading to fibroid shrinkage and decreased symptoms.[9]
- MRI-guided focused ultrasound is a new non-invasive procedure which combines high-frequency, high energy sound waves that non-invasively target and destroy fibroid's tissue, and MRI which enables monitoring of the procedure in real-time.[10]
- Myomectomy is surgical removal of the fibroid(s) which can be performed via laparotomy, laparoscopically or hysteroscopically.[1,2] Myomectomy is warranted in younger patients whose fertility is compromised by the presence of fibroids that cause significant distortion of the uterine cavity. Myomectomy may be indicated in infertility patients when the fibroids are of sufficient size or location to be a probable cause of infertility and when no more likely explanation exists for the failure to conceive.
- Hysterectomy is surgical removal of the entire uterus. Most hysterectomies are performed due to fibroids. Hysterectomy is mainly performed for symptomatic relief, but it can also be used for asymptomatic patients when the uterus is over 12 weeks' gestational size.

REFERENCES

1. Stewart EA. Uterine fibroids. Lancet. 2001;357(3252):293-8.
2. Parker WH. Uterine myomas: management. Fertil Steril. 2007;88(2):255-71.
3. Alternatives to Hysterectomy in the Management of Leiomyomas. ACOG Practice Bulletin No. 96. American College of Obstetricians and Gynecologists. Obstet Gynecol. 2008;112:201.
4. Lefebvre G, Vilos G, Allaire C, et al. The management of uterine leiomyomas. J Obstet Gynaecol Can. 2003;25(5):396-418.
5. Pritts EA, Parker WH, Olive DL. Fibroids and infertility: an updated systematic review of the evidence. Fertil Steril. 2009;91(4):1215-23.
6. Zapata LB, Whiteman MK, Tepper NK, et al. Intrauterine device use among women with uterine fibroids: a systematic review. Contraception. 2010;82(1):41-55.
7. Venkatachalam S, Bagratee JS, Moodley J. Medical management of uterine fibroids with medroxyprogesterone acetate (Depo Provera): a pilot study. J Obstet Gynaecol. 2004;24(7):798-800.
8. Lethaby A, Vollenhoven B, Sowter M. Efficacy of pre-operative gonadotrophin hormone releasing analogues for women with uterine fibroids undergoing hysterectomy or myomectomy: a systematic review. BJOG. 2002;109(10):1097-108.
9. Spies JB, Bruno J, Czeyda-Pommersheim F, et al. Long-term outcome of uterine artery embolization of leiomyomata. Obstet Gynecol. 2005;106(5 Pt1):933-9.
10. Kim HS, Baik JH, Pham LD, Jacobs MA. MR-guided high-intensity focused ultrasound treatment for symptomatic uterine leiomyomata: long-term outcomes. Acad Radiol. 2011;18(8):970-6.

CHAPTER 28

Pedunculated Uterine Fibroid and Endometriosis

Ulrich Honemeyer, Sanja Kupesic Plavsic

■ CLINICAL CASE

CR is a 34-year-old G1P1, presenting to your office with chronic pelvic pain, back pain, dysmenorrhea, and dyspareunia. Her last menstrual period was 10 days ago. Her cycles are regular, every 28 days and periods last between 5 and 6 days. Her Pap smear four months ago, at the time of her last well woman examination, was normal. Due to her complaints and because of her chronic back pain and vaginal discharge, wet mount, *Chlamydia* and gonorrhea tests were performed. The results were normal. Her laboratory findings performed one month ago were also within normal limits. The patient is unable to conceive during the course of last four years despite regular intercourse frequency with her husband, and requires further work up.

Menarche: Age 14.

Menses: 28/5–6 days.

LMP: 10 days ago.

OB history: One uncomplicated pregnancy with term delivery 8 years ago.

Sexual history: In monogamous relationship with her husband for 15 years. No history of sexually transmitted disease (STD).

Contraception: None.

Review of Systems

- No chest pain or shortness of breath
- Patient complains of premenstrual headache, chronic pelvic pain, back pain, dysmenorrhea, dyspareunia, and pain with bowel movement
- No urinary frequency, hematuria or dysuria
- *Past medical history*: History of chronic pelvic pain
- *Past surgical history*: Tonsillectomy and appendectomy
- *Vaccines*: Up to date (hepatitis B vaccine series, MMR booster and flu shot)
- *Current medications*: Ibuprofen over the counter
- *Allergies*: No known drug allergies.

- *Social history*: CR is a clerk; she does not smoke, social ETOH, no drug abuse
- *Family history*: Mother: 62 years, with no health issues. Father: 67 years, history of cirrhosis.

Physical Examination

- *Vital signs*: T 36.5°C oral; BP 125/75; P 74; BMI 26
- *Cardiac examination*: No heart murmur was detected
- *Chest examination*: Clear lungs, breathing sound was clear
- *Abdominal examination*: Within normal limits
- *Pelvic examination*: Unremarkable external genitalia. Palpation revealed enlarged, irregular uterus with decreased mobility. Tender nodules were appreciated in the cul-de-sac and on uterosacral ligaments.

■ CLINICAL QUESTIONS

1. What is the best next step in evaluation of this patient?

Ans. The most appropriate next step is to perform pelvic ultrasound (Fig. 28.1).

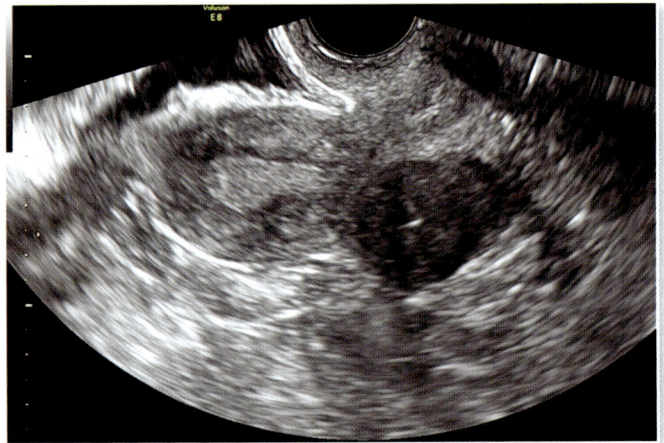

Figure 28.1: Transvaginal ultrasound revealed irregular contours of the uterus with subserosal fibroid 4 × 5 cm. There were no adnexal masses and/or free fluid in the cul-de-sac

2. What is the most likely diagnosis based on clinical and sonographic findings?

Ans. Pelvic ultrasound revealed irregular contours of the uterus and a subserosal fibroid. The adnexa were unremarkable by palpation. However, patient's symptoms (chronic pelvic pain, back pain, dysmenorrhea, dyspareunia, and pain on defecation) are suggestive of endometriosis.

3. What is the primary diagnostic modality for detection of endometriosis?

Ans. Laparoscopy is considered the primary diagnostic modality for detection of endometriosis (Figs 28.2 and 28.3).

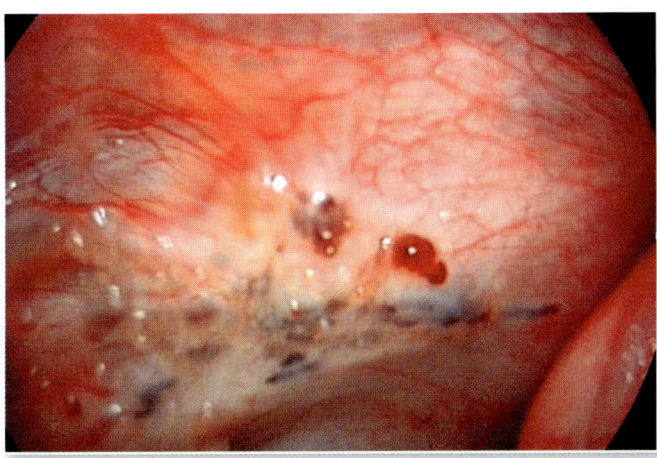

Figure 28.2: Laparoscopy revealed endometriotic lesions of the right abdominal wall, left lateral pelvic wall, left ovarian fossa, uterosacral ligaments and posterior cul-de-sac

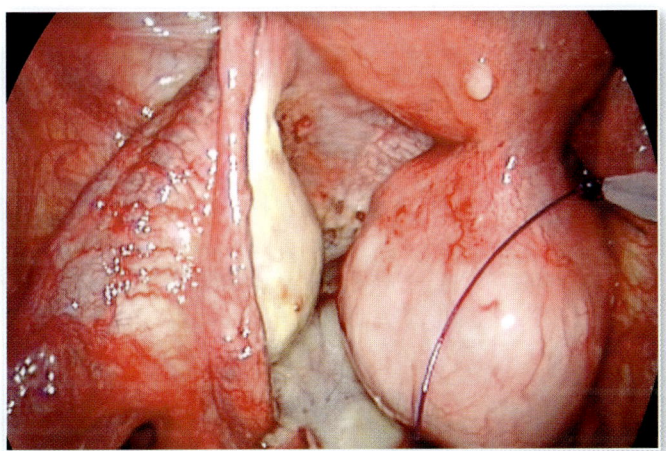

Figure 28.3: Subserous pedunculated fibroid was visualized

4. **What are the surgical options for this patient? Is removal of pedunculated fibroid required? What are the advantages of laparoscopic myomectomy?**

Ans. All visible implants of endometriosis should be excised or coagulated during laparoscopic surgery. The decision about laparoscopic myomectomy should be based on fibroid size and location, previous surgical history and the skills of the operating surgeon. Subserosal pedunculated fibroid does not cause infertility in this patient, but may be related to her back pain (Figs 28.4 and 28.5). The laparoscopic myomectomy should be reserved for experienced surgeons. In fibroids larger than 5 cm, the complication rate of laparoscopic myomectomy increases.[1] Even in larger fibroids, a skilled laparoscopic surgeon with access to modern laparoscopic instruments like electric morcellator will be able to capitalize on the advantages of laparoscopic myomectomy for the patient from reduced postoperative pain, shorter hospitalization, quick recovery to reduced blood loss.

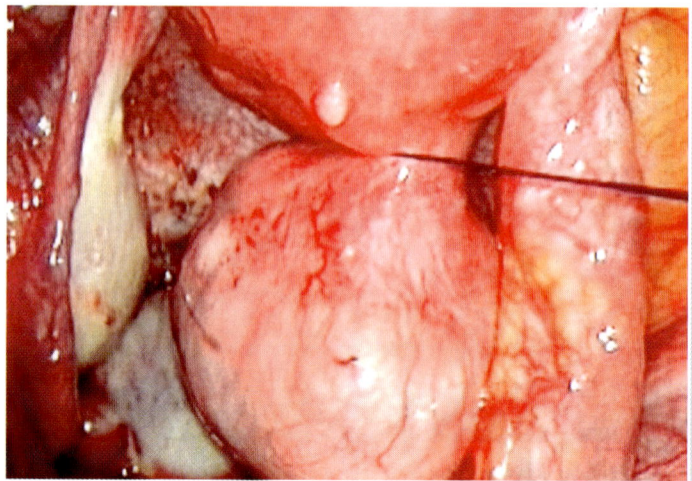

Figure 28.4: Ligation of the pedunculated fibroid was performed

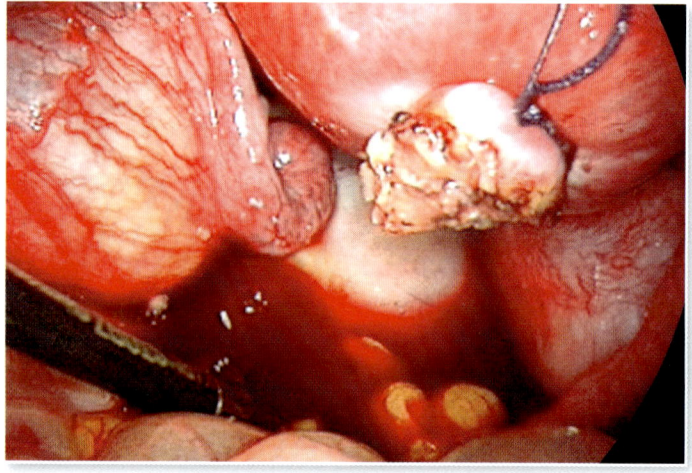

Figure 28.5: Pedunculated fibroid was dissected. The stem was cut approximately 5 mm above the ligation to prevent the knot from slipping off

5. Which instrument is used for removal of the pedunculated fibroid?

Ans. Electric morcellator is used to remove the pedunculated fibroid via small incision (Fig. 28.6). However, this innovation may lead to intraoperative injury of bowel and other nearby structures, and risk of dissemination of tissue during the morcellation process.[2] Fragments of tissue that are not retrieved may result in pain, infection and serious morbidity.[3] Of particular concern is the risk of morcellating an unidentified malignancy, with possible upstaging of the disease and worsened prognosis.

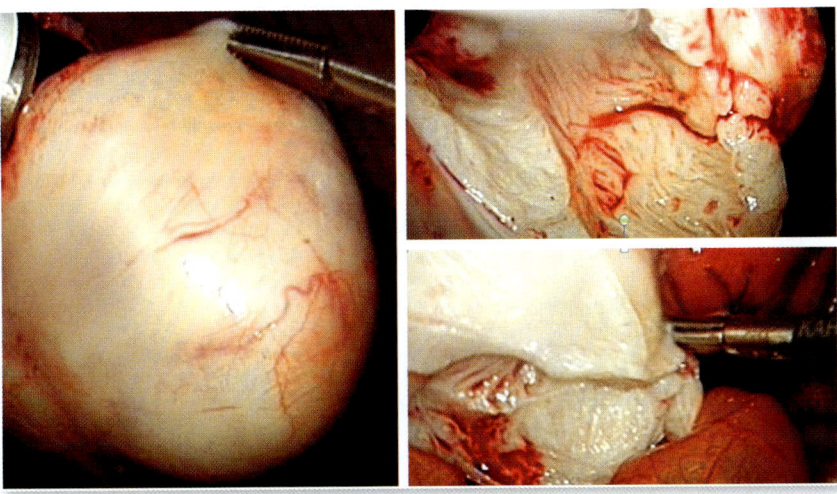

Figure 28.6: Morcellation of the pedunculated fibroid

■ TAKE-HOME MESSAGES

- Endometriosis is estrogen dependent benign condition characterized by formation and infiltration of ectopic endometrial tissue (glands and stroma), often accompanied with fibrosis and extensive scarring.[4]
- The most common symptoms of endometriosis are chronic pelvic pain, dysmenorrhea and dyspareunia.[5] There are three subtypes of endometriosis: superficial peritoneal lesions, deep infiltrating lesions and chocolate cysts (endometriomas).[4]
- It is estimated that 25–50% of women with infertility have endometriosis and about 30–50% of women with endometriosis have infertility.[6]
- Clinical examination and imaging (pelvic ultrasound and MRI) cannot provide a definitive diagnosis of endometriosis. Transvaginal ultrasonography was superior to MRI in terms of sensitivity (95% vs. 76%), specificity (98% vs. 68%) and accuracy ((97% vs. 71%).[7] However, ultrasound cannot reliably detect small endometriotic deposits (<1 cm) or depth of infiltration. Biomarkers such as CA-125 lack specificity and are not useful for routine diagnosis of endometriosis. Direct visualization by laparoscopy or histologic findings remain the gold standard for the diagnosis of endometriosis.[7,8]
- The combined oral contraceptives, oral or depot MPA (medroxyprogesterone acetate) and Mirena (levonorgestrel releasing intrauterine system) are as effective as the gonadotrophin releasing hormone (GnRH) analogs and can be used long-term for endometriosis treatment.[9]
- Surgical removal of endometriotic implants improves fertility.[10] Thus, all patients with endometriosis should have all visible implants excised during laparoscopic diagnosis.
- IVF/ET is the most appropriate next step for patients with compromised tubal function, male factor and other treatment failures.[11]
- Endometriosis is classified into one of four stages (I-minimal, II-mild, III-moderate, and IV-severe) depending on location, extent, and depth of endometriosis implants, also according to presence and severity of adhesions; and presence and size of ovarian endometriomas. Given a stage IV endometriosis, infertility is very likely.[12]
- Operation notes should include documentation of site, size, and type of endometriotic lesions to enable evaluation of treatment success during a second look.

REFERENCES

1. Olive DL, Lindheim SR, Pritts EA. Conservative surgical management of uterine myomas. Obstet Gynecol Clin North Am. 2006;33(1):115-24.
2. Lieng M, Istre O, Busund B, Qvigstad E. Severe complications caused by retained tissue in laparoscopic supracervical hysterectomy. J Minim Invasive Gynecol. 2006;13(3):231-3.
3. Leren V, Langebrekke A, Qvigstad E. Parasitic leiomyomas after laparoscopic surgery with morcellation. Acta Obstet Gynecol Scand. 2012;91(10):1233-6.
4. Hickey M, Ballard K, Farquahar. Endometriosis. BMJ. 2014;348:g1752.
5. Ballard KD, Seaman HE, de Vries CS, Wright JT. Can symptomatology help in the diagnosis of endometriosis? Findings from a national case-control study—Part 1. BJOG. 2008;115(11):1382-91.
6. Macer ML, Taylor HS. Endometriosis and infertility: a review of the pathogenesis and treatment of endometriosis-associated infertility. Obstet Gynecol Clin North Am. 2012;39(4):535-49.
7. Abrao MS, Gonçalves MO, Dias JA Jr, et al. Comparison between clinical examination, transvaginal sonography and magnetic resonance imaging for the diagnosis of deep endometriosis. Hum Reprod. 2007;22(12):3092-7.
8. Brosens I, Putemans P, Campo R, et al. Diagnosis of endometriosis: pelvic endoscopy and imaging techniques. Best Pract Res Clin Obstet Gynaecol. 2004;18(2):285-303.
9. Kennedy S, Bergqvist A, Chapron C, et al. ESHRE Special Interest Group for Endometriosis and Endometrium Guideline Development Group. ESHRE guideline for the diagnosis and treatment of endometriosis. Hum Reprod. 2005;20(10):2698-704.
10. Marcoux S, Maheux R, Berube S. Laparoscopic surgery in infertile women with minimal or mild endometriosis. Canadian Collaborative Group on Endometriosis. N Engl J Med. 1997;37(4):217-22.
11. Practice Committee of the American Society for Reproductive Medicine (ASRM). Endometriosis and Infertility. Fertil Steril. 2006;14:S156-S160.
12. Endometriosis: a guide for patients. American Society for Reproductive Medicine. https://www.asrm.org/Endometriosis_booklet/. Published; 2012.

CHAPTER 29

IUD Complications

Sanja Kupesic Plavsic

■ CLINICAL CASE

IF is a 32-year-old G2P2 presenting to the clinic with chronic abdominal and pelvic pain. She also complains of dyspareunia and vaginal spotting. Her pain started about three months ago and is getting worse. Her primary care physician performed laboratory investigations and blood tests to rule out PID and STD, and all the results came back normal. Her pregnancy test was negative. Her Pap smear was performed six months ago and was normal. She was never diagnosed with STD, and is in monogamous relationship with her husband.

Menarche: Age 14.

Menses: 25–28/7-8 days.

LMP: 2 weeks ago.

Obstetric history: Two spontaneous vaginal deliveries, six and four years ago.

Sexual history: Two male partners over her lifetime. *Chlamydia* test and Pap smear were normal.

Contraception: Four months ago a levonorgestrel (LNG) containing IUD was introduced for contraception.

Review of Systems

- No headaches, no problems with vision. No history of blood clots, DVT or PE
- No heart palpitations, no shortness of breath
- Chronic abdominal/pelvic pain for three months; Character/location: dull pain in mid-pelvis; Intensity: 4–5/10, No aggravating and alleviating factors reported
- No nausea, vomiting, constipation and/or diarrhea
- Normal urination; no symptoms of UTI
- *Past medical history*: None; no hospitalizations
- *Past surgical history*: None
- *Vaccines*: Up to date
- *Current medications*: Pain medication over the counter
- *Allergies*: None

- *Social history*: IF is a clerk. She drinks alcohol occasionally and in moderation. She does not smoke, and reports no history of substance abuse
- *Family history*: Mother: age 60, healthy. Father: age 68, diagnosed with prostate cancer. No family history of uterine, breast, ovarian or colon cancer.

Physical Examination

- *Vital signs*: T 36.8°C; BP 130/80; P 76; BMI 25
- General physical examination was normal
- *Pelvic examination*: On speculum examination, a small amount of bloody discharge was noticed. The cervix was nonerythematous, with no visible lesions. IUD strings were visualized and looked elongated. Bimanual pelvic examination revealed cervical motion and uterine tenderness. The adnexa were nonpalpable.

■ CLINICAL QUESTIONS

1. What is the most appropriate next step in evaluation of this patient?

Ans. Transvaginal ultrasound is the imaging method of choice for evaluation of this patient.[1,2] Pelvic ultrasound was performed and results are presented in Figures 29.1 to 29.3. An IUD should be visualized as centrally located bright echo within the uterine cavity. Because IUD of our patient is visualized in the lower uterine segment, the IUD is considered malpositioned. Three-dimensional ultrasound with simultaneous presentation of three orthogonal planes and the coronal view of the uterus provide superior appreciation of the IUD and its position (Fig. 29.3).[3,4] IUD located in the lower uterine segment, myometrium, cervical canal or outside the uterus is considered dislocated.

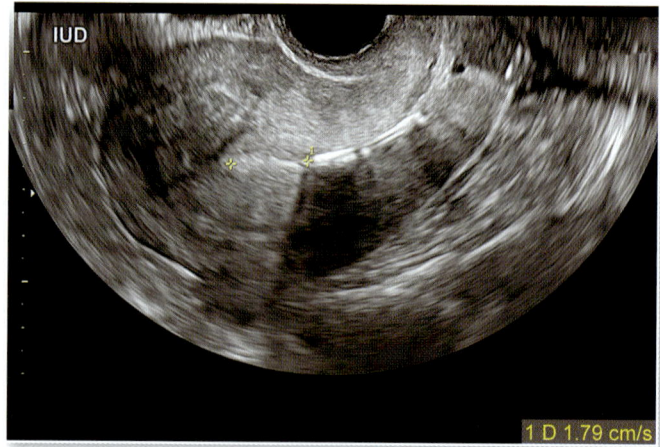

Figure 29.1: Transvaginal ultrasound demonstrates low position of IUD in a longitudinal plane, about 1.8 cm from the endometrial edge

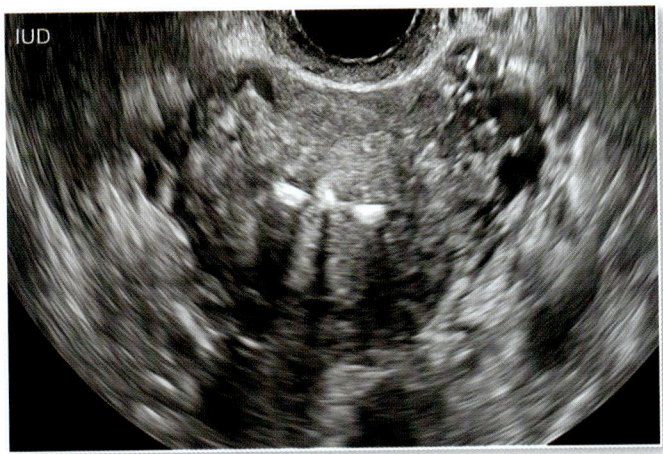

Figure 29.2: Open wings of IUD are visualized in a transverse plane

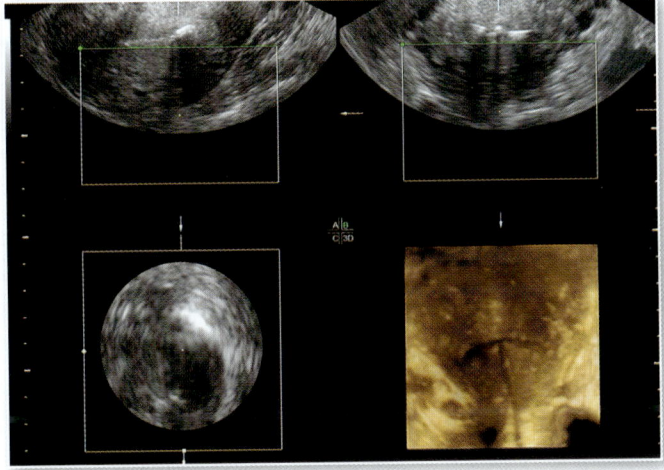

Figure 29.3: The same patient assessed by 3D ultrasound. Low position of LNG IUD is confirmed by visualization of the contraceptive device in the lower uterine segment

2. What is the frequency of malpositioned IUDs?

Ans. Studies have shown that approximately 1 in 10 IUDs is malpositioned.[5]

3. How this patient should be counseled?

Ans. Because our patient is symptomatic, and ultrasound exam showed dislocated IUD in the lower uterine segment, the IUD should be immediately removed. Because of low position of IUD the patient is at risk of becoming pregnant. To avoid a disruption in contraception, a new IUD may be placed at the same visit. New IUD may be inserted under the ultrasound guidance to ensure that a proper position is attained.[1]

4. What are the indications for the use of ultrasound in IUD placement?

Ans. The first indication for use of ultrasound in IUD placement is the suspicion of uterine anomaly on speculum or uterine sound examination. Ultrasound guidance may also be useful in patients with massive uterine fibroids and fundal fibroids interfering with IUD placement. After normal insertion, the majority of complications that require ultrasound analysis include symptomatic malposition, inability to find string on speculum examination, and spontaneous IUD expulsion reported by the patient.[1,6]

■ TAKE-HOME MESSAGES

- The IUD is the most commonly used reversible method of contraception, used by 23% of female contraceptive users worldwide.[6]
- The exact mechanism of action of the copper IUD is not completely understood. It is believed that copper IUD causes the endometrium to release leukocytes and prostaglandins. Changes in the uterine environment and cervical mucus prevent sperm migration to the fallopian tube. The LNG IUD works by thinning the endometrium as well as thickening the cervical mucus to make the entry of sperm through the cervix more difficult.[1,7]
- The copper IUD can remain inside of the uterus for approximately 10 years, and the LNG IUD can remain in the uterus for 5 years, assuming there are not associated complications, such as uterine perforation and dislocation. After this time, the device needs to be removed and/or replaced.[8]
- A number of health benefits were reported for women using the LNG IUD as a contraceptive, such as reduced menstrual bleeding, reduced dysmenorrhea, and the potential for prevention of a number of gynecological conditions in the longer-term, such as iron-deficiency anemia, endometrial hyperplasia, uterine fibroids, acute episodes of pelvic inflammatory disease, and endometriosis.[8] The LNG IUD has a potential to treat a range of preexisting gynecological conditions, such as heavy menstrual bleeding due to a wide range of underlying causes, such as endometrial hyperplasia, uterine fibroids and adenomyosis. These health benefits should be recognized in the decision-making process and counseling of the patients with specific issues.
- Although women with multiple sexual partners are at increased risk of acquiring STDs, having multiple sexual partners is not a contraindication to IUD placement. Women using IUD contraception should be advised that the concomitant use of condoms decreases the risk of acquiring STD.[2]
- Complications of intrauterine contraception can be categorized by their occurrence into the short- and long-term complications. Short-term complications include cramping, pelvic pain, PID, and uterine perforation. Long-term complications include pelvic pain, dysmenorrhea, dyspareunia, back pain, and malposition. Since perforation and dislocation may go unrecognized, many clinicians re-examine the patient 4–6 weeks after IUD insertion to ensure proper placement.[2,9] Some physicians also use ultrasound to confirm appropriate placement of an IUD at the time of insertion or one month later.
- IUD perforation occurs in about 1 in 1,000 IUD insertions and its risk is increased by practitioner's inexperience in IUD placement, retroverted uterus and uterus with anatomy defects. Patients often present with severe or chronic abdominal pain, vaginal bleeding and IUD strings that are greatly shortened or not visible.[10]

■ REFERENCES

1. Ansari AS, Tullius TG, Ross FR, Kupesic Plavsic S. The role of ultrasound in the assessment of intrauterine device complications. Donald School J Ultrasound Ob Gyn. 2012;6(3):313-20.
2. Kupesic Plavsic S. Step by Step Case Studies in Obstetrics and Gynecology. New Delhi, London, Philadelphia, Panama: Jaypee Brothers Medical Publisher. 2014, pp. 231-44.
3. Reiner JS, Brindle KA, Khati NJ. Multimodality imaging of intrauterine devices with an emphasis on the emerging role of 3-dimensional ultrasound. Ultrasound Q. 2012;28(4):251-60.

4. Benacerraf BR, Shipp TD, Bromley B. Three-dimensional ultrasound detection of abnormally located intrauterine contraceptive devices which are a source of pelvic pain and abnormal bleeding. Ultrasound Obstet Gynecol. 2009;34(1):110-5.
5. Braaten KP, Benson CB, Maurer R, Goldberg AB. Malpositioned intrauterine contraceptive devices: risk factors, outcomes, and future pregnancies. Obstet Gynecol. 2011;118(5):1014-20.
6. United Nations. World Contraceptive Use 2011. *http://www.un.org/esa/population/publications/contraceptive2011/contraceptive2011.htm*. Published 2011.
7. Lewis RA, Taylor D, Natavio MF, et al. Effects of the levonorgestrel-releasing intrauterine system on cervical mucus quality and sperm penetrability. Contraception. 2010;82(6):491-6.
8. Wu JP, Pickle S. Extended use of the intrauterine device: a literature review and recommendations for clinical practice. Contraception. 2014;89(6):495-503.
9. Thonneau P, Almont T, de La Rochebrochard E, Maria B. Risk factors for IUD failure: results of a large multicentre case control study. Hum Reprod. 2006;21(10):2612-6.
10. Gill RS, Mok D, Hudson M, et al. Laparoscopic removal of an intra-abdominal intrauterine device: case and systematic review. Contraception. 2012;85(1):15-8.

Abnormal Pap Smear and Cervical Dysplasia

CHAPTER 30

Sushila Arya, Osvaldo Padilla, Heather Pugmire, Sanja Kupesic Plavsic

■ CLINICAL CASE

JG is a 28-year-old G3P1, who was referred from her primary care physician for abnormal Pap smear assessment, colposcopy evaluation and treatment. Patient reported that her previous Pap smear was 8 years ago. No treatment was required at that time and she did not follow up until one month ago, when she had annual gynecological examination and Pap smear. She denies any postcoital bleeding and abnormal vaginal discharge. Last menstrual period was 1 week ago.

Menarche: Age 12.

Menstrual cycles: Regular (28–30/5 days), with normal flow pattern.

OB history: Two normal spontaneous vaginal deliveries and 1 spontaneous abortion (SAb) at 9 weeks.

Gynecologic history: Seven male partners over her lifetime. History of *Chlamydia* and *Trichomonas* at age of 19 years. Recent STD testing was performed one month ago, and was normal.

Contraception: Depo progesterone.

Past medical history: None, no recent hospitalizations.

Past surgical history: None.

Current medications: None.

Allergies: None.

Social history: JG is elementary school teacher. She drinks alcohol occasionally and in moderation. She reports ½ pack cigarettes daily for last 10 years; no history of substance abuse.

Family history: Significant for mother who had colon cancer at age of 61 years. No other family history of hereditary cancers or other chronic medical conditions.

Review of Systems

All other ROS is negative.

Physical Examination

- *Vital signs*: T 36.6°C oral; BP 110/76; HR 86; RR 18
- *General*: Alert, oriented to time, place and person

- Neck, heart and lungs examination is unremarkable
- *Abdomen*: Soft, no mass palpable
- *Pelvic examination*: Normal external genitalia, unremarkable cervix and vagina on speculum examination. On bimanual examination the uterus is normal size, anteverted, in mid-position and nontender; the adnexa are not palpable and non-tender
- *Urine pregnancy test*: Negative
- Evaluation of her Pap smear 8 years ago revealed ASCUS. Pap smear performed two months ago detected a high-grade dysplasia. After detailed counseling, given her noncompliance in the past and result of her most recent Pap smear and colposcopic impression consistent with high-grade dysplasia, the patient consented for "see and treat" (Figs 30.1 and 30.2). Loop electrosurgical excision procedure (LEEP) was performed without difficulty

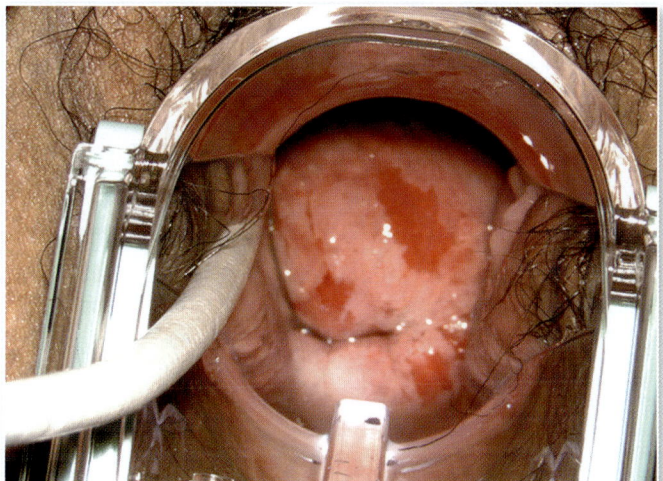

Figure 30.1: Thick, dense, opaque acetowhite and ulcerated areas extending into the endocervical canal. LEEP specimen from 12' and 3 o'clock demonstrated CIN II–III

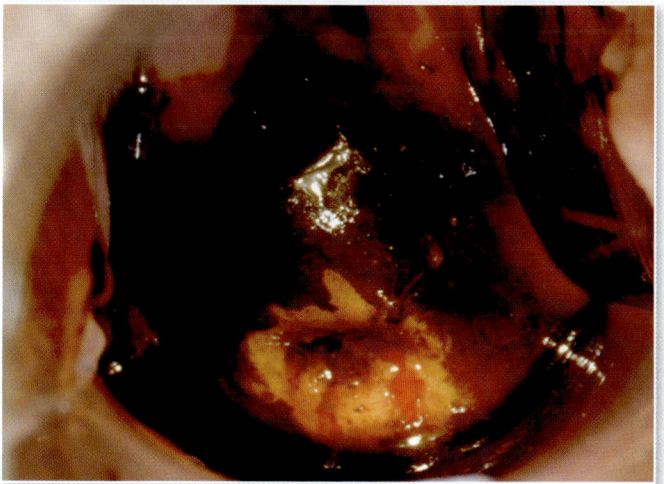

Figure 30.2: With the application of Lugol's solution normal mucosa is brown compared to pale dysplastic area

- *Final pathology of LEEP specimen were*: CIN II-III at 12 and 3 o'clock (Figs 30.3 and 30.4) and CIN I at 9 o'clock (Fig. 30.5). Margins and endocervical curettage were negative for malignancy.

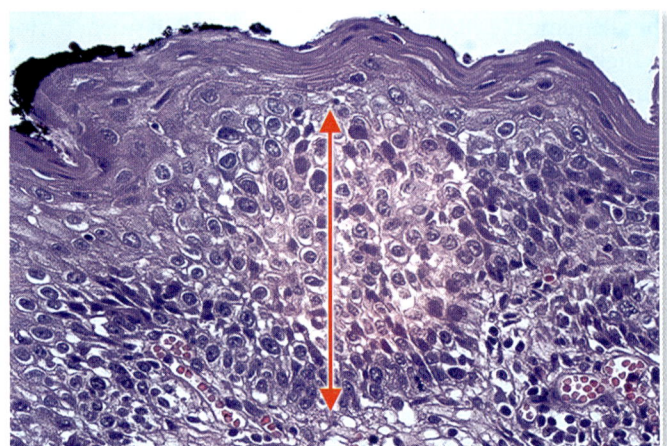

Figure 30.3: Cervical intraepithelial neoplasm II (CIN II) is present, as noted by an even thicker basal layer (red double arrow; >6 nuclei). The basal layer is more than half of the epithelial cell thickness (See an arrow). Typically, CIN II and III are grouped together as "high-grade dysplasia" to minimize intra- and interobserver variability in classifying dysplasia

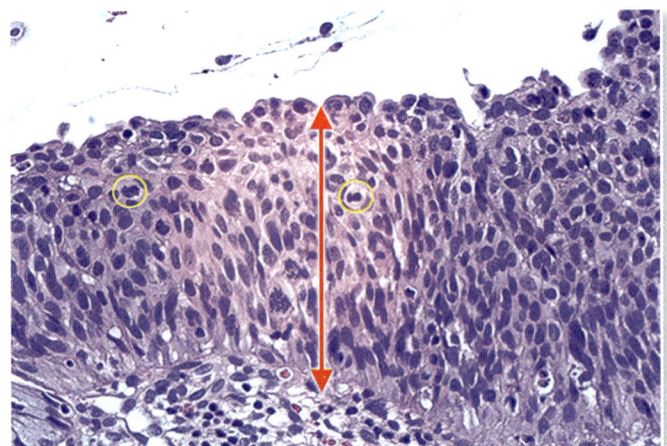

Figure 30.4: Cervical intraepithelial neoplasm III (CIN III) is present, as noted by full thickness of the basal layer (red arrow) and mitotic figures at more than half the epithelial cell thickness (yellow circles). By definition, there is no evidence of invasion, which is why CIN III is often referred to *carcinoma in situ*. Any evidence of invasion into the underlying stroma would result in a diagnosis of squamous cell carcinoma

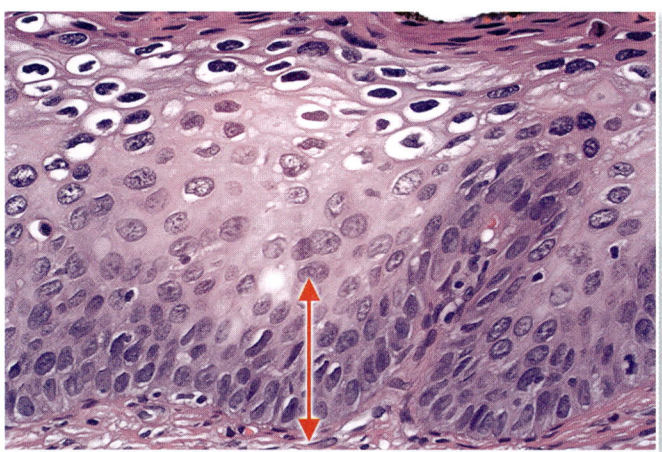

Figure 30.5: Low-grade cervical intraepithelial neoplasm (CIN I) is present, as noted by a thickened basal layer (red double arrow; 4–6 nuclei). This basal layer is less than half of the total epithelial cell thickness. In addition, there are cytologic changes (also known as koilocytic changes) consisting of enlarged nuclei, nuclear "halos", hyperchromatic nuclei, irregular nuclear contours, and multinucleation of the overlying cervical squamous cells

■ CLINICAL QUESTIONS

1. What is the progression rate of various cervical intraepithelial neoplasia (CIN)?

Ans. More advanced lesions are more likely to persist or progress to invasive cancer. If left untreated 15% of CIN III progresses to invasive cancer compared to 1% of CIN I.[1]

2. What is the accuracy of colposcopic examination?

Ans. Thin, smooth acetowhite lesions with well-demarcated, but irregular margins with or without fine punctuations and mosaic patterns make colposcopic impression of mild dysplasia. Thick, dense, opaque acetowhite areas with well-demarcated, regular margins, which sometimes may be raised and rolled out are indicative of CIN. Coarse punctuation, varying color intensity and/or mosaics within an acetowhite area are markers of a high-grade dysplasia.

Interobserver agreement, accuracy and reproducibility of colposcopic impression in diagnosing CIN II and III are fair to poor. The correlation between colposcopic impression and colpobiopsy was found to be satisfactory in 91% in CIN I, 82% in CIN II, III.[2-4] The accuracy depends on many factors; the most important is measurable physical characteristic of dysplastic epithelial lesion. Expertise of colposcopist also plays an important role.

3. What are various options to treat CIN?

Ans. Observation, cryosurgery, laser, loop electrosurgical excision procedure (LEEP), conization and hysterectomy are available options to treat CIN. The deciding factors to choose the most appropriate option are grade and extent persistence of CIN, involvement of endocervical canal, prior treatment, age, and desire for future childbearing.

4. Describe the most commonly used treatment options for CIN?

Ans. LEEP and cold knife cone biopsy (CKC) are two most common excisional procedures for cervical dysplasia. Cryotherapy and laser ablation are two most commonly used ablative therapies used in USA.

- *LEEP:* commonly done in office setting, no anesthesia is required; low cost and technically easy procedure
- *CKC:* traditional method to treat CIN. Data from the literature indicate that CKC increases the risk of preterm delivery compared to LEEP or large loop excision of the transformation zone (LLETZ).[5] There is no difference in margins positivity or residual disease with LEEP or CKC.[5,6]
- *Cryotherapy:* refrigerated CO_2 or nitrous oxide is used. The ectocervix is cooled to $-20°C$ using a cryoprobe that causes crystallization of intracellular water and destroys the lesion. More recurrence of CIN II–III is noticed with cryotherapy compared to CKC. There are more complications from CKC compared to cryotherapy, such as bleeding, infection, injury to surrounding organs, hospitalization and premature deliveries
- *Laser ablation:* Using colposcopic guidance laser is directed to the cervical lesions. Intracellular water absorbs laser and cell is destroyed. A 2 mm spot size is used to destroy a lesion and 5 mm is used for hemostasis. The depth of the cervical ablation should be at least 4.8 mm. CO_2 Laser ablation should be performed by a trained specialist.[1]

■ TAKE-HOME MESSAGES

- Human papilloma virus (HPV) causes most cervical cancers (99.7%). HPV 16 and 18 are responsible for 70% of all cervical cancers.[1] HPV can cause some cancers of the vagina, vulva, penis, anus, rectum, and oropharynx.
- High risk HPV viral proteins E6 and E7 cause reduced cell apoptosis and unregulated cell growth.[7]
- Majority (90%) of HPV infection are cleared by young women in 1–2 years.[8]
- Since the introduction of cervical cytology cervical cancer related mortality and morbidity were significantly reduced. In the USA the cervical cancer was reduced from 36.3 to 7.2 per 100,000 women from 1930 to 1990.[9]
- Cytology has 51% (30–87%) sensitivity and 98% (86–100%) specificity.[9,10]
- Due to poor sensitivity of cytology alone, cotesting for high risk (hr) HPV was approved by Food and Drug Administration (FDA) in 1999.[10]
- Cotesting (cytology + hr HPV) has higher sensitivity and reproducibility with 99% negative predictive value to rule out CIN II/III.[11] HPV cotesting also improves detection of adenocarcinoma, which accounts for 15–25% cervical cancers.[12]
- The colposcopy diagnosis of cervical dysplasia depends on the recognition of four main features: Intensity (color tone) of acetowhitening, margins and surface contours of acetowhite areas, vascular features and color changes after iodine application.[1] Using a scoring system such as Reid's colposcopic index may guide colposcopic interpretation and diagnosis.

■ REFERENCES

1. Creasman WT. Preinvasive Disease of the Cervix. In: Di Saia PJ, Creasman WT (Eds). Clinical Gynecologic Oncology: Eighth Edition ; Philadelphia, PA: Elsevier; 2012. p. 1-30.
2. Ferris DG, Litaker MS. Prediction of cervical histologic results using an abbreviated Reid Colposcopic Index during ALTS. Am J Obstet Gynecol. 2006;194(3):704-10.
3. Ferris DG, Litaker M. Interobserver agreement for colposcopy quality control using digitized colposcopic images during the ALTS trial. J Low Genit Tract Dis. 2005;9(1):29-35.

4. Ferris DG, Litaker MS. Cervical biopsy sampling variability in ALTS. J Low Genit Tract Dis. 2011;15(2):163-8.
5. Santesso N, Mustafa RA, Wiercioch W, Kehar R, Gandhi S, Chen Y, et al. Systematic reviews and meta-analyses of benefits and harms of cryotherapy, LEEP, and cold knife conization to treat cervical intraepithelial neoplasia. Int J Gynecol Obstet. 2016;132(3):266-71.
6. Li L, Chen C-X, Jiang Y-M. Meta-analysis of cold-knife conization versus loop electrosurgical excision procedure for cervical intraepithelial neoplasia. OncoTargets and Therapy. 2016;9:3907-15.
7. Beaudenon S, Huibregtse JM. HPV E6, E6AP and cervical cancer. BMC Biochem 2008;9 (Suppl 1):S4.
8. Plummer M, Schiffman M, Castle PE, Maucort-Boulch D, Wheeler CM. A 2-year prospective study of human papillomavirus persistence among women with a cytological diagnosis of atypical squamous cells of undetermined significance or low-grade squamous intraepithelial lesion. Journal Infectious Dis. 2007;195:1582-9.
9. Wingo PA, Cardinez CJ, Landis SH, Greenlee RT, Ries LAG, Anderson RN, et al. Long-Term Trends in Cancer Mortality in the United States, 1930-1998. Cancer. 2003;97(12):3133-275.
10. Lees BF, Erickson BK, Huh WK. Cervical cancer screening: Evidence behind the guidelines. Am J Obstet Gynecol 2016;214(4):438-43.
11. Huh WK, Ault KA, Chelmow D, Davey DD, Goulart RA, Garcia FAR, et al. Use of primary high-risk human papillomavirus testing for cervical cancer screening: Interim clinical guidance. Gynecol Oncol. 2015;136(2):178-82.
12. Silverberg SG, Loffe OB. Pathology of Cervical Cancer. Cancer J. 2003;9(5):335-47.

CHAPTER 31

Condylomata Acuminata

Sushila Arya, Sireesha Y Reddy, Sanja Kupesic Plavsic

■ CLINICAL CASE

PN is 4.5-year-old patient, accompanied by her mother, who was referred by her pediatrician for multifocal vulvar lesions. Her mother reports history of "bumpy lesions" on her daughter's vulva since age 4; gradual increase in size and spread of the lesions was noted. By inspection, various small vulvar lesions have coalesced together. Patient complaints of itching and oozing with small amount of blood while wiping after urination and bowel movement. She denies any vaginal bleeding or urinary symptoms.

Physical examination revealed no breast development and absence of pubic or axillary hair. Patient and mother were separately questioned about history of sexual abuse, and no history or evidence of sexual abuse was encountered.

Primary care health prevention: She is up-to-date with her vaccines.

Past medical history: None.

Past surgical history: None.

Current medications: Denies.

Allergies: None.

Family history: Mother has cold knife cone biopsy for cervical dysplasia prior to conception with PN.

Social history: Doing very well in pre-school. She loves biking, which is restricted due to discomfort in perineal area from these vulvar lesions. She lives with her parents.

Review of Systems

It is negative except states above in history of present illness.

Physical Examination

- Normal vital signs
- *General:* Well-developed, well nourished, in no apparent distress
- *Neck:* Supple, no lymphadenopathy, no thyroid enlargement

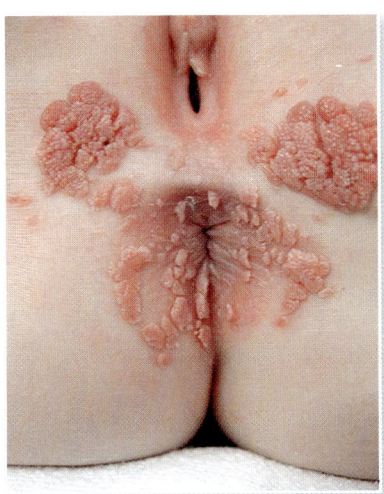

Figure 31.1: Multifocal lobulated vulvar lesions in a 7.5-year-old patient

- *Abdomen:* Soft, no mass or tenderness, no rigidity or guarding
- *Genitourinary:* Multiple soft raised lobulated vulvar masses (Fig. 31.1). No evidence of abnormal discharge or bleeding from the vulvar lesions.

Laboratory Tests

- *Urinalysis:* Negative for leukocyte esterase and nitrites
- It is likely that our patient contracted a disease from her mother during parturition. The patient was treated with Imiquimod 5% ointment, three times a day for 12 weeks, with monthly follow-up. Complete resolution was noted at the completion of treatment.

CLINICAL QUESTIONS

1. What is clinical presentation of condylomata acuminata?

Ans. Most of HPV virus infections are subclinical. Condylomata acuminata or venereal/genital warts are benign proliferative epidermal or mucosal lesions caused by HPV type 6 or 11, but coinfections with high-risk subtype exist. HPV is the most common STI. Common presenting symptoms are multiple multifocal painless bumps, pruritus, discharge or bleeding. Commonly affected areas are perineal, vaginal, cervix, oral, and laryngeal regions. Perianal warts are the most common.[1,2]

2. What is the typical appearance of condylomata acuminata?

Ans. Condylomata acuminata are soft, raised masses with smooth, verrucous ends.[1]

3. What are the treatment options for condylomata acuminata?

Ans. Most of the times these lesions are treated with topical therapy. None of the treatment leads to complete clearance rate, and none of the treatments can permanently remove HPV virus. Surgical excision is usually reserved for high-risk condylomata, in patients in whom topical therapy failed or is unfeasible due to location and/or size. Table 31.1 reviews therapeutic options for condylomata acuminata.[3-10]

Table 31.1 Therapeutic options for condylomata acuminata

Therapeutic option	Mode of action / Technique of application	Clearance rate	Recurrence rate	Common side effects	Advantages	Use during pregnancy
Imiquimod 5% topical cream (Aldara)[3-5]	• Cell immunity modification by inducing significant production of interferon alpha • Three times a week; application at bedtime until clearance of lesions for maximum 16 weeks	35–68%[2,4]	6–26%[2]	Pain, erythema, ulceration, and skin irritation	Home therapy	Contraindicated
Podophyllotoxin (0.15% cream or 0.5% solution)[5]	• Antimitotic • Twice daily for three days followed by 4 rest days	45–83%[5] within 3–6 weeks	6–100%[5]	Burning, tenderness, erythema, ulcerations	Home therapy	Contraindicated
Sinecatechins ointment[6,7]	• Green tea extracts catechins • Antiproliferative • Three times a day until complete resolution for maximum of 16 weeks	47–59%[6,7]	7–11%[6,7]	Redness, burning, itching and pain	Home therapy	Unknown
Trichloroacetic acid (TCA) 80–90%[4]	Cauterizes skin, keratin Applied weekly	56–81%[4]	36%[4]	Damage to surrounding skin, ulcerations	Less local symptoms and low cost	Safe during pregnancy
Cryotherapy[8,10]	• Liquid nitrogen • Mixture of dimethyl ether and propane gas at a temperature of −57°C • Weekly; applied with spray or cotton tipped applicator for 10-20 seconds	44–75%[8,10]	21–42%[8,10]	Rare scarring or depigmentation	Simple to use and low cost	Safe during pregnancy
Surgical[1,9,10]	Electrocautery, laser or curettage	60–90%[1,9,10]	19–29%[1,9,10]	Bleeding, infection, stenosis of the cervix	Precision, cost-benefit	Contraindicated in pregnancy

4. What are treatment options for condylomata acuminata in pediatric patients?

Ans. There is no FDA approved treatment for pediatric patients.[11] Center for Disease Control and Prevention (CDC) has recently released guidelines to treat condylomata acuminata in pediatric patients using various options (Podophyllotoxin, TCA, Imiquimod, cryotherapy, laser, and surgical excision), previously tested and approved for adult population.[13,14] Most pediatric warts resolve if untreated, most pediatric warts resolve within 2 years. However, intervention prevents the autoinoculation and decreases the duration of lesions.[15] Age of the child, symptoms, extent and location of the lesions are major factors determining the treatment. Cryotherapy with liquid nitrogen is commonly used, but can be traumatic for a child due to pain.

■ TAKE-HOME MESSAGES

- Low risk HPV subtypes 6, 11, 42, 43 and 44 are isolated from 90% of genital warts.[11]
- Average age to develop genital warts in pediatric patients is between 2.8 and 5.6 years.[11,12]
- Mechanisms proposed for perinatal and postnatal transmission are vertical transmission, autoinoculation, sexual transmission and direct contamination through infected objects/surfaces.[12]
- Rate of vertical transmission to the neonate from a mother who does not have clinically evident disease is 1–18% versus 5–72% from a mother with detectable HPV during pregnancy.[12] Although most of pediatric patients with condyloma acuminata contract a disease from the mother, it is important to rule out sexual abuse. With increasing child's age, sexual abuse is more prevalent as a mode of transmission compared to congenital.
- In about 90% of cases HPV virus infection is cleared by cell-mediated immunity. Approximately 10% will have persistent disease with evident sequelae.[13,14]
- Primary prevention of HPV using nonavalent HPV vaccine is a key component in decreasing the burden of disease. Gardasil 9 protects against HPV 6, 11, 16, 18, 31, 33, 45, 52, and 58, and is determined to be 97% effective in preventing cervical, vulvar and vaginal cancers.[15]

■ REFERENCES

1. Léonard B, Kridelka F, Delbecque K, Goffin F, Demoulin S, Doyen J, Delvenne P. A clinical and pathological overview of vulvar condyloma acuminata, intraepithelial neoplasia and squamous cell carcinoma. Biomed Res Int. 2014;2014:480-573. doi: 10.1155/2014/480573.
2. Komericki P, Akkilic-Materna M, Strimitzer T, Aberer W. Efficacy and safety of imiquimod versus podophyllotoxin in the treatment of anogenital warts. Sex Transm Dis. 2011;38(3):216-8.
3. Arican O, Guneri F, Bilgic K, Karaoglu A. Topical imiquimod 5% cream in external anogenital warts: a random-ized, double-blind, placebo-controlled study. Journal of Dermatol. 2004;31(8):627-31.
4. Sherrard J, Riddell L. Comparison of the effectiveness of commonly used clinic-based treatments for external genital warts. Int J STD AIDS. 2007;18(6):365-8.
5. Lacey CJN, Goodall RL, Ragnarson Tennvall G, et al. Randomised controlled trial and economic evaluation of podophyl-lotoxin solution, podophyllotoxin cream, and podophyllin in the treatment of genital warts. Sex Transm Infections. 2003;79(4):270-5.
6. Meltzer SM, Monk BJ, Tewari KS. Green tea catechins for treatment of external genital warts. Am J Obstet Gynecol. 2009;200(3):233.e1-233.e7.
7. Gross G, Meyer KG, Pres H, Cieler H, Taw K, Mescheder A. A randomized, double-blind, four-arm parallel- group, placebo-controlled Phase II/III study to investigate the clinical efficacy of two generic formulations of Polyphenon E in the treatment of external genital warts. JEADV. 2007;21(10):1404-12.
8. Gilson RJC, Ross RJ, Maw D, Rowen C, Sonnex D, Lacey CJN. A multicentre, randomised, double-blind, placebo con- trolled study of cryotherapy versus cryotherapy and podophyl-lotoxin cream as treatment for external anogenital warts. Sex Transm Infections. 2009;85(7):514-9.

9. Forcier M, Musacchio N. An overview of human papillomavirus infection for the dermatologist: disease, diagnosis, management, and prevention. Dermatol Ther. 2010;23(5):458-76.
10. Safi F, Bekdache O, Al-Salam S, Alashari M, Mazen T, El-Salhat H. Management of peri-anal giant condyloma acuminatum - a case report and literature review. Asian J Surg. 2013;36(1):43-52.
11. Thornsberry L, English JC, III. Evidence-based treatment and prevention of external genital warts in female pediatric and adolescent patients. J Pediatr Adolesc Gynecol. 2012;25(2):150-4.
12. Leclair E, Black A, Fleming N. Case report imiquimod 5% cream treatment for rapidly progressive genital condyloma in a 3-year-old girl. J Pediatr Adolesc Gynecol. 2012;25(6):e119-e121.
13. Moresi JM, Herbert CR, Cohen BA. Treatment of anogenital warts in children with topical 0.05% podofilox gel and 5% imiquimod cream. Pediatr Dermatol. 2001;18:448.
14. Stefanaki C, Barkas G, Valari M, et al. Condylomata acuminata in children. Pediatr Infect Dis J. 2012;31(4):422-4.
15. Ornstein A, Hatchette T. Human papillomavirus and anogenital warts in children. CMAJ. 2012;184(3):321.

CHAPTER 32

Primary Amenorrhea

Sushila Arya, Sireesha Y Reddy, Sanja Kupesic Plavsic

■ CLINICAL CASE

SM is a 12-year-old adolescent girl who was referred to the pediatric gynecologist for what the pediatrician noted as a "labial fusion." She reports several months of cyclical colicky abdominal and pelvic pain lasting for three days each month. At times when the pain occurs, she has urinary urgency. She denies any history of urinary tract infections. She reports breast development, as well axillary and pubic hair growth. She denies having any menstrual bleeding. Her sister started menses at age 11. She denies any family history of gynecological concerns.

Primary care health prevention: She received all three doses of the HPV vaccine, Gardasil at age 11 years, and is up-to-date with her other vaccines.

Past medical history: Attention deficit hyperactivity disorder (ADHD).

Surgical history: None.

Current medications: Denies.

Allergies: None.

Family history: Mother has depression, anxiety, and DM.

Social history: SM lives with both of her parents. She is in the seventh grade. She reports receiving good grades in her classes. She is active in sports.

Review of Systems

Negative, except abdominal/pelvic discomfort mentioned in history of present illness.

Physical Examination

- Normal vital signs
- *General*: Well-developed, well-nourished, in no apparent distress.
- *Neck*: supple, no lymphadenopathy, no thyroid enlargement
- *Breast*: Tanner stage III

- *Abdomen*: Soft, no mass or tenderness, no rigidity or guarding
- *Genitourinary*: Normal pubic hair distribution, no change in skin texture or color. No excoriation or marks or scratching. Hymen was noticed to be imperforated with slight bulge and normal color (Fig. 32.1). Rectal examination revealed a palpable tense bulging, fluctuant mass in the pelvis.
- *Urinalysis*: Normal
- *Laboratory tests*: WBC 8.9, Hb/Hct 13.4/39
- Ultrasound findings are presented in Figures 32.2 and 32.3.
- Our patient has imperforated hymen, demonstrated as slight bulge at the vaginal opening and was scheduled for standard surgical treatment (hymenectomy). The procedure was done under general anesthesia. The patient was placed into the lithotomy position; urethra was catheterized prior to making the hymenal incision. After cruciate incision was made,

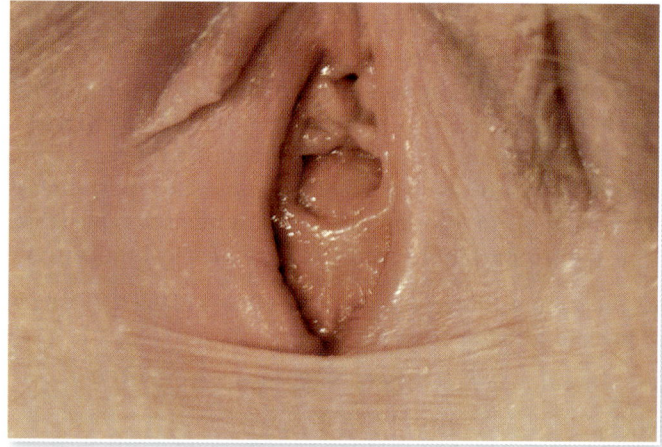

Figure 32.1: Image of imperforate hymen. Note that vaginal orifice is bulging and covered by hymen

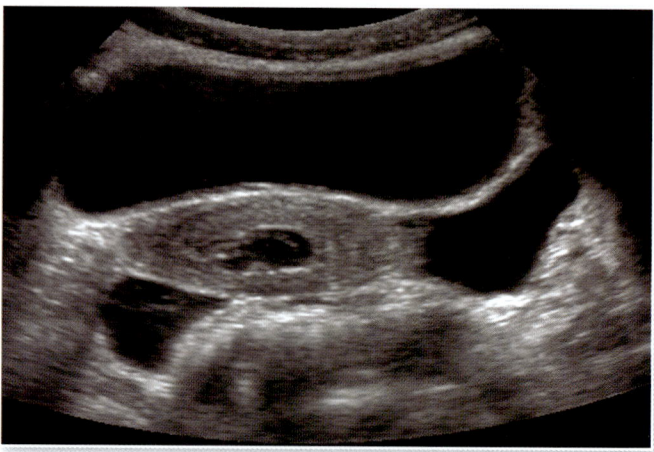

Figure 32.2: Transabdominal ultrasound of a patient with imperforate hymen. Note accumulation of intracavitary fluid (hematometra) and presence of free fluid in the cul-de-sac

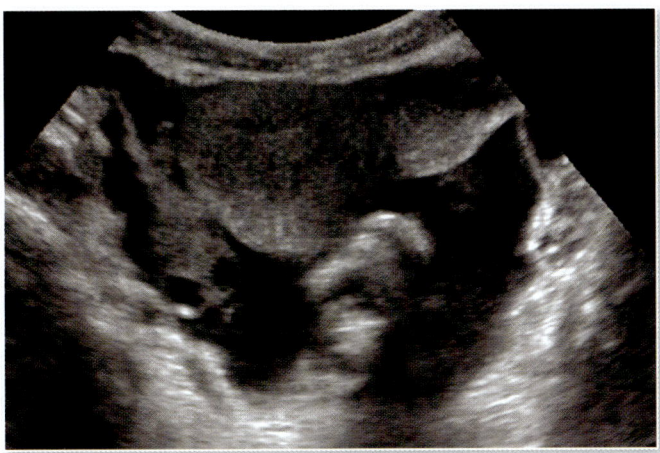

Figure 32.3: The same patient. Normal size right ovary is floating in the free fluid

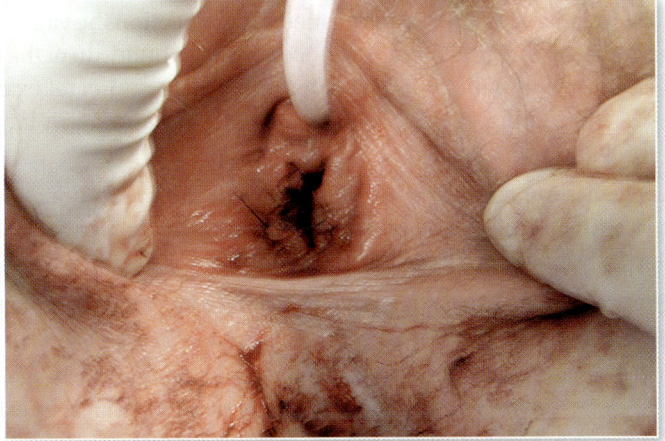

Figure 32.4: Postprocedure: hymen edges plicated with 2–0 vicryl

200 cc of old blood was drained using suction tip (Fig. 32.4). The edges were everted and plicated using 2-0 vicryl. She had followed up in the clinic at one and 5 weeks. Complete healing of the edges was noticed and the patient reported normal menstrual period after the procedure.

CLINICAL QUESTIONS

1. What is primary amenorrhea?

Ans. The definition of primary amenorrhea is:
- No period by age 14 in the absence of secondary sexual characteristics, or
- No period by age 16 regardless of growth and development.

We should not hold on to the appropriate evaluation until the ages stated above if history and physical examination is informative of a diagnosis (for example, obvious stigmata of Turner syndrome or imperforate hymen[1]).

2. What are the most common reasons of primary amenorrhea?

Ans. Gonadal dysgenesis, endocrinological and Müllerian abnormalities are the major causes of primary amenorrhea. Imperforate hymen is the most common obstructive urogenital anomaly.[1,2] Hymen is a mesodermal membrane that is formed through the fusion of caudal end of paramesonephric ducts and urogenital sinus. Usually the central portion of this membrane is resorbed and absence of that process leads to imperforate hymen. Though imperforate hymen is most common genital tract anomaly, its incidence is only 0.014–0.1%.[2] Mean age of presentation is 13.2 years (range from 11–16 years).[3-5] Rare presentation can be during newborn and early childhood due to collection of uterovaginal secretion.[6-8]

3. How is imperforate hymen diagnosed?

Ans. The diagnosis is based on clinical evaluation. Extensive laboratory and radiologic investigations are not required routinely.[4] If doubt exists transabdominal, transperineal or transrectal ultrasound should be performed. On inspection the vaginal orifice is closed. After menarche bluish bulging membrane occurs due to build-up of the menstrual blood, which is seen in 60% of patients with imperforate hymen.[4] Rectal examination reveals distended soft fluctuating vagina. In patients with hematometra large uterus can be palpated during abdominal and rectal examination.

Recurrent cyclical lower abdominal/pelvic pain is the most common presentation (60% of patients), as was in our case. Late presentation or missed diagnosis causes complications like endometriosis, infection (pyocolpos), hematocolpos, ruptured hematosalpinx, etc.[3,4]

4. What are other conditions associated with imperforate hymen or other obstructive cause of amenorrhea?

Ans. Imperforate hymen is usually not associated with other genital or extragenital anomalies.[2,3] Rarely, it is associated with genitourinary tract anomalies (renal agenesis) or rare genetic disorder ectrodactyly ectodermal dysplasia-clefting syndrome.[9,10]

5. What is the treatment of imperforate hymen?

Ans. Surgical hymenectomy can be performed by different incisions like T, X, cruciate or X incision with or without removal of excessive hymenal segments. The free edges are everted and plicated using 2-0 vicryl sutures to avoid refusion as shown in Figure 32.4. In a case series report, serial dilatation for microperforate hymen was done with success.[11]

■ TAKE-HOME MESSAGES

- Thorough history and physical examination are crucial in patients with primary amenorrhea. Further work up depends upon the development/presence of breast and uterus.
- Gonadal dysgenesis is the most common cause of primary amenorrhea (30–40%) followed by Müllerian anomalies and agenesis.[1]
- Imperforate hymen should be suspected in all pubertal girls presenting with amenorrhea, low abdominal, pelvic or lower back pain, tenesmus and urinary tract obstruction.

- The majority of patients with chromosomal abnormalities have primary amenorrhea (50% of X0 and 25% of patients with mosaicism such as X0 /XY).[1]
- Streak gonads are seen in pure gonadal dysgenesis, while testicular tissue is seen with mixed gonadogensis.[1] Gonadectomy is suggested after pubertal development (~18 years) when Y chromosome or hyperandrogenism is present, because of future risk of gonadoblastoma.[12]
- Imperforate hymen should be differentiated from low transverse septum. Transverse septum is usually accompanied by other upper genital tract anomalies and is typically thicker than imperforate hymen. With Valsalva's maneuver in patients with transverse septum, no distention is noticed due to greater thickness of transverse septum compared to imperforate hymen.[1]
- In patients with uterus and absent breast development an astute physician should evaluate CNS-hypothalmic-pituitory disorder and gonadal development, by performing E2, FSH and LH.
- Women with hypergonadotropic hypogonadism (FSH >30 mIU/mL) require karyotyping. Those with XX karyotype require electrolyte and serum progesterone levels to rule out 17 alpha hydroxylase deficiencies.
- In patients with hypogonadotropic hypogonadism, prolactin and head CT scan or MRI should be performed to rule out CNS lesion.
- Lack of uterus and vagina leads to the diagnosis of Müllerian agenesis. Absence or hypoplasia of the uterus and vagina is seen. Approximately 1/3rd of these patients have urinary tract anomalies and 12% have skeletal anomalies.[1]
- Androgen insensitivity is suspected in patients with blind vagina and absent uterus.[12]

REFERENCES

1. Fritz MA, Speroff L. Chapter 11: Amenorrhea. Clinical Gynecologic Endocrinology and Infertility: 7th (seventh) Edition. Philadelphia, PA: Walters Kluwer/Lippincott Williams and Wilkins; 2010.
2. Nagai N, Murakami Y, Nagatani K, et al. Life threatening acute renal failure due to imperforate hymen in an infant. Paediatrics International. 2012;54(2):280-2.
3. ane C, Dane B, Erginbas M, Cetin A. Imperforate hymen-a rare cause of abdominal pain: two cases and review of the literature. J Pediatr Adolesc Gynecol. 2007;20(4):245-7.
4. Lui CT, Chan TWT, Fung HT, Tang SYH. A retrospective study on imperforate hymen and hematocolpos in a regional hospital. Hong Kong J Emerg Med. 2010;17(5):435-40.
5. Liang CC, Chang SD, Soong YK. Long-term follow-up of women who underwent surgical correction for imperforate hymen. Arch Gynecol Obstet. 2003;269:5-8.
6. Ayaz UY, Dilli A, Api A. Ultrasonographic diagnosis of congenital hydrometrocolpos in prenatal and newborn period: a case report. Medical ultrasonography. 2011;13(3):234-6.
7. Ercan CM, Karasahin KE, Alanbay I, Ulubay M, Baser I. Imperforate hymen causing hematocolpos and acute urinary retention in an adolescent girl. Taiwan J Obstet Gynecol. 2011;50(1):118-20.
8. Abu-Ghanem S, Novoa R, Kaneti J, Rosenberg E. Recurrent urinary retention due to imperforate hymen after hymenotomy failure: a rare case report and review of the literature. Urology. 2011;78:180-2.
9. Posner JC, Spandorfer PR. Early detection of imperforate hymen prevents morbidity from delays in diagnosis. Pediatrics. 2005;115(4):1008-12.
10. Kumar A, Mittal M, Prasad S, Sharma JB. Haematocolpos--an uncommon cause of lower abdominal pain in adolescent girls. J Indian Med Assoc. 2002;100(4):240-1.
11. Segal TR, Fried WB, Krim EY, Parikh D, Rosenfeld DL. Treatment of microperforate hymen with serial dilation: a novel approach. J Pediatr Adolesc Gynecol. 2015;28(2):e21-2.
12. Lobo RA. Primary and secondary amenorrhea and precocious puberty: etiology, diagnostic evaluation, management (Chapter 38). In: Lentz GM, Lobo RA, Gershenson DM, Katz VL, eds. Comprehensive Gynecology; 6th ed. Philadelphia, PA: Elsevier Mosby; 2012.

CHAPTER 33

Labia Minora Hypertrophy

Ann M Dobry, Sireesha Y Reddy

■ CLINICAL CASE

AL is a 12-year-old premenarchal patient who presented to adolescent clinic accompanied by her mother for concerns of an abnormal size of the labia minora. Her mother states that AL has had "larger" labia since a young age. Their pediatrician reassured them that there was nothing abnormal. However, they wanted a second opinion. AL reports occasional itching and some discomfort when she is wearing tight jeans. Her daily activities are not affected. She denies history of UTIs or yeast infections.

Menarche: Age 11.

Menstrual cycle: Regular menses, every 28 days, lasting for 4 days. She is virginal.

Past medical history: Hx of Langerhans histiocytosis currently in remission. She sees oncology biannually for monitoring.

Surgical history: Biopsy of arm for Langerhans histiocytosis.

Current medications: Denies.

Vaccines: Up to date. She received all three doses of the HPV vaccine, Gardasil.

Allergies: None. Not known drug allergies (NKDA).

Family history: Mother (42 years) has hypertension. Father (45 years) with history of nephrolithiasis.

Social history: AL is in seventh grade, enjoys school, and sings in choir. She lives with her parents.

Review of Systems

Negative other than in the history of present illness.

Physical Examination

- *General*: Well-developed, well-nourished, no apparent distress
- *Breast*: Tanner stage III

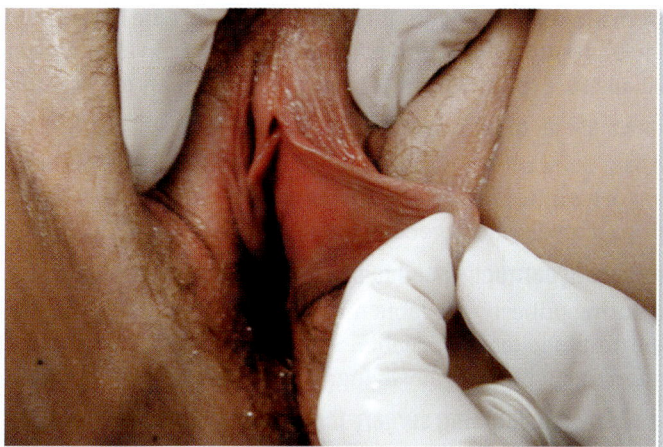

Figure 33.1: Asymmetric labia on the left. The appearance of right labia is normal. The left labia extend about 4 cm from the midline to the lateral edge of the labia

- *Genitourinary examination*: Normal pubic hair distribution, no lesions or masses, no hyperpigmentation; labia minora are unilaterally enlarged, extending 3 cm from midline to the lateral edge of the labia minora. Figure 33.1 shows that the labia minora on the left are enlarged and extend about 4 cm from the midline to lateral surface. Tanner stage III. Vagina is patent. Hymen is thin, and shows some signs of being estrogenized.
- *Urinalysis*: Normal.
- *Beta-hCG*: Negative.

■ CLINICAL QUESTIONS

1. How would you describe these clinical findings to the mother and her daughter?

Ans. The labia minora may have some enlargement. The labia minora are protuberant and tend to project outward beyond the midline. Labia minora have normal variants and there is no definitive statement whether this finding is considered abnormal.

2. How is labia minora hypertrophy diagnosed?

Ans. It is a clinical diagnosis, noticed incidentally by a gynecologist or pediatrician. The definition of labia minora hypertrophy varies in the literature. It has been described anywhere from 3–5 cm from midline to the lateral edge of the labia minora.[1-3]

3. Are the symptoms of this patient expected or are they are incidental?

Ans. Symptoms such as itching and discomfort are general symptoms that can occur when there is no association with labial hypertrophy. Sometimes, perineal discomfort is caused by emotional (psychological) factors caused by perception of abnormal anatomy (somatization). Patients can present with complaints that there is a bulge in their underclothes, discomfort with activities, such as biking, dancing, running, chronic irritation, and pain. Increased risk of infections, such as UTIs, dyspareunia, and emotional disturbance may also be reported.[4-7] Another issue to consider is that patients who present with labial minora hypertrophy should be assessed for psychological symptoms that may be related to the perception of an abnormality. In extreme cases, the patient may even suffer from body dysmorphic disorder.[4,6] Adolescents given their concerns of appearance can be especially susceptible to stress if they perceive that they are different.

4. What is the mechanism of labia minora hypertrophy?

Ans. The mechanism is unknown. Current theories include that it is due to hormones, or a manifestation of lymphedema.[6] Labial hypertrophy has been associated with spina bifida, meningocele and myelomeningocele.

5. Does labia minora hypertrophy need to be corrected with surgery?

Ans. Sometimes, during puberty, the labia majora may also enlarge, making the labia minora which is hypertrophied less noticeable. Surgery is not recommended unless it interferes with the patient's activities of daily living.[4,7]

6. What are the risks of undergoing surgery for labia minora hypertrophy?

Ans. The surgery to help reduce labial hypertrophy is called a labiaplasty. The usual risks of any surgery include infection, bleeding, and risks involving anesthesia. A unique risk for labiaplasty is neural damage affecting sexual arousal. Another complication is being disappointed with the results.[4-6] Patients should be aware that there may be complications associated with scarring leading to chronic vulvar pain, dyspareunia or decreased sexual satisfaction.

7. What are the indications for labiaplasty?

Ans. Labiaplasty is considered an elective procedure that is done for aesthetic reasons, but can have functional impairments associated with it.[5-7]

8. If surgery is offered, at what age is appropriate to have labiaplasty performed?

Ans. Surgery is not recommended for aesthetic reasons only, and is still controversial. It should be postponed as long as hypertrophy is not interfering with patient's activities of daily living.[5] At any age, reasons for surgery, and expectations should be discussed with the patient.[4,6]

9. If surgery is not offered, what therapy can you offer this patient?

Ans. Initial approaches should include counseling with reassurance. Self care and hygiene instructions should be offered, such as use of mild soaps, cotton underwear, avoiding bubble baths and tight clothing.

■ TAKE-HOME MESSAGES

- Labial hypertrophy is a normal variant of the size of the labia. There is no consensus on the definition but has been described as hypertrophic when greater than 3–5 cm from the midline lateral edge of labia minora.
- Patients should be counseled and reassured about this condition as long as the labial size does not interfere with patient's activities of daily living. Offering conservative self-care options should be first step.
- If this condition does affect patients' lives either by irritation in common activities, or by increased infections, such as UTIs, surgery can be offered.
- Surgical risks from labiaplasty should be explained. The nature of the surgery is elective and for aesthetic reasons. The risks can include pain, scarring and losing sensation in the genital area.

REFERENCES

1. Freidrich EG. Vulvar Disease, 2nd ed, WB Saunders, Philadelphia. 1983.
2. Rouzier R, Louis-Sylvestre C, Paniel BJ, Haddad B. Hypertrophy of labia minora: experience with 163 reductions. Am J Obstet Gynecol. 2000;182(1 Pt 1):35.
3. Munhoz AM, Filassi JR, Ricci MD, Aldrighi C, Correia LD, Aldrighi JM, Ferreira MC. Aesthetic labia minora reduction with inferior wedge resection and superior pedicle flap reconstruction. Plast Reconstr Surg. 2006;118(5):1237.
4. Motakef S, Rodriguez-Feliz J, Chung MT, Ingargiola MJ, Wong VW, Patel A. Vaginal labiaplasty: current practices and a simplified classification system for labial protrusion. Plast Reconstr Surg. 2015;135(3):774-88.
5. Oranges CM, Sisti A, Sisti G. Labia minora reduction techniques: a comprehensive literature review. Aesthet Surg J. 2015; 35(4):419-31.
6. Reddy J, Laufer MR. Hypertrophic labia minora. J Pediatr Adolesc Gynecol. 2010;23(1):3-6.
7. Wu JA, Braschi EJ, Gulminelli PL, Comiter CV. Labioplasty for hypertrophic labia minora contributing to recurrent urinary tract infections. Female Pelvic Med Reconstr Surg. 2013;19(2):121-3.

CHAPTER 34

Lichen Sclerosus

Sushila Arya, Sireesha Y Reddy, Sanja Kupesic Plavsic

■ CLINICAL CASE

JS is a 9-year-old patient who presents to the clinic with complaints of perianal itching and pain for a duration of 4 months. Her symptoms are gradually worsening. She also complains of pain with urination. She denies any onset of menses. Her mother reports some pubertal development to include changes in breast appearance and some pubic hair growth. She denies any sexual abuse.

Primary care health prevention: She is up-to-date with her vaccines and nutritional status is appropriate.

Past medical history: Vitiligo.

Past surgical history: None.

Current medications: Denies.

Allergies: None.

Family history: Mother has hypothyroidism. Father does not report any health issues.

Social history: Doing very well in school, in 4th grade. She is physically active and lives with her parents.

Review of Systems

Negative other than in the history of present illness.

Physical Examination

- Normal vital signs
- *General*: Well-developed, well nourished, in no apparent distress
- *Upper extremities*: Vitiligo lesions noted on both hands
- *Neck*: Supple, no lymphadenopathy, no thyroid enlargement
- *Abdomen*: Soft, no mass or tenderness, no rigidity or guarding

- *Genitourinary examination*: Hypopigmentation and thinned skin noticed around clitoris and vaginal orifices (Fig. 34.1). Marks of itching; small fissure noted in perianal area. Mucous membranes are not involved. No abnormal discharge or bleeding from the hypopigmented lesion
- *Urinalysis*: Negative for leukocyte esterase and nitrites.

Biopsy was deferred since diagnosis was clinically made. 0.05% clobetasol ointment was started and patient followed up in 3 months with remarkable improvement (Fig. 34.2).

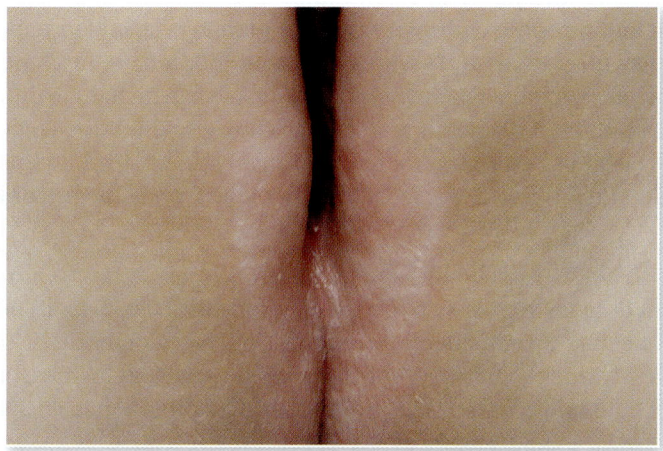

Figure 34.1: Hypopigmented erythematous area around vaginal and anal orifices leading to typical "hourglass" appearance of lichen sclerosus

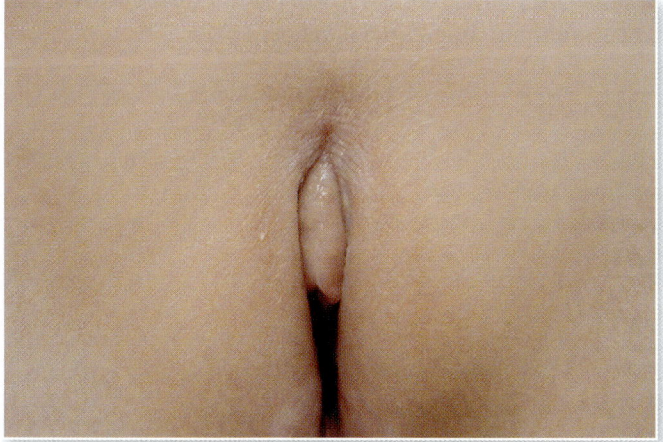

Figure 34.2: Improvement of lichen sclerosus three months after initiation of the treatment with clobetasol ointment

CLINICAL QUESTIONS

1. What is clinical presentation of lichen sclerosus (LS)?

Ans. Excessive itching in anogenital area, more at night, pain, dyspareunia and urinary hesitancy due to pain with urination are common symptoms of lichen sclerosus. Fissures and scars form if left untreated.[1,2] Scarring in anogenital area can cause narrowing of the introital and anal orifices, and hence dyspareunia and dyschezia.

2. How is the diagnosis of LS established?

Ans. Thorough history and physical examination is important. On inspection anogenital area is pale and atrophic with ivory colored plaques ("crinkled paper appearance"), hyperkeratosis, ulcerations and fissures.[3,4] Among children, redness and depigmentation are common presentation as shown in Figure 34.1. It can be hard to differentiate LS from vitiligo and eczema. If diagnosis is not clear clinically then histologic confirmation is suggested. The biopsy is taken prior to initiating treatment. In children biopsy should be deferred, rather referral to a specialist (dermatologist, gynecologist, or urologist) should be made.

3. What is the first-line treatment for LS?

Ans. Ultra or high potency steroid (clobetasol or halobetasol 0.05% in an ointment base) for 12 weeks is needed to gain adequate control. Topical calcineurin is 2nd line, probably less effective treatment option.[1,2] Topical treatment and general measures (avoidance of friction with tight and synthetic clothes, etc.) lead to remission in 93.3% of patients.[3]

4. How do you follow a patient with LS?

Ans. After initial treatment a follow-up in 3 months is advisable.[5,6] Patient should be educated to be vigilant to observe affected skin changes like plaques or ulcerations.

5. What is differential diagnosis of LS?

Ans. Erosive form of lichen planus, vitiligo, psoriasis, chronic vulvovaginal candidiasis, and eczema are most common differential diagnoses of LS.[4,7-10]

TAKE-HOME MESSAGES

- LS is a chronic inflammatory condition, and is considered a lifelong disease. The cause of LS is unknown; 10% patients have familial predisposition.
- Loss of androgen receptors in LS lesions has been noted.[5] Hormonal influence may play a role that probably explains bimodal age distribution of this disease, in early childhood and after menopause.[6] Most common presenting symptoms are itching and pain.
- Prevalence of LS is from 0.1% to 3%, and is more common in females than males. Most common site is anogenital area, while prevalence of extragenital LS in submammary area is estimated to 6–20%. Extragenital LS is not as symptomatic and there is no increased risk of malignancy.[7]
- 20–30 % of LS patients have autoimmune disease; thyroid disease (12–16%), vitiligo, psoriasis, irritable bowel disease, alopecia, rheumatoid arthritis, and pernicious anemia are most common coexisting disorders.[7-9]
- Often underdiagnosed and undertreated LS elevates the risk of malignancy and is associated with greater scarring.[4]
- In adult patients diagnosis of LS should be confirmed with skin biopsy. Indurated plaques or unhealing ulcers warrant biopsy to rule out malignant transformation.[3,7]

- First-line treatment are high potency topical corticosteroids as early as possible (to prevent scarring which is irreversible), for initial 3 months. This treatment significantly improves LS in 75–90%.[1,4]
- Lifetime risk of squamous cell carcinoma is 4–5%.[2,7] Chronic inflammation and oxidative DNA damage are likely mechanism of malignant transformation.[10]
- Early and compliant treatment and regular follow up reduce the development of malignancy and scarring.[3]

REFERENCES

1. Chi CC, Kirtschig G, Baldo M, et al. Topical interventions for genital lichen sclerosus. Cochrane Database Syst Rev. 2011;12 CD008240.
2. Kirtschig G, Becker K, Günthert A, et al. Evidence-based (S3) guideline on (anogenital) Lichen sclerosus. J Eur Acad Dermatol Venereol. 2015;10:e1-e43.
3. Lee A, Bradford J, Fischer G. Long-term management of adult vulval lichen sclerosus. A prospective cohort study of 507 women. JAMA Dermatol. 2015;151(10):1061-7.
4. Kirtschig G, Habil M. Review Article. Lichen Sclerosus - Presentation, Diagnosis and Management Dtsch Arztebl Int 2016; 113(19): 337-43.
5. Taylor AH, Guzail M, Al-Azzawi F. Differential expression of oestrogen receptor isoforms and androgen receptor in the normal vulva and vagina compared with vulval lichen sclerosus and chronic vaginitis. Br J Dermatol. 2008;158:319-28.
6. Friedrich EG, Kalra PS. Serum levels of sex hormones in vulvar lichen sclerosus, and the effect of topical testosterone. N Engl J Med. 1984;310:488-491.
7. Wallace HJ. Lichen sclerosus et atrophicus. Transactions's of the St. John's Hospital Dermatological Society. 1971;57:9-30.
8. Kreuter A, Kryvosheyeva Y, Terras S, et al. Association of autoimmune diseases with lichen sclerosus in 532 male and female patients. Acta Derm Venereol. 2013;93:238-41.
9. Simpkin S, Oakley A. Clinical review of 202 patients with vulval lichen sclerosus: A possible association with psoriasis. Australas J Dermatol. 2007;48:28-31.
10. Wang SH, Chi CC, Wong YW, Salim A, Manek S, Wojnarowska F. Genital verrucous carcinoma is associated with lichen sclerosus: a retrospective study and review of the literature. J Eur Acad Dermatol Venereol. 2010;24:815-9.

SECTION 2
OBSTETRICS

Section Outline

35. Early Pregnancy Loss
36. Residual Products of Conception
37. Preterm Labor
38. Cervical Insufficiency
39. Multifetal Gestation
40. Intrauterine Growth Restriction
41. Oligohydramnios
42. Placenta Previa
43. Placenta Percreta
44. Fetal Malpresentation
45. Gestational Hypertensive Disorders
46. Operative Delivery
47. Cesarean Section
48. Caudal Regression Syndrome
49. Fetal Hydronephrosis
50. Asymptomatic Adnexal Mass in Pregnancy
51. Adnexal Mass and Pelvic Pain in Pregnancy
52. Appendicitis in Pregnancy
53. Congenital Heart Disease in Pregnancy
54. Deep Venous Thrombosis in Pregnancy
55. Gallstones in Pregnancy
56. Liver Disease in Pregnancy
57. Kidney Stones in Pregnancy
58. Thyroid Nodule in Pregnancy
59. Gestational Trophoblastic Disease
60. Postpartum Tubal Ligation

CHAPTER

Early Pregnancy Loss

35

Melissa D Mendez

■ CLINICAL CASE

MS, a 32-year-old G1 at 10 weeks gestation by last menstrual period (LMP) presents to your office for a new obstetrical visit. She is complaining of some cramping that woke her early this morning. She had a positive home pregnancy test a couple of weeks ago. She denies nausea and vomiting. She states she had breast tenderness earlier in the pregnancy, but does not have breast tenderness now. Her last Pap smear was one year ago and was normal.

Menarche: Age 11.

Menses: 28/5.

LMP: 12 weeks ago.

Sexual history: In a monogamous relationship with her husband of 5 years. No history of sexually transmitted diseases.

Contraception: None.

Review of Systems

- No chest pain or shortness of breath
- No diarrhea or constipation
- No urinary frequency, no hematuria or dysuria
- *Past medical history*: Noncontributory
- *Past surgical history*: Appendix removed at age 9
- *Vaccines*: Up-to-date
- *Current medications*: Prenatal vitamins which she started taking three months before actual conception
- *Allergies*: No known drug allergies
- *Social history*: She does not smoke, no drug use, has occasional alcohol intake on weekends
- *Family history*: Noncontributory.

Physical Examination

- *Vital signs*: T36.9°C oral, BP 118/65, P 75, BMI 26
- *Cardiac examination*: Regular rate and rhythm, no heart murmur
- *Chest examination*: Lungs clear to auscultation bilaterally
- *Abdomen*: Non-distended, non-tender. Fetal heart tones cannot be auscultated
- *Pelvic examination*: Normal appearing cervix, no discharge, cervix is closed, uterus feels anteverted and 8 week size
- The patient undergoes a transabdominal and transvaginal ultrasound for further evaluation. You visualize a yolk sac (Fig. 35.1), but the crown rump length (Fig. 35.2) is lagging and measuring approximately 6 weeks. M-mode and color Doppler ultrasound reveal no fetal cardiac activity (Figs 35.3 and 35.4).

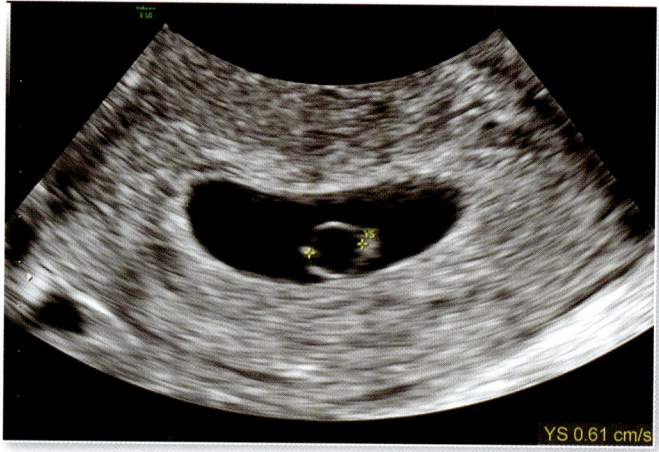

Figure 35.1: A gestational sac with a yolk sac is demonstrated on transvaginal ultrasound. Embryonic pole is visualized adjacent to the yolk sac

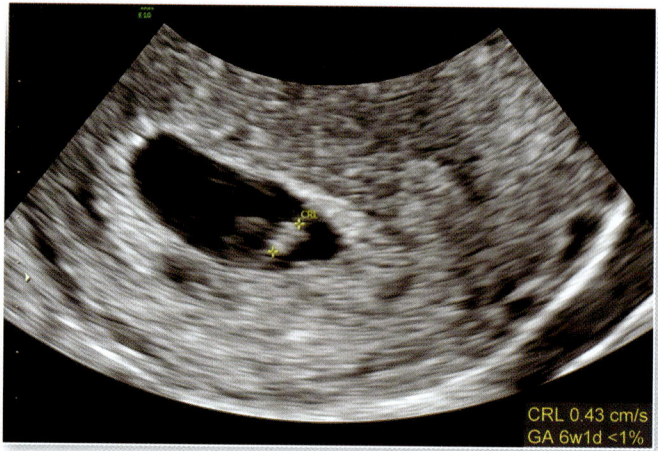

Figure 35.2: A transvaginal ultrasound measuring a crown–rump length (CRL) at 0.43 cm, consistent with a six weeks intrauterine pregnancy

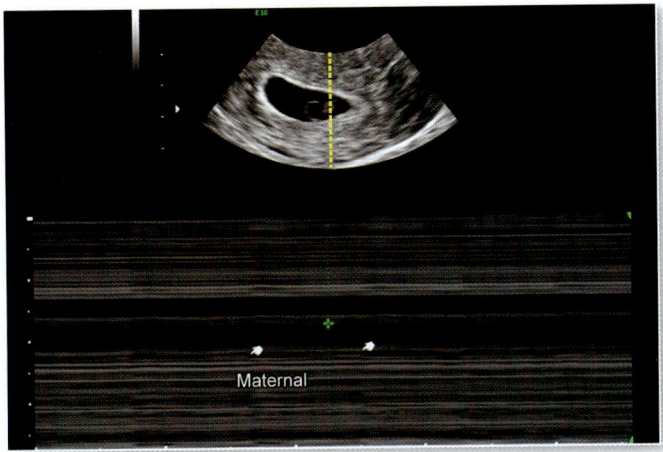

Figure 35.3: M-mode demonstrating absent fetal cardiac activity

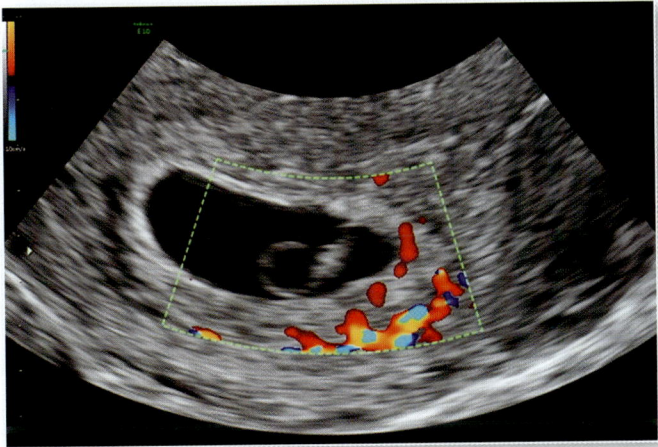

Figure 35.4: Color Doppler ultrasound demonstrating absence of embryonic flow

■ CLINICAL QUESTIONS

1. What are the risk factors for having an early pregnancy loss or first trimester miscarriage?

Ans. It is estimated that about 20–25% of all women will experience a miscarriage. Up to 70% of miscarriages may be associated with karyotype abnormalities.[1,2] Miscarriage is also associated with advanced maternal age, prior early pregnancy loss, African racial heritage, smoking, and increased body mass index (BMI).[1,2]

2. What ultrasound characteristics are seen with an early pregnancy loss?

Ans. Early pregnancy failure may be diagnosed on ultrasound by failure to visualize a yolk sac, yolk sac greater than 5.6 mm, failure to visualize a fetal pole or heart motion or a discordance between the mean sac diameter and CRL.[3-5]

3. What is the best way to treat a missed abortion?

Ans. There are three acceptable management plans for treatment of missed abortion. This includes expectant management, medical management or surgical management. Various studies and a Cochrane Review have found that all three options are safe and effective and the physician should take into account the patient's preferences.[1,2] Rates of complete resolution vary from study to study. Expectant management of missed abortion results in complete resolution up to 75% of the time, there may be a need for emergency surgical management and hospitalization. Surgical management may be more effective, associated with less pain and less bleeding; however, it has a higher rate of infection than medical or expectant management.[7-9]

4. What are some of the most common complications of missed abortion treatment?

Ans. Dilation and curettage (D and C) with suction and sharp curettage may be associated with the trauma and small risk (1–4%) for need for additional attempt to remove retained products of conceptions. Manual vacuum extraction (MVA) has less risk than D and C due to anesthesia risks. Medical and expectant management[6] have a high rate of resolution; however, they have the risk of additional hospitalization due to bleeding, need for blood transfusion, pain, and/or need for surgical management to remove retained products of conception (RPOC).[7-9]

■ TAKE-HOME MESSAGES

- Approximately 20–25% of all pregnancies result in miscarriage.[1,2] Up to 70% of miscarriages are associated with karyotype abnormalities.[3] Women may benefit from karyotyping of the products of conception.[3]
- Transvaginal ultrasonography is currently the method of choice to evaluate an early pregnancy.[3]
- Early pregnancy failure may be diagnosed on ultrasound by failure to visualize a yolk sac, yolk sac greater than 5.6 mm, failure to visualize a fetal pole or heart motion or a discordance between the mean sac diameter and CRL.[3-5]
- Acceptable management of miscarriage includes expectant management, medical management or surgical management.[1,2]
- Women often need further support with a social worker, clinical psychiatry and spiritual guidance for the emotional support in dealing with their loss.[5]
- Expectant management has been shown to be effective in 25–85% and can be managed in the community without the need for hospitalization or with minimal need for hospitalization, analgesia, antibiotics or blood transfusion.[3,6]
- Rate of complete resolution of early pregnancy loss or missed abortion with expectant management vary from study to study and may take up to two weeks.[7]
- Expectant management may be associated with bleeding requiring hospital admission and unplanned surgical evacuation.[7]
- Medical management may be achieved with misoprostol, a prostaglandin E1 analog. There are many different regimens, most commonly used is 800 µg one dose vaginally and then repeated in 24 hours, although more recent trials show that you can use 600 or 400 µg with similar effects.[10,11]
- Surgical management of first trimester pregnancy loss has risks associated with anesthesia, uterine perforation, intrauterine adhesions, cervical trauma, infection, and need for additional surgery in about 1–4% for evacuation of RPOC.[7-9]
- Surgical management can also be achieved with manual vacuum aspiration which can be done in a clinic, emergency room or hospital setting. It is also associated with less risk than a sharp curettage, is quicker and more cost effective than suction or sharp curettage.[6,9]

REFERENCES

1. Rafi J and Khalil H. Expectant Management of Miscarriage in View of NICE Guideline 154. J of Pregnancy. 2014;2014:824527.
2. ACOG Practice Bulletin Number 150 Early Pregnancy Loss. Obstetrics and Gynecology. 2015;125:1248-67.
3. Salamanca A, Fernandez-Salmeron P, Beltran E, Mendoza N, Florido J, Mozas J. Early embryonic morphology sonographically assessed and its correlation with yolk sac in missed abortion. Arch Gynecol Obstet. 2013;287:139-42.
4. Tan S, Ipek A, Pektas MK, Arifoglu M, Teber MA, Karaoglanoglu M. Irregular yolk sac shape: is it really associated with an increased risk of spontaneous abortion? J Ultrasound Med. 2011;30:31-6.
5. Papaioannou GI, Syngelaki A, Maiz N, Ross JA, Nicolaides KH. Ultrasonographic prediction of early miscarriage. Human reproduction. 2011;26:1685-92.
6. Nanda K, Peloggia A, Grimes D, Lopez I, Nanda G. Expectant care versus surgical treatment for miscarriage. Cochrane Database Syst Rev. 2006;19;(2):CD003518.
7. Nadarajah R, Quek YS, Kuppannan K, Woon SY, Jeganathan R. A randomized controlled trial of expectant management versus surgical evacuation of early pregnancy loss. Euro J Obstet Gynecol Repro Bio. 2014;178:35-41.
8. Al-Maani W, Solomayer E, Hammadeh M. Expectant versus surgical management of first-trimester miscarriage: A randomized controlled study. Arch Gynecol Obstet. 2014;289:1011-5.
9. Choobun T, Khanuengkitkong S, Pinjaroen S. A Comparative study of cost of care and duration of management for first trimester abortion with manual vacuum aspiration (MVA) and sharp curettage. Arch Gynecol Obstet. 2012;286(5):1161-4.
10. Barcelo F, DePaco C, Lopez-Espin JJ, Silva Y, Abad L, and Parrilla JJ. The management of missed miscarriage in an outpatient setting: 800 versus 600µg of vaginal misoprostol. Aust N Z J Obstet Gynaecol. 2012;52(1):39-43.
11. Peterson SG, Perkins A, Gibbons K, Bertolone J, Devenish-Meares P, Cave D, et al. Can we use a lower intravaginal dose of misoprostol in the medical management of miscarriage? A randomised controlled study. Aust N Z J Obstet Gyneaecol. 2013;53:63-73.

CHAPTER 36

Residual Products of Conception

Sanja Kupesic Plavsic, Osvaldo Padilla

■ CLINICAL CASE

SC is a 32-year-old woman, G2P1, who was referred to the clinic with symptoms of continuous vaginal bleeding for three weeks after D and C for incomplete abortion at 12 weeks gestation. Her history is significant for two consecutive courses of methylergonovine treatment (5 days each). Despite therapy the patient failed to stop the vaginal bleeding. Pelvic ultrasound was performed and findings are presented in Figures 36.1 to 36.3. The patient also complains of a lower abdominal and pelvic pain (severity 3–4), and has no fever or chills.

Menarche: Age 13.

Menses: 28/5 days, regular.

LMP: 17 weeks ago; reports continuous bleeding for three weeks following D and C.

Pregnancy: One uncomplicated pregnancy six years ago.

Delivery: One normal vaginal term delivery.

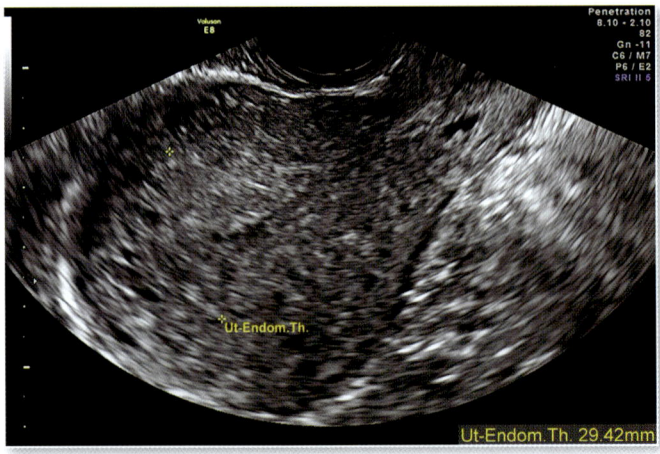

Figure 36.1: Gray-scale transvaginal ultrasound shows thickened endometrium (29.4 mm) and heterogeneous content within the uterine cavity

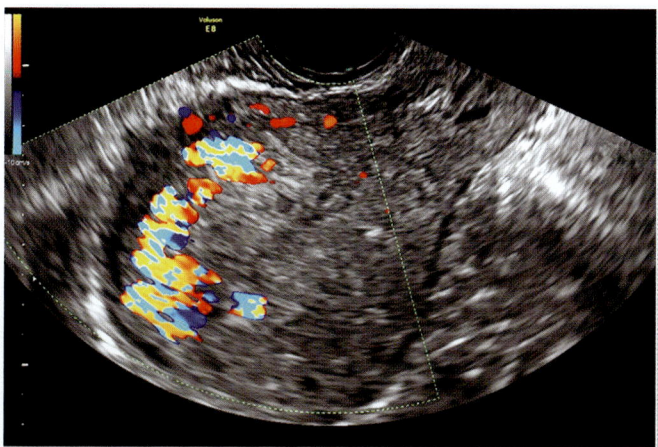

Figure 36.2: The same patient assessed with color Doppler ultrasound. Note abundant blood flow signals beneath the endometrium and within the proximal myometrial layer

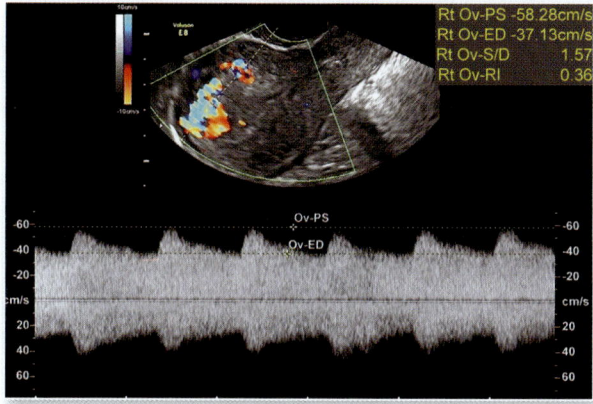

Figure 36.3: Low resistance blood flow signals (RI 0.36) are indicative of residual products of conception, which was later confirmed by histopathologic report

Sexual history: In monogamous relationship with her husband for 7 years.

Contraception: She was using condoms prior to the current pregnancy.

Review of Systems

- No chest pain or shortness of breath
- No headache, no fever
- The patient complains of vaginal bleeding and uterine contractions. There is no evidence of purulent vaginal discharge
- No diarrhea or constipation
- No hematuria or dysuria
- *Past medical history:* Noncontributory

- *Past surgical history:* None
- *Vaccines:* Up to date (hepatitis B vaccine series, MMR booster and flu shot)
- *Current medications:* None. Two cycles of five days of methylergonovine two and one week ago
- *Allergies*: No known drug allergies
- *Social history*: She is a high school teacher; does not smoke, social ETOH, no drug abuse
- *Family history:*
  - *Mother:* 54 years, with no health issues
  - *Father:* 55 years, history of essential hypertension

Physical Examination

- The patient is pale and in moderate distress due to vaginal bleeding and pelvic pain
- *Vital signs*: Temp 36.6°C oral, BP 110/80, P 95, BMI 28
- *Cardiac examination*: Normal
- *Chest examination*: Clear lungs
- *Abdominal examination*: Soft, non-tender
- *Pelvic examination*: Vaginal bleeding that fills the upper vagina during the examination. Blood clot extruding from the cervical os is visualized in speculum. The large cotton swab was easily passed into the uterine cavity; the internal cervical os is dilated. Bimanual examination does not reveal cervical motion tenderness. However, mild uterine tenderness is detected. There are no adnexal masses and tenderness.

■ CLINICAL QUESTIONS

1. What is the best next step for the diagnosis?

Ans. Laboratory studies are often normal in patients with bleeding following miscarriage. However, following laboratory tests are recommended: complete blood count (CBC), differential, hemoglobin (Hb), hematocrit (HCT), and qualitative human chorionic gonadotropin (hCG). A single hCG concentration is not useful because hCG remains positive for weeks after miscarriage. An elevated white blood cell (WBC) count supports the diagnosis of uterine infection; rising neutrophil count associated with elevated number of bands is suggestive of an infectious process.[1] Ultrasound examination with color and pulsed Doppler imaging is a sensitive tool to rule out residual products of conception (RPOC).

2. What is the average duration of bleeding after miscarriage?

Ans. Prospective studies report an average 10–14 bleeding days after identification of miscarriage. The average number of bleeding days following medical treatment of miscarriage is between 9 and 12 days. Vaginal bleeding is reported to be significantly shorter after surgical evacuation of the uterus.[2] Note that our patient reported bleeding during the course of 3 weeks following D and C.

3. What are the typical sonographic findings of RPOC?

Ans. Thickened endometrium and visualization of hyperechogenic or complex (heterogeneous) uterine mass within the uterine cavity in a patient with prolonged bleeding following miscarriage, pregnancy termination, preterm or term delivery are suggestive of RPOC (Fig. 36.1). However, necrotic decidua and blood clots can mimic residual trophoblastic tissue. Color and pulsed Doppler ultrasound is beneficial for detection of abundant low resistance flow beneath the endometrium and/or within the myometrium (Figs 36.2 and 36.3), indicative of RPOC.

4. What is the most appropriate management of patients with RPOC?

Ans. Management of patients with RPOC depends on their clinical presentation, physical examination findings and results of laboratory and imaging studies. Hemodynamically unstable patients should be stabilized with fluid and blood products before uterine evacuation. Medically stable patients with endometritis and no evidence of RPOC on color Doppler ultrasound should be treated with broad spectrum antibiotics.

■ TAKE-HOME MESSAGES

- RPOC refers to placental and/or fetal tissue that remains in the uterus after a spontaneous pregnancy loss (miscarriage), pregnancy termination, preterm or term delivery (Figs 36.4 and 36.5).[1] The characteristic symptoms of RPOC are uterine bleeding, pelvic pain, fever and/or uterine tenderness.
- The patient should be asked about the details of pregnancy: gestational age at the time of miscarriage, timing/course of tissue passage, and management option (surgical, medical or expectative).[2,3] The amount and duration of vaginal bleeding should be determined, as well as associated symptoms, such as pain (ask about the intensity, pattern and location of associated pain), fever, chills, vaginal discharge, etc.
- Physical examination should assess blood pressure, pulse, respiratory rate, and mental status changes.[4] Evaluation of abdomen should determine distension, rigidity and involuntary guarding, all suggestive of inflammatory disease.
- Speculum examination should assess the amount and character of uterine bleeding, presence of purulent discharge, evidence of fetal parts, villi and/or membranes, and opening of the cervical os.[4]
- Bimanual pelvic examination should evaluate cervical motion tenderness, uterine enlargement and tenderness, and adnexal masses and tenderness.[5]
- Laboratory studies should include: CBC, differential, Hb, HCT, and qualitative hCG.[1] Endometrial cultures and blood cultures are not performed routinely because they are not cost-effective.

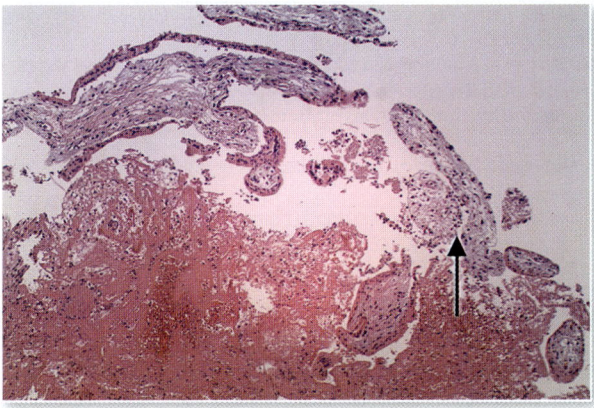

Figure 36.4: These retained products of conception demonstrate chorionic villi with infiltration by acute inflammatory cells (arrow) as well as necrotic chorionic villi with partially, denuded cytotrophoblastic cells

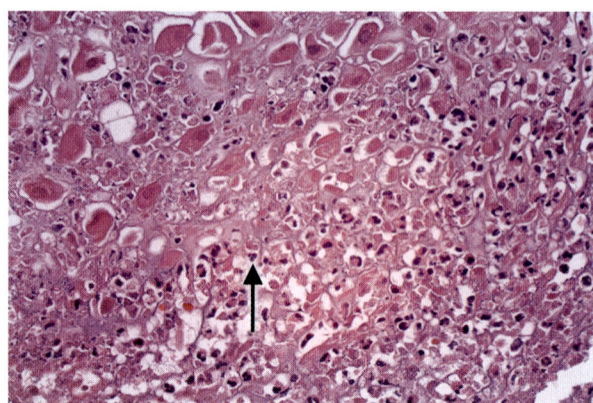

Figure 36.5: Necrotic decidua with acute inflammatory cells is also present, which is consistent with endometritis

- The best test for prediction of RPOC is pelvic ultrasound with color Doppler imaging.[6] The presence of abnormal endometrial thickness and/or heterogeneous intracavitary mass with abundant low impedance blood flow signals is typical for RPOC.[7-9]
- Hemodynamically unstable and septic patients with RPOC on US/Doppler imaging should undergo immediate surgical evacuation. Infection/sepsis should be treated with broad spectrum antibiotics (e.g., cefotetan 2 g iv plus doxycycline 100 mg iv or orally every 12 hours, or ceftriaxone 250 mg IM. in a single dose plus doxycycline 100 mg orally every 12 hours for 14 days, with or without metronidazole 500 mg orally every 12 hours for 14 days).[1] Medically stable patients with no signs of RPOC on US, should be treated with antibiotics. Patients complaining of prolonged vaginal bleeding lasting more than three weeks should be treated with surgical evacuation.[10]
- The decision to intervene should be based on clinical presentation, physical and pelvic examination findings, laboratory and imaging studies.

■ REFERENCES

1. Crusi DA. Residual products of conception. UpToDate. http://cursoenarm.net/UPTODATE/contents/mobipreview.htm?22/47/23280?source=see_link.
2. Trinder J, Brocklehurst P, Porter R, et al. Management of miscarriage: expectant, medical or surgical? Results of randomized controlled trial. BMJ. 2006;332:1235.
3. Bagratee JS, Khullar V, Regan L, et al. A randomized controlled trial comparing medical and expectant management of first trimester miscarriage. Hum Reprod. 2004;19:266.
4. Hakim Elahi E, Tovell HM, Burnhill MS. Complications of first trimester abortions: a report of 170,000 cases. Obstet Gynecol. 1990;76:129.
5. Maslovitz S, Almong B, Mimouni GS, et al. Accuracy of diagnosis of residual products of conception after dilatation and curettage. J Ultrasound Med. 2004;23:749.
6. Kupesic Plavsic S, Kurjak A. Zafar N. Color Doppler and 3D ultrasound imaging in normal and abnormal pregnancy. In: Kupesic Plavsic S (Ed). Color Doppler, 3D and 4D Ultrasound in Gynecology, Infertility and Obstetrics, 2nd edition. New Delhi: Jaype Publisher. 2011; pp. 146-65.
7. Ben-Ami I, Schneider D, Maymon R, et al. Sonographic vs. clinical evaluation as predictors of residual trophoblastic tissue. Hum Reprod. 2005;20:1107.
8. Sawyer E, Ofuasia E, Ofili-Yebovi D, et al. The value of measuring endometrial thickness and volume on transvaginal ultrasound scan for the diagnosis of incomplete miscarriage. Obstet Gynecol. 2007;29:205.
9. Abbasi S, Jamal A, Eslamian L, Marsousi V. Role of clinical and ultrasound findings in the diagnosis of retained products of conception. Ultrasound Obstet Gynecol. 2008;32:704.
10. Van den Bosch T, Daemen A, Van Schoubroeck D, et al. Occurrence and outcome of residual trophoblastic tissue: a prospective study. J Ultrasound Med. 2008;27:357.

CHAPTER

Preterm Labor

37

Melissa D Mendez, Naima Khamsi, Diego Ramirez, Sanja Kupesic Plavsic

■ CLINICAL CASE

NK is a 33-year-old G2P0 at 18 weeks by her LMP and a 6 week sonogram. She is in your clinic to establish prenatal care. She denies vaginal bleeding, contractions or loss of fluid. She has not yet started to feel the baby move. Her last Pap smear was last year and was normal.

Menarche: Age 12.

Menses: 28/5.

LMP: 20 weeks ago.

Pregnancy: Her first pregnancy was complicated by preterm premature rupture of membranes (PPROM) at 35 weeks. She delivered an otherwise healthy baby boy; however, he was admitted to the NICU for 5 days for respiratory distress.

Sexual history: In a monogamous relationship with her husband for 8 years. No history of sexually transmitted diseases.

Contraception: Oral contraception pills in between her pregnancies. This was a planned pregnancy.

Review of Systems

- No chest pain or shortness of breath
- No diarrhea or constipation
- No urinary frequency, no hematuria or dysuria
- *Past medical history*: Noncontributory
- *Past surgical history*: Cholecystectomy at age 29
- *Vaccines*: Up to date
- *Current medications*: Prenatal vitamins with iron
- *Allergies*: No known drug allergies
- *Social history*: She does not smoke, no drug use, has occasional alcohol intake on weekends
- *Family history*: Mother died of endometrial cancer at 59. Father 66, healthy.

Physical Examination

- *Vital signs*: T36.9°C oral, BP 105/65, P 75, BMI 29
- *General*: Alert and oriented, no apparent distress
- *Cardiac examination*: Regular rate and rhythm, no heart murmur
- *Chest examination*: Lungs clear to auscultation bilaterally
- *Abdomen*: Non-distended, non-tender. Fetal heart tones auscultated at 140 beats per minute
- *Pelvic examination*: Normal appearing cervix, no discharge; cervical os is closed and uterus feels
- 18-week size
- Pelvic ultrasound reveals normal fetal biometry. Cervix is closed; cervical length >35 mm.

■ CLINICAL QUESTIONS

1. What are risk factors for preterm birth?

Ans. In 2014, 9.6% of all live births were preterm in the United States.[1] Preterm birth is defined as birth between 20 and 0/7 weeks of gestation and 36 and 6/7 weeks of gestation.[2] The annual cost of preterm birth in the Unites States is estimated to be 26.2. billion.[2] There are many risk factors for preterm birth, including uterine anomalies, history of previous preterm birth, multiple gestation, polyhydramnios, history of cervical surgery, sexually transmitted infections, periodontal disease, vaginal bleeding, substance abuse, smoking, maternal age less than 18 and more than 40, African American ethnicity, poor nutrition, and anemia.[3]

2. How can we predict preterm birth?

Ans. Identifying women with preterm labor who ultimately will give birth preterm can be difficult. Approximately 30% of preterm labor spontaneously resolves and 50% of patients hospitalized for preterm labor actually give birth at term.[3] The best strategy to detect patients at risk for preterm labor is to take a detailed history and perform transvaginal ultrasound for cervical length, with or without the use of fetal fibronectin (Figs 37.1 to 37.4).[4-6]

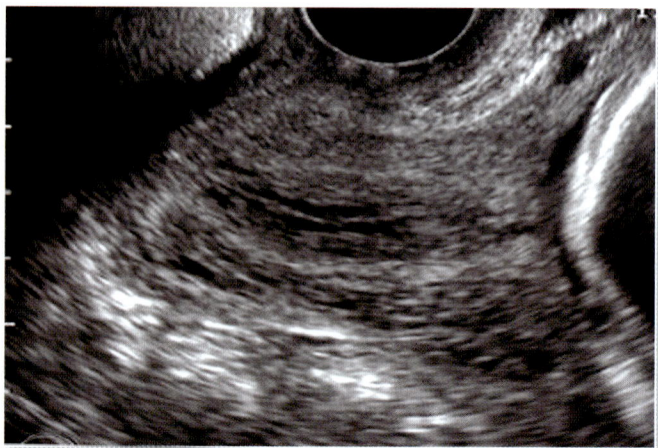

Figure 37.1: Transvaginal ultrasound of closed, T-shaped cervix. Internal os is closed and there is no funneling

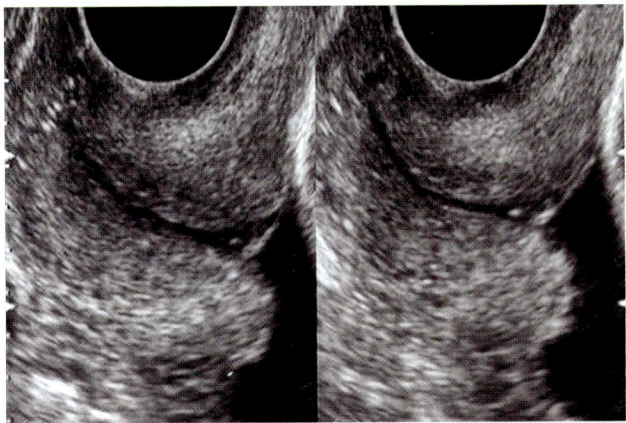

Figure 37.2: Transvaginal ultrasound of the progressive shortening of the cervix. As the cervix effaces, the relationship between the cervical canal and the lower uterine segment changes to Y shape

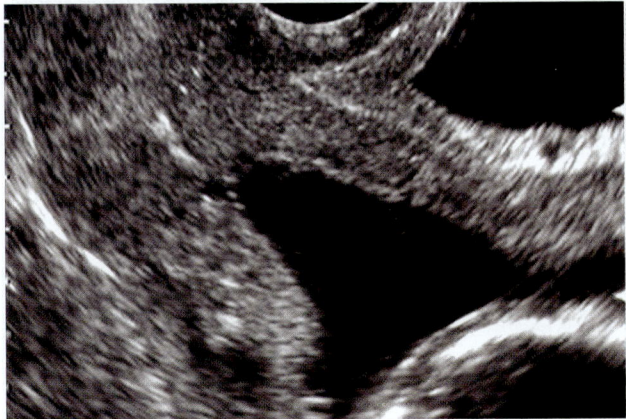

Figure 37.3: Further enhancement leads to V shape of the cervix. Cervical canal is shortened to 1 cm

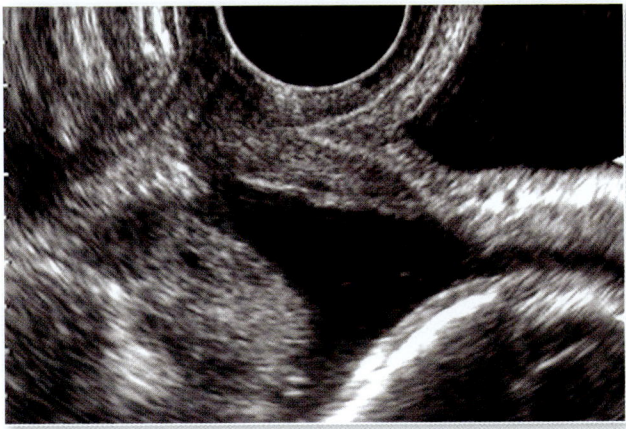

Figure 37.4: Transvaginal ultrasound shows a short (3 mm) cervix

3. Is there a role for tocolysis in preterm labor?

Ans. Tocolytic therapy is effective for up to 48 hours, and should be administered together with antenatal corticosteroids for fetal lung maturity. In general, tocolytics are not indicated for use before neonatal viability. There is no evidence to support the use of prophylactic tocolytic therapy in women with contractions but no cervical change. Women with preterm contractions without cervical changes, especially those with a cervical dilation of less than 2 cm, generally should not be treated with tocolytics.[7-9]

4. What are the most beneficial interventions for prevention of preterm labor?

Ans. The most beneficial intervention for improvement of neonatal outcomes among patients who give birth preterm is the administration of antenatal corticosteroids. Betamethasone and dexamethasone are the most widely studied corticosteriods.[10] Treatment with corticosteroids for less than 24 hours is still associated with significant reduction in neonatal morbidity and mortality, including respiratory distress syndrome, cerebroventricular hemorrhage, necrotizing enterocolitis, and intensive care admissions. Therefore, a first dose of antenatal corticosteroids should still be administered even if the ability to give the second dose is unlikely, based on the clinical scenario.[11]

Magnesium sulfate may reduce the severity and risk of cerebral palsy in surviving infants if administered when birth is anticipated before 32 weeks of gestation.[12] 17-hydroxyprogesterone weekly injections reduce preterm delivery in patients with singleton gestations. Injections should start at 16 weeks and go through 36 weeks.[13]

■ TAKE-HOME MESSAGES

- In 2014, 9.6% of live births were preterm birth in the United States.[1] Preterm labor preceded approximately 50% of these preterm births.[2]
- Preterm birth costs the US health care system greater than 26 billion in 2005 or greater $51,000 per premature infant.[2,3]
- There are multiple risk factors for preterm labor. The biggest predictor of preterm delivery is a prior history of preterm delivery.[2]
- Transvaginal ultrasound for cervical length with or without the use of fetal fibronectin may assist in establishing the risk for preterm labor.[4-6]
- Tocolytics are usually given along with glucocorticoid injection. Steroids are administered between 23 and 34 weeks of gestation.[7-9]
- Antenatal corticosteroids have been shown to have significant reduction in neonatal morbidity and mortality.[10]
- 17-hydroxyprogesterone weekly injections reduce preterm delivery in patients with singleton gestations. Injections should start at 16 weeks and go through 36 weeks.[13]

■ REFERENCES

1. March of Dimes Premature Birth Report Card 2015. *www.marchofdimes/org/reportcard*.
2. American College of Obstetrics and Gynecologist. Practice Bulletin number 159: Management of Preterm Labor. Obstet Gynecol. 2016;127(1):190-1.
3. American College of Obstetrics and Gynecology. Practice Bulletin number 130: Prediction and Prevention of Preterm Birth. Obstet Gynecol. 2012;120(4):964-73.
4. Skoll A, St Louis P, Amiri N, Delisle MF, Lalji S. The evaluation of the fetal fibronectin test for prediction of preterm delivery in symptomatic patients. J Obstet gynecol Can. 2006;28:206-13.

5. Doyle NM, Monga M. Role of ultrasound in screening patients at risk for preterm delivery. Obstet Gynecol Clinic North Am. 2004;31:125-39.
6. Fuchs IB, Henrich W, Osthues K, Dudenhausen JW. Sonographic vertical length in singleton pregnancies with intact membranes presenting with threatened preterm labor. Ultrasound Obstet Gynecol. 2004;24:554-7.
7. Van Vilet EO. Boormans EM, de Lange TS, Mol BW, Oudik MA. Preterm labor: current pharmacotherapy for tocolysis. Expert Opin Pharmacother. 2014;15(6):787-97.
8. Hosli I, Sperschneider C, Drack G, Zimmermann R, Surbek D, Irion O. Tocolysis for preterm labor: Expert Opinion. Arch Gynecol Obstet. 2014;289(4):903-9.
9. Vogel JP, Nardin JM, Dowswell T, West HM, Oladapo OT. Combination of tocolytic agents for inhibiting preterm labour. Cochrane Database Syst Rev. 2014;7:CD006169. doi: 10.1002/14651858.CD006169.pub2.
10. Melamed N, Shah J, Soraisham A, Yoon EW, Lee SK, Shah PS, Murphey KE. Association between antenatal corticosteroid administration-to-birth interval and outcomes of preterm neonates. Obstet Gynecol. 2015;125(6):1377-84.
11. Sotiriadis A, Tsiami A, Papatheodorou S, Bashat AA, Sarafidis K, Makrydimas G. Neurodevelopmental outcome after a single course of antenatal steroids in children born preterm. Obstet Gynecol. 2015;125(6):1385-95.
12. Crowther CA, Brown J, McKinlay CJ, Middleton P. Magnesium sulphate for preventing preterm birth in threatened preterm labour. Cochrane Database Syst Rev. 2014;8:CD001060. doi: 10.1002/14651858.CD001060.pub2.
13. Meis PJ, Klebenoff M, Thorn E, Dombrowski MP, Sibai B, Moawad AH, Spong CY, Hauth JC, Miodovnik M, Varner MW, Leveno KJ, Caritis SN, Iams JD, Wapner RJ, Conway D, O'Sullivan MJ, Carpenter M, Mercer B, Ramin SM, Thorp JM, Peaceman AM. Prevention of recurrent preterm delivery by 17-alpha-hydroxyprogesterone caproate. NEJM. 2003;348:2379-85.

CHAPTER

Cervical Insufficiency

38

Diego Ramirez, Melissa D Mendez, Sireesha Y Reddy

■ CLINICAL CASE

NM is a 35-year-old G2P1 at 27 weeks 2 days by LMP, consistent with a 20 weeks 1 day sonogram. She presented to the office complaining of pelvic pressure. A transvaginal ultrasound revealed a cervical length of <1.0 cm, with evidence of funneling (Fig. 38.1). Patient was not contracting at the time of diagnosis. Her obstetrical history is significant for a 36 week labor induction for intrauterine growth restriction (IUGR) resulting in a vaginal delivery. She reported that she had painless, preterm cervical dilation discovered at 24 weeks of gestational age in her first pregnancy. Her anatomical scan is normal. She reports a transabdominal ultrasound showing a "normal cervix." (Fig. 38.2).

Menarche: Age 10.

Menses: 28/5.

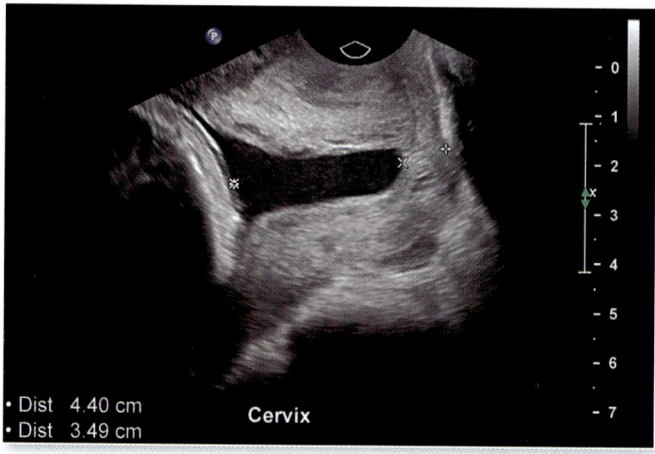

Figure 38.1: A transvaginal ultrasound demonstrates a cervical length of <1.0 cm with funneling

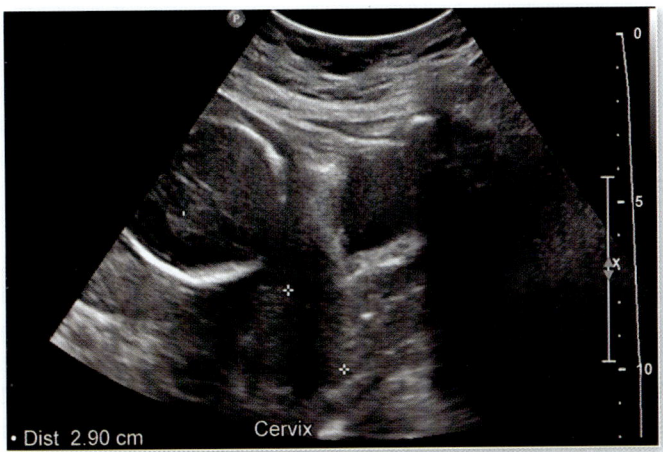

Figure 38.2: Transabdominal ultrasound of the same patient

LMP: 29 weeks ago.

Gynecological history: Denies any history of abnormal cervical cancer screening and sexually transmitted diseases.

Review of Systems

- Denies shortness of breath, nausea, and vomiting
- Denies pain, vaginal bleeding or loss of fluid. She feels the baby moves
- Denies urinary frequency or dysuria
- *Past medical history*: Chronic hypertension
- *Past surgical history*: None
- *Vaccines*: Received the influenza vaccine one month ago and is due for her TDap
- *Current medication*: Nifedipine 20 mg three times daily
- *Allergies*: None known drug allergies
- *Social history*: She denies tobacco, alcohol or drugs now or at the time of conception. She works as a secretary at a school
- *Family history*: Noncontributory.

Physical Examination

- *Vital signs:* Temp 37.1°C oral; BP 145/95; P 92; BMI 28
- *General:* Well nourished, well developed in no acute distress
- *Lungs:* Clear to auscultation bilaterally, good breathing sounds
- *Cardiac:* Regular rate and rhythm, no murmurs noted
- *Abdomen:* Non-tender, gravid uterus
- *Extremities:* Without clubbing, cyanosis or edema. 2+ deep tendon reflexes

- *Psychiatric:* Alert and oriented to all spheres
- *Fetal heart tones:* 140s reassuring tracing
- *Tocometer:* No contractions seen
- *Ultrasound cervicometry:* Demonstrates funneling with a functional length of 0.83 cm.

■ CLINICAL QUESTIONS

1. What is cervical insufficiency?

Ans. Cervical insufficiency is the inability of the uterus to retain pregnancy in the absence of signs of labor. A short cervix is very suggestive but not diagnostic of cervical insufficiency. Known risk factors include: cervical surgery, mechanical dilation, obstetric laceration, and Müllerian duct anomalies. Patients with cervical insufficiency are usually asymptomatic, but they may present with vague complaints, such as pelvic pressure, cramping, back pain or increased vaginal discharge. They may have bulging membranes, preterm/premature rupture of membranes or rapid delivery of a previable infant with rare or absent uterine contractions.[1]

2. According to ACOG Practice Bulletin No. 142 who is the most appropriate candidate for a cerclage placement?

Ans. Cerclage placement may be effective in the following setting: Singleton pregnancy with prior spontaneous preterm birth at less than 34 weeks of gestation, and short cervical length (<25 mm) before 24 weeks of gestation. Cerclage is performed either vaginally or abdominally. Vaginal cerclage includes Shirodkar technique which is dissecting the vesicocervical mucosa and putting the suture below the mucosa. The McDonald cerclage is a single purse like suture in cervicovaginal junction.[1,2]

3. What is the best approach to screen for cervical insufficiency in future pregnancies?

Ans. Performing a transvaginal ultrasound assessment of the cervical length (CL) between 16–24 weeks is the best approach to detect cervical insufficiency. Having a CL <25 mm is considered a risk of going into preterm labor. In this case, this patient had a fetal anatomy (transabdominal) scan at 20 weeks gestation showing a "normal" cervix (Fig. 38.2). Transabdominal ultrasound setting is suboptimal to evaluate the cervical length.[1-4]

4. Based on cervical findings in Figure 1, what is the next best intervention to improve fetal outcome in this patient?

Ans. A course of antenatal corticosteroids (ANCS), usually betamethasone 12 mg IM every 24 hours is recommended. The risk of preterm birth with cervical shortening and history of preterm delivery is 15–20% before 28 weeks of gestation, 25–30% before 32 weeks and 50–60% before 37 weeks.[5]

5. What is the best intervention for this patient to prevent preterm labor?

Ans. Progesterone supplementation, either vaginal progesterone gel 90 mg or vaginal progesterone suppositories 200 mg per night for the remaining of pregnancy. A rescue cerclage is not indicated in this scenario since the cervix although short, is still closed.[6,7] An example of an abdominal cerclage using a laparoscopic approach at 14 weeks is demonstrated in Figure 38.3.

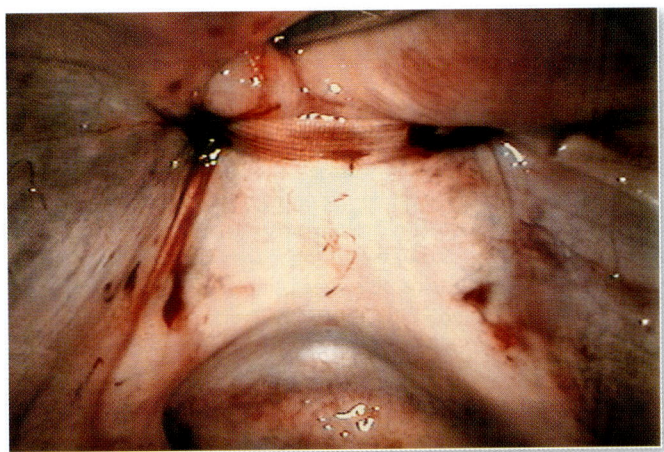
Figure 38.3: An abdominal cerclage using a laparoscopic approach at 14 weeks

■ TAKE-HOME MESSAGES

- Cervical insufficiency is the inability of the uterus to retain pregnancy in the absence of signs of labor. A short cervix is very suggestive but not diagnostic of cervical insufficiency.[1]
- Indications for cerclage (should be tailored to each individual patient) and include:
  - History of second trimester pregnancy loss with painless cervical dilatation
  - Prior cerclage placement for cervical insufficiency
  - History of spontaneous preterm birth (prior to 34 weeks gestation) and short cervical length (i.e. <25 mm) prior to 24 weeks' gestation, and
  - Painless cervical dilatation on physical examination in the second trimester.[7–10]
- Contraindications for a cervical cerclage include infection, preterm labor, an incidental short cervix less than 20 mm before 24 weeks without history of preterm delivery. Other contraindications include multifetal gestation, prior cervical surgery and Müllerian duct anomalies.[7,8,10,11]
- There is no evidence that cerclage is an effective intervention for preventing preterm births and reducing perinatal deaths or neonatal morbidity in twin gestations.[12]
- The decision to place a cerclage based on a history of 2nd trimester loss alone needs to be individualized and is not a general rule or a universal intervention.
- Cervical length screening should be performed at 16–24 weeks.[1,10]
- Ultrasound findings suggestive of cervical insufficiency include:
  - Dilatation of internal os: >5 mm dilated 33% risk of preterm delivery vs. 3.5% if the internal os was closed $P <0.01$[10]
  - Transfundal pressure was the most predictive with sensitivity, specificity, PPV and NPV of 83.3%; 97.2%; 88.2%; and 95.8%, respectively[10]
  - Shortening of the cervix: cervical length ≤10th centile (22 mm) or funneling was associated with a significantly higher probability of delivery within two to four weeks of examination or before 35 weeks of gestation (33% vs. 0%, $P = 0.01$); (67% vs. 0%, $P <0.001$); (100% vs. 19%, $P <0.001$), respectively.[10]
- Activity restriction including bed rest or pelvic rest are not recommended.[11] Rescue cerclage has been shown to have improved results vs. bed rest.[11]

- A woman with a singleton gestation and a prior spontaneous preterm singleton birth should be offered progesterone supplementation starting at 16–24 weeks of gestation, regardless of transvaginal ultrasound cervical length, to reduce the risk of recurrent spontaneous preterm birth.[3,12] An incidental finding of a short cervix in a singleton pregnancy before week 24 should be treated with either vaginal progesterone gel 90 mg or vaginal progesterone suppositories 200 mg nightly for the remaining of pregnancy.[3,5]
- Vaginal progesterone is recommended as a management option to reduce the risk of preterm birth in asymptomatic women with a singleton gestation without a prior preterm birth with an incidentally identified very short cervical length less than or equal to 20 mm before or at 24 weeks of gestation.[3] Vaginal progesterone in the context of a short cervix with history of preterm delivery has only shown to improve preterm birth before 33 weeks. Therefore, it may still be helpful when cerclage is not an option.[5]
- Patients with history of a single preterm birth but no evidence of cervical shortening and/or funneling should be offered weekly 250 mg of 17 OH-P-C (hydroxyprogesterone caproate) starting at 16–20 weeks until 36 weeks of gestation.[6]

REFERENCES

1. American College of Obstetricians and Gynecologists; ACOG Practice Bulletin No. 142: Cerclage for the management of cervical insufficiency. Obstet Gynecol. 2014;123(2 Pt 1):372-9.
2. Alfirevic Z, Stampalija T, Roberts D, Jorgensen, AL. Cervical stitch (cerclage) for preventing preterm birth in singleton pregnancy Cochrane Database Syst Rev. 2012; issue 4. doi 10.1002/14651858.CD008991.pub2.
3. The American College of Obstetricians and Gynecologists. Practice bulletin no. 130: prediction and prevention of preterm birth. Obstet Gynecol. 2012;120(4):964-73.
4. Werner EF, Han CS, Pettker CM, et al. Universal cervical-length screening to prevent preterm birth: a cost-effectiveness analysis. Ultrasound Obstet Gynecol. 2011;38(1):32-7.
5. Combs CA. Vaginal progesterone or cerclage to prevent recurrent preterm birth? Am J Obstet Gynecol. 2013;208(1):1-2.
6. Haram K, Mortensen JH, Morrison JC. Cerclage, progesterone and α-hydroxyprogeterone caproate treatment in women at risk for preterm delivery. J Matern Fetal Neonatal Med. 2014;27(16),1710-5.
7. Rush RW, McPherson K, Jones L, et al. A randomized controlled trial of cervical cerclage in women at high risk of spontaneous preterm delivery. Br J Obstet Gynaecol. 1984;91(8):724-30.
8. Lazar P, Gueguen S, Dreyfus J, et al. Multicentred controlled trial of cervical cerclage in women at moderate risk of preterm delivery. Br J Obstet Gynaecol. 1984;91(8):731-5.
9. Rafael TJ, Berghella V, Alfirevic Z. Cervical stitch (cerclage) for preventing preterm birth in multiple pregnancy. Cochrane Database Syst Rev. 2014; issue 9. DOI10.1002/14651858.CD009166.pub2
10. Rozenburg P, Gillet A, Ville Y. Transvaginal sonographic examination of the cervix in asymptomatic pregnant women: review of the literature. Ultrasound Obstet Gynecol. 2002;19(3):302-11.
11. Skupski DW, Lin SN, Reiss J, Eglinton GS. Extremely short cervix in the second trimester: bed rest or modified Shirodkar cerclage? J Perinat Med. 2014; 42(1), 55-9.
12. Iams JD. Identification of candidates for progesterone: why, who, how, and when? Obstet Gynecol. 2014;123(6):1317-26.

CHAPTER 39

Multifetal Gestation

Melissa D Mendez, Carla Martinez

■ CLINICAL CASE

RL is a 34-year-old G2P1 at 32 weeks gestation by her LMP and an 8 week ultrasound who presents to the office for her routine prenatal care visit. She has a monochorionic diamniotic twin gestation. She denies contractions, loss of fluid or vaginal bleeding. She states she can feel both fetuses moving. She would like to know if she can have a vaginal delivery.

Menarche: Age 12.

Menses: Every 32 days lasting 4 days.

LMP: 34 weeks ago.

Pregnancy: Her previous baby was born 3 years ago at 39 weeks via an uncomplicated spontaneous delivery. The baby weighed 3,610 g.

Sexual history: In a monogamous relationship with her husband for 7 years. She has a history of *Chlamydia* that was treated 10 years ago.

Contraception: None.

Review of Systems

- No chest pain or shortness of breath
- No diarrhea or constipation
- No urinary frequency, no hematuria or dysuria
- No headaches, visual changes or abdominal pain
- *Past medical history:* Noncontributory
- *Past surgical history:* None
- *Vaccines:* Up to date
- *Current medications:* Prenatal vitamins, ferrous sulfate
- *Allergies:* No known drug allergies
- *Social history:* She does not smoke; no drug use, and no alcohol use. She works in an office for a box company
- *Family history:* Noncontributory.

Physical Examination

- *Vital signs*: Height 5'6", weight 180 lbs; BMI 29.05 T 36.9°C oral, BP 110/65, P 85
- Urine dip negative for protein, ketones, and glucose
- *General*: She is alert and oriented, in no apparent distress, well groomed
- *Cardiac examination*: Regular rate and rhythm, grade 2/6 systolic heart murmur
- *Chest examination*: Lungs clear to auscultation bilaterally
- *Abdomen*: Nontender, both fetal heart tones are 140 beats per minute.

■ CLINICAL QUESTIONS

1. What is the prevalence of multiple gestation?

Ans. The rate of multifetal pregnancies is currently 33.3 per 1000 births.[1] The multifetal pregnancy rate has increased in recent decades most likely due to increasing maternal age and increasing use of assisted reproductive technology (ART).[1]

2. How is chorionicity and amnionicity determined?

Ans. Ultrasound performed early in pregnancy, late first trimester or early second trimester, is the best time to determine chorionicity. Number of placentas, presence or absence of the intertwin membrane, characterization of the membrane, twin peak or lambda sign (intervening placenta between membranes), thickness of the membrane dividing the sacs, and fetal gender all aid in differentiating dichorionic and monochorionic pregnancies. These signs become less reliable as the pregnancy progresses.[2,3] Figure 39.1 shows a dichorionic–diamniotic gestation at. Figure 39.2 shows a dichorionic diamniotic twin placenta after delivery. Figure 39.3 shows a 9-week triplet gestation.

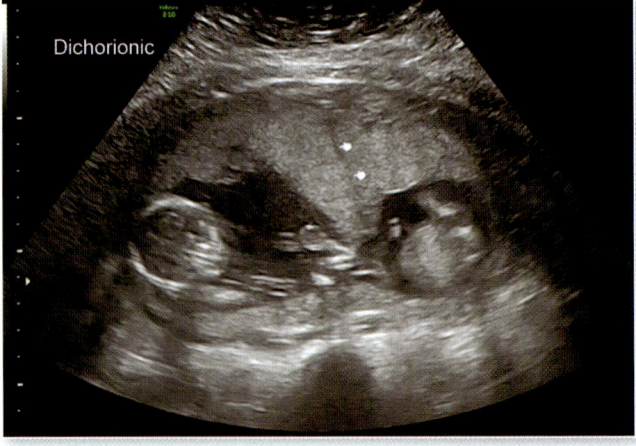

Figure 39.1: A dichorionic diamniotic twin gestation on transabdominal ultrasound. The arrows point to the dividing membrane between two placentas. There is one fetus per gestational sac

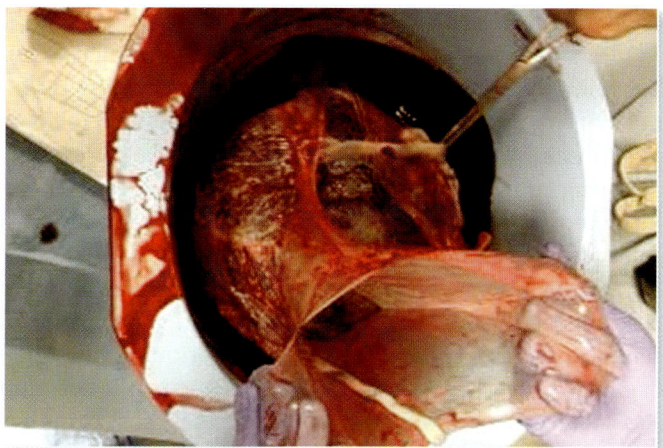

Figure 39.2: A dichorionic–diamniotic twin gestation placenta after delivery: each sac is clearly seen with separate cord insertions

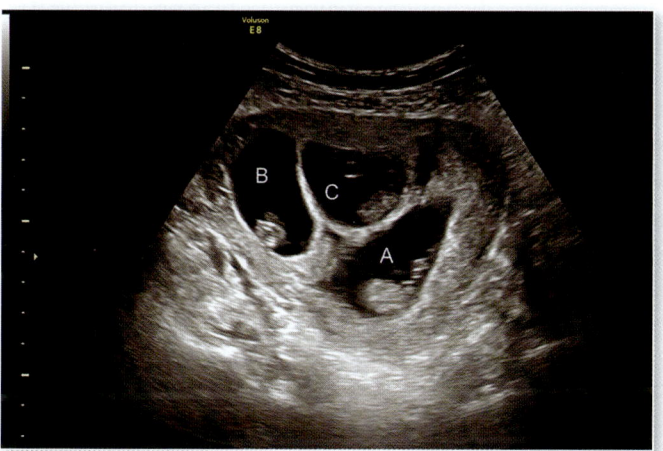

Figure 39.3: A 9-week triplet gestation showing three distinct gestational sacs each with its own distinct fetus

3. What are some of the complications that can occur with multiple gestations?

Ans. While dichorionic twins have separate placental circulations, monochorionic twins share circulation 95% of the time.[5] Monitoring for fetal growth disturbances is recommended for all twins. Complications that can occur with monochorionicity are twin-twin transfusion syndrome, selective fetal growth restriction, twin anemia polycythemia syndrome, twin reversed arterial perfusion sequence, and discordant anomalies. Death of one twin can result in the death or permanent disability of the other twin.[5] Monochorionic–monoamniotic twins may be complicated with a perinatal mortality rate of 17%.[5] This may be due to umbilical cord entanglement, congenital anomalies, preterm delivery, intrauterine growth restriction and placental vascular anastomotic events.[6]

4. How are multiple gestations monitored during pregnancy?

Ans. Recommendations for surveillance differ based on chorionicity. Once chorionicity is established, dichorionic pregnancies should have an ultrasound at 18–22 weeks to evaluate the twin fetal anatomy, amniotic fluid, and placentation with follow-up evaluation for growth every 4–6 weeks. As monochorionic pregnancies have more risks it is recommended to begin monitoring for twin-to-twin transfusion starting at 16 weeks and repeated every two weeks. Each ultrasound should include a maximum vertical pocket and assessment of fetal bladder status.[2,3] Some institutions may choose to also follow middle cerebral artery (MCA) Doppler to assess for twin anemia polycythemia. A complete anatomic scan should be performed at 18–22 weeks. Monochorionic pregnancies have a 3 to 5 fold higher rate of congenital anomalies than singletons or dichorionic twins. The fetuses should be evaluated for growth every 4 weeks.[2,3] In addition, all uncomplicated monochorionic twins should receive a fetal echocardiogram at 18–22 weeks as these twins have a higher rate of congenital heart defects.[2]

5. When should multiple gestations be delivered?

Ans. There is a significant risk for perinatal mortality in twin pregnancies after 38 weeks of gestation. Uncomplicated dichorionic diamniotic twin pregnancies it is recommended to undergo delivery at 38 weeks.[1] Consider elective delivery of uncomplicated monochorionic twins between 36 and 0/7 and 37 and 6/7 weeks of gestation.[1,3,6] The American College of Obstetricians and Gynecologists recommends delivery between 34 and 0/7 and 37 and 6/7 weeks of gestation. Monochorionic monoamniotic twin gestations are recommended to be delivered by 32–34 weeks.[1,6]

6. What is the preferred mode of delivery for twin gestations?

Ans. For uncomplicated diamniotic dichorionic twins and uncomplicated diamniotic monochorionic twins, there is no increased risk for vaginal delivery if the first twin is vertex and the twins are not more than 20% growth discordant. Monoamnionitic twins are usually recommended to be delivered at 32–34 weeks via cesarean section (CS) due to risks with cord entanglement. Higher order multiples usually require CS as well.[8]

■ TAKE-HOME MESSAGES

- The rate of multifetal gestation has been rising over the past few decades.[1]
- Consultation with maternal fetal medicine specialist is recommended.[2]
- Determine chorionicity as soon as possible, preferably in the first trimester.[3]
- Monochorionic twin gestations should be monitored with ultrasound every two weeks starting at 16 weeks.[3]
- Perform anatomical survey at 18–22 weeks.[3]
- Perform fetal echocardiography at 18–22 weeks.[3]
- Perform growth of each fetus every four weeks.[3]
- Consider delivery of uncomplicated dichorionic twins at 38 weeks.[1] Consider delivery of uncomplicated monochorionic twins between 36 and 0/7 and 37 and 6/7 weeks.[3]
- Expectant management to term is warranted after the death of one twin.[4]
- Monochorionic monoamniotic twin gestations are recommended to be delivered by 32–34 weeks.[6]

- For uncomplicated dichorionic diamniotic or monochorionic–diamniotic twins there is no increased risk for vaginal delivery.[7,8]
- Monochorionic monoamnionitic twins are usually recommended to be delivered at or by 32–34 weeks via CS due to risks with cord entanglement.[7,8]
- Higher order multiples usually require CS as well.[8]

REFERENCES

1. American College of Obstetricians and Gynecologists. Practice Bulletin number 169. Multiple gestation: Twin, triplet, and higher-order multifetal pregnancies. Obstet Gynecol. 2016;128:e131-46.
2. Bahtiyar MO, Emery SP, Dashe JS, Wilkins-Haug LE, Johnson A, Paek BW, et al. The North American fetal therapy network consensus statement. Prenatal surveillance of uncomplicated monochorionic gestations. Obstetrics Gynecol. 2015;125: 118-23.
3. Emery SP, Bahtiyar MO, Dashe JS, Wilkins-Haug LE, Johnson A, Paek BW, et al. The North American fetal therapy network consensus statement. Prenatal management of uncomplicated monochorionic gestations. Obstetrics Gynecol. 2015;125(5) 1236-43.
4. Emery SP, Bahtiyar MO, Dashe JS, Moise KJ. The North American fetal therapy network consensus statement. Prenatal management of complicated monochorionic gestations. Obstetrics Gynecol. 2015;126(3):575-84.
5. Lewi L, Deprest J, Hecher K. The vascular anastomoses in monochorionic twin pregnancies and their clinical consequences. AJOG. 2013;p19-30.
6. Murata M, Ishii K, Kamitomo M, Murakoshi T, Takahashi Y, Sekino M, et al. Perinatal outcome and clinical features of monochorionic monoamniotic twin gestation. J Obstet Gynececol Res. 2013;39(5):922-5.
7. Breathnach F, McAuliffe, F, Geary M, Daly S, Higgins JR, Dornan J, et al. Optimum timing for planned delivery of uncomplicated monochorionic and dichorionic twin pregnancies. Obstet Gynecol. 2012;119(1):50-9.
8. American College of Obstetrics and Gynecology. Committee Opinion number 560. Medically indicated late-preterm and early term deliveries. Obstet Gynecol. 2013;121(4):908-10.

CHAPTER

Intrauterine Growth Restriction

40

Melissa D Mendez, Carla Martinez, Osvaldo Padilla

CLINICAL CASE

AB is a 25-year-old G antenatal and postnatal 1P0 who presents to your office for routine obstetrical care. Her last menstrual period was 10 weeks prior and ultrasound confirms a 10-week intrauterine pregnancy with cardiac activity. At 13 weeks, she undergoes another ultrasound for nuchal translucency, which is normal. Her sequential screen test returns as low risk for trisomy 18, 21 and open neural tube defects. At 20 weeks, she undergoes a full anatomy ultrasound. The fetus is noted to be male with no anatomical abnormalities noted. The fetus at this time is noted to be in the 15% percentile for growth. You continue to follow her during her pregnancy. At 25 weeks, the patient undergoes another ultrasound assessment. At this time, it is noted that the fetus in the 6% for growth, as seen in Figure 40.1. Currently, at 29 weeks, a subsequent growth ultrasound shows the fetus to be in the 1% for growth with normal heart action, good fetal movement, AFI of 5 and uterine artery Doppler with elevated systolic/diastolic ratio (Fig. 40.2).

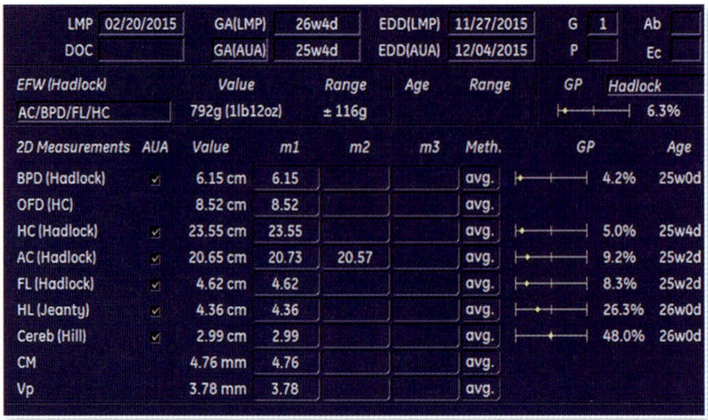

LMP	02/20/2015	GA(LMP)	26w4d	EDD(LMP)	11/27/2015	G	1	Ab	
DOC		GA(AUA)	25w4d	EDD(AUA)	12/04/2015	P		Ec	

EFW (Hadlock)	Value	Range	Age	Range	GP	Hadlock
AC/BPD/FL/HC	792g (1lb12oz)	± 116g				6.3%

2D Measurements	AUA	Value	m1	m2	m3	Meth.	GP	Age
BPD (Hadlock)	✓	6.15 cm	6.15			avg.	4.2%	25w0d
OFD (HC)		8.52 cm	8.52			avg.		
HC (Hadlock)	✓	23.55 cm	23.55			avg.	5.0%	25w4d
AC (Hadlock)	✓	20.65 cm	20.73	20.57		avg.	9.2%	25w2d
FL (Hadlock)	✓	4.62 cm	4.62			avg.	8.3%	25w2d
HL (Jeanty)	✓	4.36 cm	4.36			avg.	26.3%	26w0d
Cereb (Hill)	✓	2.99 cm	2.99			avg.	48.0%	26w0d
CM		4.76 mm	4.76			avg.		
Vp		3.78 mm	3.78			avg.		

Figure 40.1: Intrauterine growth restriction (IUGR) report demonstrating the biometric measurements for head circumference (HC), abdominal circumference (AC), and femur length (FL) are all less than the 10th percentile, and overall is at the 6th percentile which is consistent with IUGR

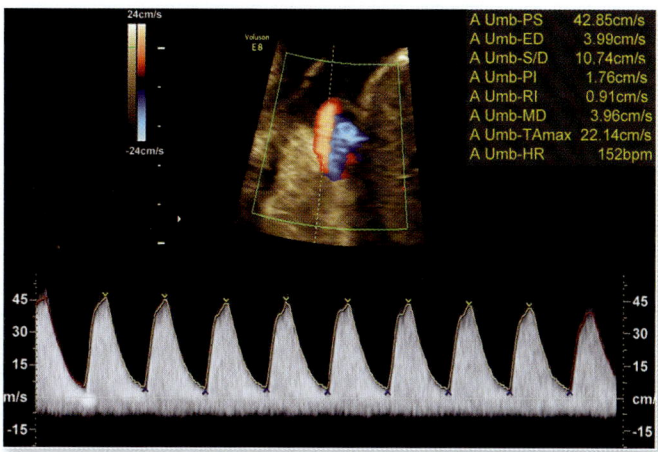

Figure 40.2: Elevated systolic/diastolic ratio (S/D) of the umbilical artery Doppler waveforms

Past gynecologic history: The patient has a history of abnormal uterine bleeding due to an endometrial polyp. The polyp was removed hysteroscopically two years ago. She used oral contraceptives until she was ready to conceive and achieved pregnancy within three months of trying. She has no history of STIs. Patient had an abnormal Pap smear 3 years prior. Colposcopy and biopsies were normal. She received three doses of the HPV vaccine, and her subsequent Pap smears were normal.

Menarche: Age 13.

Menses: 28/4.

LMP: 12 weeks ago.

Pregnancy: As above.

Sexual history: In a monogamous relationship with her husband for 5 years. No history of STI.

Contraception: As above.

Review of Systems

- No chest pain or shortness of breath
- No diarrhea or constipation
- No urinary frequency, no hematuria or dysuria
- *Past medical history*: Noncontributory
- *Past surgical history*: Hysteroscopy, dilation, and curettage and polypectomy two years ago
- *Vaccines*: Up to date
- *Current medications*: Prenatal vitamins which she started taking three months before actual conception
- *Allergies*: No known drug allergies
- *Social history*: She does not smoke, no drug use, has occasional alcohol intake on weekends
- *Family history*: Noncontributory.

Physical Examination

- *Vital signs*: T36.9°C oral, BP 118/65, P 75, BMI 26
- *Cardiac examination*: Regular rate and rhythm, no heart murmur
- *Chest examination*: Lungs clear to auscultation bilaterally
- *Abdomen*: Gravid, non-tender, fundal height measures 24 weeks
- *Pelvic examination*: Normal appearing cervix, no discharge, os is closed and uterus feels 24 week size.
- *Extremities*: No swelling, 2+ deep tendon reflexes
- *Non-stress test (NST)*: 140s baseline, no accelerations, has one spontaneous decal for one minute
- *Tocometer*: No contractions
- The patient is admitted to labor and delivery for continuous fetal monitoring and antenatal corticosteroids for fetal lung maturity in case early delivery is required. On hospital day #3, the patient had increasing numbers of deep prolonged late decelerations and was taken for an urgent CS. She had a classical uterine incision and delivered a baby boy weighing 765 g who was intubated and admitted to the neonatal intensive care unit. The gross anatomy of the placenta is presented in Figure 40.3.

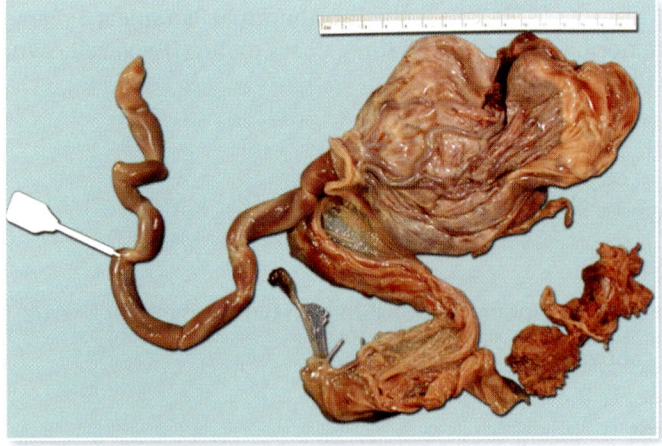

Figure 40.3: Placenta weighs 202 grams, which is less than 3rd percentile weight for gestational age

■ CLINICAL QUESTIONS

1. What are causes of IUGR?

Ans. Fetal intrauterine growth restriction (IUGR) is defined as an estimated fetal weight of less than the 10th percentile.[1] There are many causes of IUGR. Maternal disorders that cause IUGR include pregestational diabetes mellitus, renal insufficiency, autoimmune disorders, pregnancy-related hypertensive disorders, antiphospholipid syndrome and substance use of tobacco, alcohol or narcotics.[1,2] Fetal disorders include multiple gestation, teratogen exposure, such as to antiepileptic medications or antineoplastic medications, infectious diseases and genetic disorders.[1,2] Placental disorders associated with IUGR include single umbilical artery, abnormal cord insertions and bilobed placenta.[1,2] Fetal growth restriction has been associated with intrauterine fetal demise, neonatal morbidity, and neonatal death.[1] When a fetus is at or below the 10% for weight, the risk of fetal death is approximately 1.5%. When a fetus weighs less than 5% for weight, the risk of stillbirth increases to 2.5%.[1] Every fetus is screened for IUGR at prenatal visits between 24–38 weeks for fundal height. Ultrasonography can be used to assess fetal growth. Fetal anatomy should also be assessed.[1]

2. What is the management of IUGR?

Ans. Once the diagnosis of IUGR is made, fetal umbilical artery Doppler velocimetry should be evaluated. The umbilical artery Doppler is assessed near the abdominal cord insertion and the systolic/diastolic (S/D) ratio, resistance and/or pulsatility indices measured. Absent or reversed end-diastolic flow is associated with severe IUGR, less than 3% weight and an increased risk for fetal demise.[3] Use of umbilical artery Doppler evaluation in an IUGR fetus has been shown to decrease the induction rate, decrease the number of cesarean deliveries and decrease neonatal deaths.[3] Both the middle cerebral artery and ductus venosus have been studied, but there is currently not enough evidence to show their use decreases neonatal deaths.[3] Fetuses may be monitored with serial growth ultrasounds every 3–4 weeks. They may have nonstress tests or biophysical profiles twice weekly once viable; however, a specific recommendation has not been determined.[3] Once absent or reverse diastolic flow in umbilical artery is noted, admission to the hospital for close monitoring and administration of corticosteroids should be considered.[2,3] Umbilical artery Doppler is not useful as a stand-alone screening test for IUGR, even when used in conjunction with maternal characteristics.[4]

3. Is there a role for antenatal corticoid steroids in IUGR?

Ans. If less than 34 weeks, consider administration of antenatal corticosteroids for fetal lung maturity. There is some evidence that administering antenatal corticosteroids in a severely growth restricted fetus (<3%) may cause deterioration of the fetus and should be given with caution.[5] Some sheep models of IUGR have shown to have decreased blood flow to the brain and increased peripheral vasoconstriction which can cause elevated blood pressure at the time of birth.[6] Antenatal glucocorticoids may severely compromise the mechanism established in the IUGR fetus to maintain blood pressure and cerebral blood flow.[6] Some authors stated they too did not find improved neonatal outcomes with antenatal steroids in severe IUGR fetuses and that delivery should not be delayed when indicated in this population to allow time for the steroid administration.[7]

4. When should a fetus with IUGR be delivered?

Ans. Delivery is based on a combination of gestational age, Doppler velocimetry of the umbilical artery, biophysical profile (BPP) score and/or nonstress test (NST). Every IUGR fetus should be evaluated with Doppler velocimetry. If normal, this may constitute a small for gestational age fetus and the pregnancy can continue with weekly or biweekly NSTs and or BPP.[8] Interpretation of the biophysical profile score should be within the context of the gestational age. However, if the fetus has absent or reverse flow Doppler velocimetry, and abnormal NST and/or BPP score, fetal central nervous system depression including fetal acidosis should be considered. A BPP of 4 and NST with repetitive decelerations are considered abnormal and the risk of fetal asphyxia within 1 week is high if there is no intervention.[8] If less than 32 weeks, magnesium sulfate for neuroprotection prior to delivery should be considered. Late onset IUGR is the underlying reason for up to 50% of stillbirths at term. To prevent this, delivery is recommended between 37 weeks and for IUGR fetuses with normal testing parameters.[8] American College of Obstetrics and Gynecology recommends delivery of the IUGR fetus at 34–37.6 weeks gestation if there are concurrent complicating conditions and at 38–39 weeks if otherwise uncomplicated.[9]

5. How would you counsel a woman with IUGR on subsequent pregnancy outcomes?

Ans. If a woman's first pregnancy was affected with IUGR, she is about 20–28% likely to have a second pregnancy that is also affected by intrauterine growth restriction.[10] This is especially true if the first pregnancy was also complicated by hypertensive disorder of pregnancy.[10] Fetuses that are born small for gestational age are at increased risk of adverse events in the antenatal and postnatal period, as well as at increased risk of certain diseases in adult life.[11] If the infant was born IUGR and premature, the outcomes are worse.[11] Maternal factors that can be controlled for subsequent pregnancies should be addressed and corrected before she achieves pregnancy again, such as for autoimmune disease, diabetes, renal disease and preeclampsia.[11] Antiplatelet agents to prevent preeclampsia and balanced protein/energy supplementation may benefit future pregnancies.[11]

■ TAKE-HOME MESSAGES

- Fetal IUGR is defined as an estimated fetal weight of less than the 10th percentile.[1]
- There are many causes of IUGR and include maternal, fetal and placenta disorders.[1]
- Fetal growth restriction has been associated with intrauterine fetal demise, neonatal morbidity and neonatal death.[1]
- Once the diagnosis of IUGR is made, fetal umbilical artery Doppler should be performed. Absent or reversed end-diastolic flow is associated with severe IUGR, less than 3% weight and an increased risk for fetal demise.[3]
- Fetuses may be monitored with serial growth ultrasounds every 3–4 weeks. They may have NST or BPP twice weekly once viable; however, a specific recommendation has not been determined.[3]
- If less than 34 weeks, consider administration of antenatal corticosteroids for fetal lung maturity; however, antenatal corticosteroids in a severely growth restricted fetus (<3%) may cause deterioration of the fetus and should be given with caution.[5]
- American College of Obstetrics and Gynecology recommends delivery of the IUGR fetus at 34–37.6 weeks gestation if there are concurrent complicating conditions and at 38–39 weeks if otherwise uncomplicated.[9]
- Prior to 34 weeks, the IUGR fetus should be evaluated with Doppler velocimetry and followed with NST or BPP, and a decision to continue the pregnancy or deliver a preterm fetus is based on these testing. There are no set guidelines to these tests.[9]
- Fetuses that are born small-for-gestational age are at increased risk of adverse events in the antenatal and postnatal period as well as at increased risk of certain diseases in adult life.[10,11]
- Antiplatelet agents to prevent preeclampsia and balanced protein/energy supplementation may benefit future pregnancies.[11]

REFERENCES

1. American College of Obstetricians and Gynecologists. ACOG Practice Bulletin no. 134: fetal growth restriction. Obstet Gynecol. 2013;121(5):1122-33.
2. Copel JA, Bahtiyar MO. A practical approach to fetal growth restriction. Obstet Gynecol. 2014;123(5):1057-69.
3. Society for Maternal-Fetal Medicine Publications Committee. Doppler assessment of the fetus with intrauterine growth restriction. Am J Obstet Gynecol. 2012;206(4):300-8.
4. Seravalli V, Block-Abraham DM, Turan OM, et al. Second-trimester prediction of delivery of a small-for-gestational neonate: integrating sequential Doppler information, fetal biometry, and maternal characteristics. Prenat Diagn. 2014;34(11):1037-43.
5. Vidaeff AC, Blackwell SC. Potential risks and benefits of antenatal corticosteroid therapy prior to preterm birth in pregnancies complicated by severe fetal growth restriction. Obstet Gynecol Clin North Am. 2011;38(2):205-14.
6. Morrison JL, Botting KJ, Soo PS, et al. Antenatal steroids and the IUGR fetus: Are exposure and physiological effects on the lung and cardiovascular system the same as normally grown fetuses? J Pregnancy 2012; Article ID 839656, 15 pages, 2012. Doi:10.1155/2012/839656.
7. Mitsiakos G, Kovacs L, Papageorgiou A. Are antenatal steroids beneficial to severely growth restricted fetuses? J Matern Fetal Neonatal Med. 2013;26(15):1496-9.
8. Galan HL. Timing delivery of the growth-restricted fetus. Semin Perinatol. 2011;35(5):262-9.
9. American College of Obstetricians and Gynecologists. ACOG committee opinion no. 560: Medically indicated late-preterm and early term deliveries. Obstet Gynecol. 2013;121(4):908-10.
10. Voskamp BJ, Kazemier BM, Ravelli AC, et al. Recurrence of small for gestational age pregnancy: analysis of first and subsequent singleton pregnancies in The Netherlands. Am J Obset Gynecol. 2013;208(5):374,e1-6.
11. Morris RK, Oliver EA, Malin G, et al. Effectiveness if interventions for the prevention of small-for-gestational age fetuses and perinatal mortality: a review of the systematic reviews. Acta Obstet Gynecol Scand. 2013;92(2):143-51.

CHAPTER 41

Oligohydramnios

Melissa D Mendez, Sanja Kupesic Plavsic

■ CLINICAL CASE

PM is a 39-year-old G1P0 at 35 weeks gestation by her LMP that was consistent with a first trimester ultrasound, who presents to the clinic for her routine obstetrical visit. Patient has no acute complaints and denies any leakage of fluid, vaginal bleeding/discharge or uterine contractions. Her blood pressure was 128/74. Fetal heart tones were measured at 156 bpm. Fundus was below umbilicus. Her quad screen was negative as well as the rest of the prenatal laboratory findings. Results were discussed with the patient. Targeted ultrasound was ordered to assess fetal anatomy and interval fetal growth. Figures 41.1 and 41.2 illustrate head and abdominal circumference, femur length and estimated fetal weight compared to their respective centile ranks.

Menarche: Age 13.

Menses: 28/5.

LMP: 37 weeks ago.

Pregnancy: As above.

Sexual history: In a monogamous relationship with her husband of 3 years. No history of sexually transmitted diseases.

Contraception: None.

Review of Systems

- No chest pain or shortness of breath
- No diarrhea or constipation
- No urinary frequency, no hematuria or dysuria
- *Past medical history*: Non-contributory
- *Past surgical history*: None
- *Vaccines*: Up to date.
- *Current medications*: Prenatal vitamins

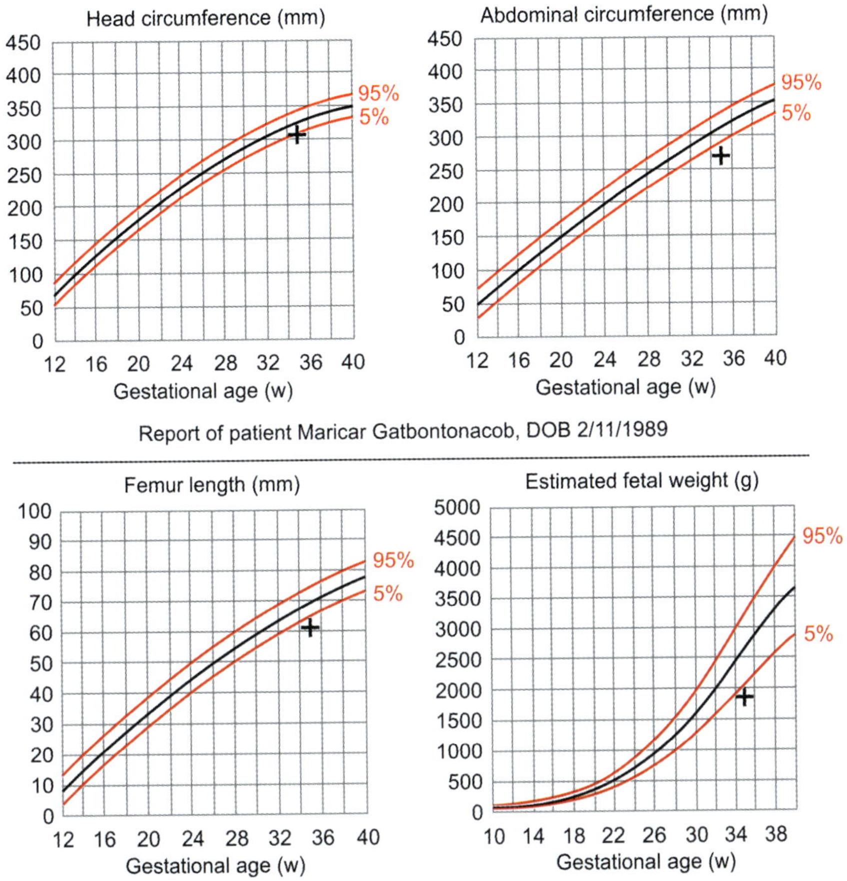

Figure 41.1: Comparison of head and abdominal circumference, femur length and estimated fetal weight indicate an asymmetric intrauterine growth restriction

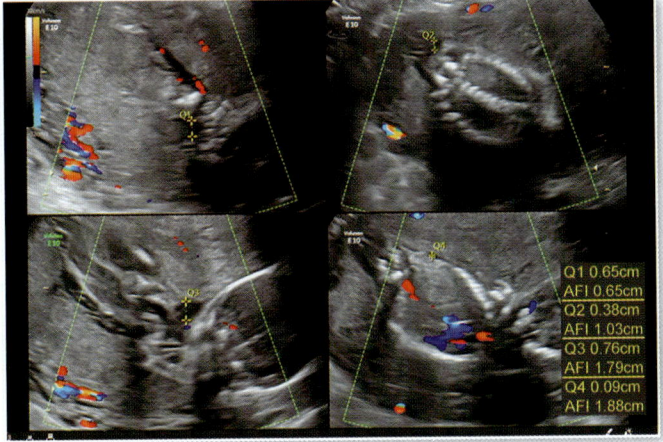

Figure 41.2: Color Doppler image of the same patient indicating severe oligohydramnios

- *Allergies*: No known drug allergies
- *Social history*: She does not smoke, no drug use, no alcohol use
- *Family history*: Non-contributory

Physical Examination

- *Vital signs:* T36.8°C oral, BP 128/74, P 78
- *Cardiac examination:* Regular rate and rhythm, no heart murmur
- *Chest examination:* Lungs clear to auscultation bilaterally
- *Abdomen:* Fundus below umbilicus, non-tender. Fetal heart tones auscultated at 156 beats per minute.

■ CLINICAL QUESTIONS

1. How is amniotic fluid made?

Ans. Fetal kidneys start making amniotic fluid at the end of the first trimester and its production continues until term gestation, representing the main source of amniotic fluid.[1] Fetal lungs also produce fluid that exit the mouth and is added to the amniotic fluid volume. The fluid flowing into and out of the amniotic sac ultimately determines the amniotic fluid volume.[2,3]

2. What are the common causes of oligohydramnios?

Ans. The majority of women with oligohydramnios or borderline/low normal amniotic fluid volume have no identifiable cause. The most likely etiologies of oligohydramnios vary according to the trimester in which it is diagnosed. In early second trimester oligohydramnios generally reflects a fetal or placental abnormality. In patients with oligohydramnios, a detailed patient history should be obtained and rupture of membranes should always be excluded. When oligohydramnios is diagnosed in late second or in the third trimester, it more likely is associated with rupture of membranes, fetal-growth restriction, a placental abnormality, or a maternal complication. Oligohydramnios has also been associated with exposure to drugs that block the renin–angiotensin system.

3. What is the role of the amniotic fluid?

Ans. Amniotic fluid is necessary for the proper development of the gastrointestinal tract, lungs and musculoskeletal systems. Amniotic fluid guards against umbilical cord compression and protects the fetus from trauma. Early onset oligohydramnios is associated with anatomical and functional abnormalities, such as skeletal deformations, contractures and pulmonary hypoplasia.[3,4]

4. What tests should be performed in a patient with oligohydramnios?

Ans. First of all, rupture of membranes should be ruled out. The patient should be questioned for any history consistent with rupture of membranes, leakage of fluid or wetness of the underwear. Sterile speculum examination should be performed to obtain fluid that can be investigated for evidence of rupture. Target ultrasound should assess fetal anatomy, determine the amount of amniotic fluid, and examine the interval growth. Umbilical artery Doppler is indicated when growth restriction is identified.

5. How amniotic fluid index (AFI) is performed and what is the sonographic diagnosis of oligohydramnios?

Ans. To determine the AFI the uterus is divided into four imaginary quadrants using linea nigra and umbilicus as the vertical and horizontal axis. The deepest pocket not including fetal parts and umbilical cord is measured in the vertical dimension. Measurement of the four pockets in centimeters is summed up and AFI is expressed. Normal AFI values range from 5-25 cm. AFI lower than 5 cm is considered as oligohydramnios, while AFI exceeding 25 cm are considered as polyhydramnios.[4]

6. What is the management of a pregnancy complicated by oligohydramnios?

Ans. The fetal/neonatal prognosis depends on the cause, severity, gestational age at onset and duration of oligohydramnios. In the first trimester, reduced amniotic fluid appears to be an ominous finding and pregnancy generally aborts. In the second trimester prognosis and management depend upon the underlying etiology and severity. Before 36 weeks, expectant management with increased fetal surveillance can be considered if normal fetal anatomy and growth are observed. When there is evidence of fetal or maternal compromise, delivery may be indicated overriding the potential complications from preterm delivery. Given the potential high risk of adverse outcome, in pregnancies at term with oligohydramnios delivery is indicated.

■ TAKE-HOME MESSAGES

- Fetal urine is the main source of amniotic fluid. Fetal kidneys begin to make urine before the end of the first trimester. Throughout gestation, the fetal lung produces fluid that is either swallowed, or leaves the mount, and enters the amniotic compartment adding to the fluid volume.[1,2]
- Amniotic fluid permits fetal swallowing which is essential for gastrointestinal tract development and fetal breathing, necessary for lung development.[3]
- An adequate volume of amniotic fluid guards against umbilical cord compression and protects the fetus from trauma. Also creates physical space, allowing normal fetal growth and movement, which are critical for normal musculoskeletal development.[3]
- The sonographic diagnosis of oligohydramnios is usually based on an amniotic fluid index (AFI) ≤5 cm or on a single deepest pocket of amnionic fluid ≤2 cm.[4]
- The term borderline AFI or borderline oligohydramnios is somewhat controversial. It usually refers to AFIs between 5 and 8 cm.[5]
- The term *anhydramnios* is used when no measurable pocket of amniotic fluid is identified. The incidence of oligohydramnios varies depending on which definition is used, with a general reporting rate of 1–3% and a much higher incidence (19–20%) reported in pregnancies with high-risk conditions.[1]
- When oligohydramnios is identified, rupture of membranes should be excluded. Common symptoms are: leakage of fluid, vaginal bleeding or uterine contractions.[3]
- Noninvasive tests performed to diagnose rupture of membranes include examining for microscopic ferning, checking for a neutral pH on nitrazine paper, looking pooling in the posterior vagina and Amniosure test.[6,7]
- Early-onset (from early second trimester) oligohydramnios is generally caused by impaired placental perfusion or a fetal abnormality that prevents normal urination. Evaluation includes targeted sonography to assess for fetal abnormalities (e.g. renal agenesis or polycystic kidneys).[3]
- When decreased amnionic fluid is first identified before the mid-second trimester, pulmonary hypoplasia is a significant concern with a perinatal, mortality rates approaching 100%.[1,3]

- Oligohydramnios in the late second or third trimester is commonly the result of conditions associated with uteroplacental insufficiency causing impaired fetal growth and reduced fetal urine production, including fetal–growth restriction, placental abnormalities, or maternal complications, such as preeclampsia or vascular disease.[1,3]
- Investigation of third-trimester oligohydramnios generally includes evaluation to rule out rupture of membranes, sonography to assess growth and umbilical artery Doppler studies, if growth restriction is identified.[3]
- Amniotic fluid volume decreases by approximately 8% per week beyond 40 weeks. Oligohydramnios is commonly identified in *postterm* pregnancies and has been associated with nonreassuring fetal heart rate patterns and adverse pregnancy outcomes.[5]
- Also, there are *indirect causes* of oligohydramnios resulting from other organ systems anomalies, aneuploidy, and other genetic syndromes.[3]
- Selected renal abnormalities that lead to absent fetal urine production include bilateral *renal agenesis*, bilateral *multicystic dysplastic kidney,* unilateral renal agenesis with contralateral multicystic dysplastic kidney, and the infantile form of *autosomal recessive polycystic kidney disease.* [3] The following fetal abnormalities cause oligohydramnios secondary to fetal bladder outlet obstruction: *posterior urethral valves, urethral atresia* or *stenosis*, or the *megacystis microcolon intestinal hypoperistalsis syndrome*.[3]
- Oligohydramnios has been associated with exposure to drugs that block the renin–angiotensin system, including angiotensin-converting enzyme (ACE) inhibitors creating hypotension, renal hypoperfusion and ischemia, with subsequent anuric renal failure; and nonsteroidal anti-inflammatory drugs (NSAIDs) associated with fetal ductus arteriosus constriction and with decreased fetal urine production.[8,9]
- Oligohydramnios is associated with higher rates of fetal stillbirth, growth restriction, nonreassuring heart rate pattern, meconium aspiration syndrome, spontaneous or medically indicated preterm birth, cesarean delivery for fetal distress and a fivefold risk for an Apgar score <7 at 5 minutes, even in the absence of fetal abnormalities.[1,5,10]
- Pregnancies <36 weeks with normal fetal anatomy and growth complicated with oligohydramnios should be managed expectantly. In cases with evidence of fetal or maternal compromise, delivery is planned depending on the underlying etiology.[3,6,7]

REFERENCES

1. Gabbe SG Obstetrics: Normal and problem pregnancies (Sixth edition.). Philadelphia, PA: Elsevier/Saunders; 2012.
2. American College of Obstetricians and Gynecologists: Ultrasonography in pregnancy. Practice Bulletin No. 101, February 2009, Reaffirmed 2011.
3. Cunningham F. Gary. Williams Obstetrics. 24th edition. New York: McGraw-Hill Education; 2014.
4. Magann EF, Bass JD, Chauhan SP, et al. Amniotic fluid volume in normal singleton pregnancies. Obstet Gynecol. 1997; 90(4):524-8.
5. Petrozella LN, Dashe JS, McIntire DD, et al. Clinical significance of borderline amniotic fluid index and oligohydramnios in preterm pregnancy. Obstet Gynecol. 2011;117(2):338, 2011.
6. American College of Obstetricians and Gynecologists: Premature Rupture of Membranes, Practice Bulletin No. 160, January 2016.
7. American College of Obstetricians and Gynecologists: Antepartum fetal Surveillance, Practice Bulletin No. 9, October 1999, Reaffirmed 2012.
8. Guron G, Friberg P. An intact renin-angiotensin system is a prerequisite for normal renal development. J Hypertens 2000; 18(2):123-37.
9. Bullo M, Tschumi S, Bucher BS. Pregnancy outcome following exposure to angiotensin-converting enzyme inhibitors or angiotensin receptor antagonists: a systematic review. Hypertension. 2012; 60:444-50.
10. Chauhan SP, Sanderson M, Hendrix NW, et al: Perinatal outcome and amniotic fluid index in the antepartum and intrapartum periods: a meta-analysis. Am J Obstet Gynecol. 1999;181(6):1473-8.

CHAPTER 42

Placenta Previa

Melissa D Mendez

■ CLINICAL CASE

SL is a 31-year-old G2P1 at 36 weeks gestation by LMP and 15 weeks ultrasound who presents to OB triage complaining of leaking of fluid and vaginal bleeding. She is also complaining of some cramping that woke her early this morning. She had good prenatal care with you and she is aware that she was diagnosed with a placenta previa at 20 weeks. The fetal heart rate tracing is reassuring.

Menarche: Age 10.

Menses: 28/4.

LMP: 38 weeks ago.

Pregnancy: Her first pregnancy was 2 years ago; she had a CS at term for breech presentation.

Sexual history: In a monogamous relationship with her husband of 7 years. No history of sexually transmitted diseases.

Contraception: Previously used a copper intrauterine device (IUD).

Review of Systems

- No chest pain or shortness of breath
- No diarrhea or constipation
- No urinary frequency, no hematuria or dysuria
- She has good fetal movement, no contractions, but has leaking of bloody fluid
- *Past medical history:* A1 gestational diabetes—good control on diet only
- *Past surgical history:* One previous CS as above
- *Vaccines:* Up to date
- *Current medications:* Prenatal vitamins and calcium.
- *Allergies:* No known drug allergies
- *Social history:* She does not smoke, no drug use, has occasional alcohol intake on weekends, but not during her pregnancy. She is a stay at home mom
- *Family history:* Noncontributory

Physical Examination

- *Vital signs*: T37.1°C oral, BP 110/60, P 85, BMI 28
- *Cardiac examination*: Regular rate and rhythm, no heart murmur
- *Chest examination*: Lungs clear to auscultation bilaterally
- *Abdomen*: Non-distended, non-tender. Fetal heart tones 150 beats per minute
- *Pelvic examination*: Cervical os appears closed on speculum examination. There is bright red blood in the vault
- You suspect bleeding from the placenta previa. A transvaginal ultrasound reveals a closed cervix with the placenta completely covering the internal cervical os as seen in Figure 42.1.

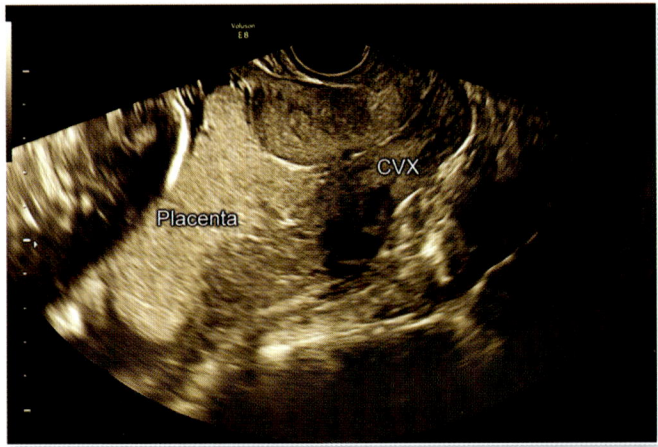

Figure 42.1: Transvaginal ultrasound shows a closed cervical os completely covered by the placenta

■ CLINICAL QUESTIONS

1. How often does a placenta previa occur?

Ans. Placenta previa is defined as a placenta that covers the endocervical os. If the placenta is near the cervical os, within 2 cm but not overlying the cervical os, this is called a low-lying placenta. Placenta previa occurs in approximately 1 in 200 pregnancies.[1] The incidence is increased with CS, any other uterine surgeries, previous pregnancy terminations and/or spontaneous abortions.[1] Approximately 80–90% of all placenta previa cases diagnosed at 20 weeks will resolve by the late third trimester, as the placenta "moves away" from the cervix.[2]

2. How do you diagnose a placenta previa?

Ans. Most women in the United States undergo routine screening for placental location using transabdominal ultrasonography. This is typically done at the mid-trimester anatomy scan. In cases where the placenta is suspicious to be low-lying or a previa, the patient should undergo a transvaginal ultrasound. Transvaginal ultrasound can be repeated in the late third trimester to confirm placental location.[3-5] Low-lying placentas found in mid-trimester resolve by 32 weeks in 90% of cases.[6]

3. What are some of the complications that can occur with a placenta previa?

Ans. Women with a placenta previa are at an increased risk for antepartum vaginal bleeding. This may be due to the placenta separating from the underlying decidua resulting from contractions or cervical effacement and dilation.[6] The vaginal bleeding may increase the need for a maternal blood transfusion, hysterectomy, intensive care admission, septicemia and even maternal death. Fetal complications include premature birth and small for gestational age.[7]

4. How do you clinically manage a placenta previa?

Ans. If the placenta is found to be 2 cm away from the os in the third trimester, or low-lying, then the woman can have a trial of labor. If there continues to be a placenta previa, the optimal treatment is a CS.[8,9] Stable patients with a placenta previa may be delivered after 36 weeks with no prior amniocentesis. Unstable patients may warrant earlier delivery, depending on the amount of significant bleeding.[10,11]

■ TAKE-HOME MESSAGES

- Placenta previa is defined as a placenta that covers the endocervical os.[1]
- A low-lying placenta is defined as a placenta that is within 2 cm of the cervical os.[1]
- The incidence is increased with CS, any other uterine surgeries, previous pregnancy terminations and/or spontaneous abortions.[1]
- Transabdominal ultrasound may be used to screen women for placenta previa and transvaginal ultrasound is used to confirm the diagnosis.[3]
- Maternal complications from a placenta previa may include vaginal bleeding, maternal blood transfusion, hysterectomy, intensive care admission, septicemia and even maternal death.[6]
- Fetal complications include premature birth and small for gestational age.[7]
- Stable patients with a placenta previa may be delivered after 36 weeks with no prior amniocentesis.[11]
- Unstable patients may warrant earlier delivery, depending on the amount of significant bleeding.[10,11]

■ REFERENCES

1. Silver RM. Abnormal Placentation. Clinical Expert Series. Obstet Gynecol. 2015;126(3):654-68.
2. Becker RH, Vonk R, Mende BC, Ragosh V, Entezami M. The relevance of placental location at 20–23 gestational weeks for the prediction of placenta previa at delivery: evaluation of placenta previa at delivery: evaluation of 8650 cases, Ultrasound Obstet Gynecol. 2001;17:496-501.
3. Quant HS, Friedman AM, Wang E, Parry S, Schwartz N. Transabdominal ultrasonography as a screening test for second-trimester placenta previa. Obstet Gynecol. 2014;123:628-33.
4. Robinson AJ, Muller PR, Allen R, Ross R, Baghurst PA, Keirse MJNC. Precise mid-trimester placental localization: Does it predict adverse outcomes? ANZOG. 2012;52(2):156-60.
5. Kapoor S, Thomas JT, Peterson SG, Gardener GJ. Is the third trimester repeat ultrasound for placental localization needed if the placenta is low lying but clear of the os at mid-trimester morphology scan? ANZJOG. 2014;54(5):428-32.
6. Heller HT, Mullen KM, Gordon RW, Reiss RE, Benson CB. Outcomes of pregnancies with a low-lying placenta diagnosed on second-trimester sonography. J Ultrasound Med. 2014;33:691-6.
7. Raisanen S, Kancheria V, Kramer MR, Gissler M, Heinonen S. Placenta previa and the risk of delivering a small-for-gestational age newborn. Obstet Gynecol. 2014;124(2):285-91.
8. Rao KP, Belogolovkin V, Yankowitz J, Spinnato JA. Abnormal Placentation: Evidence—based diagnosis and management of placenta previa, placenta accreta, and vasa previa. Obstetrical and Gynecology Survey. 2012;67(8):503-19.
9. Fitzpatrick KE, Sellers S, Spark P, Kurinczuk JJ, Brocklehurst P, Knight M. The management and outcomes of placenta accreta, increta, and percreta in the UK: a population-based descriptive study BJOG. 2014;121(1):62-7.
10. Blackwell SC. Timing of delivery for women with stable placenta previa. Semin Perinatology. 2011;35:249-51.
11. American College of Obstetricians and Gynecologists. Medically indicated late-preterm and early term deliveries. Committee opinion No.560. Obstet Gynecol. 2013;121:908-10.

CHAPTER 43

Placenta Percreta

Melissa D Mendez, Shaked Laks, Osvaldo Padilla, Sanja Kupesic Plavsic

CLINICAL CASE

JM is a 30-year-old G3P1 at 26 weeks gestation by her LMP and a 19 week ultrasound. She presents to OB triage for cramping and vaginal bleeding. She states the cramping woke her up early this morning and when she went to the restroom she noted some vaginal bleeding and a small clot. She denies nausea, vomiting, constipation, or diarrhea. She feels the baby moving. She denies leaking of fluid.

Menarche: Age 11.

Menses: 30/5.

LMP: 28 weeks ago.

Pregnancy: Her previous baby was born 2 years ago at 41 weeks via low transverse CS for failed induction of labor. There were no complications and the baby weighed 3,805 g.

Sexual history: In a monogamous relationship with her husband of 10 years. No history of sexually transmitted diseases.

Contraception: None.

Review of Systems

- No chest pain or shortness of breath
- No diarrhea or constipation
- No urinary frequency, no hematuria or dysuria
- *Past medical history*: Noncontributory
- *Past surgical history*: None
- *Vaccines*: Up-to-date
- *Current medications*: Prenatal vitamins, iron sulfate
- *Allergies*: No known drug allergies

- *Social history*: She does not smoke, no drug use, has occasional alcohol intake on weekends
- *Family history*: Noncontributory.

Physical Examination

- *Vital signs*: Temperature 37.2°C oral, BP 110/55, P 75
- *Cardiac examination*: Regular rate and rhythm, no heart murmur
- *Chest examination*: Lungs clear to auscultation bilaterally
- *Abdomen*: Non tender, fetal heart tones are 140 beats per minute
- *Pelvic examination*: On speculum examination, you see scant bright red blood in the vaginal vault, no clots. Bleeding appears to be coming from the os and the os appears closed. You do not perform a cervical examination as the patient has a known placenta previa, which was noted on her previous ultrasound
- Pelvic ultrasound images are presented in Figures 43.1 to 43.4. Figure 43.1 shows the patient's cervix with the placenta covering the entire internal os, which is known as a placenta previa. Figure 43.2 shows color Doppler ultrasound of the placenta extending upward to the anterior wall. There are few vascular lacunae noted. However, since the patient has a previous CS and now has placenta previa she should be further screened with an MRI for placenta accreta or percreta. Figure 43.3. shows the MRI image of a placenta percreta.
- The patient underwent a cesarean hysterectomy at 36 weeks gestation. Figures 43.4 and 43.5 show gross specimen of the uterus with placenta extended to the outer serosal surface of the uterus.

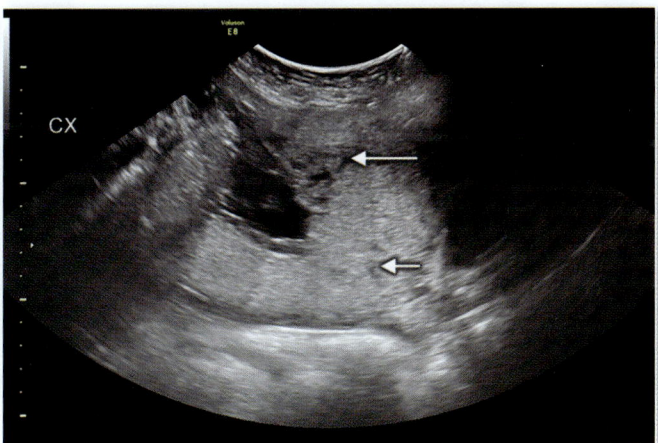

Figure 43.1: Transabdominal ultrasound demonstrates the placenta (long arrow) fully covering the cervical os (short arrow) consistent with placenta previa. A finding of placenta previa should elicit a detailed evaluation of placenta accreta, including color Doppler imaging. Note multiple tortuous hypoechoic structures within the placenta

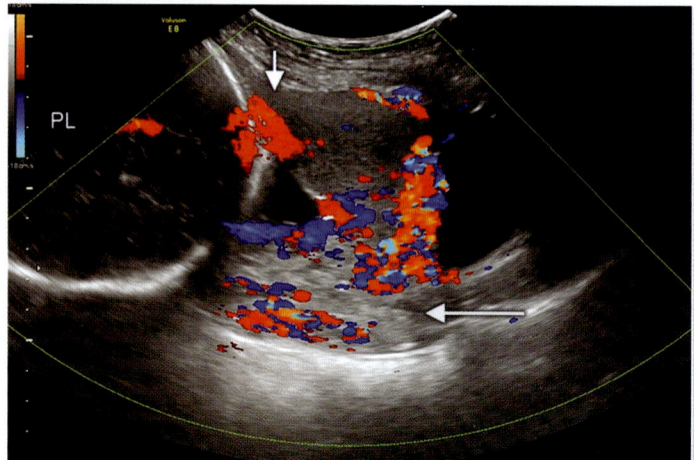

Figure 43.2: Transabdominal color Doppler ultrasound demonstrates the placenta covering the cervical os (long arrow), and extending over the anterior uterine wall, to the level of the cesarean section scar (short arrow). Color Doppler confirms that the hypoechoic areas are vascular, and therefore represent placental lacunae. Note that placenta is extending to the bladder margin without any intervening myometrium. You are concerned about a placenta accrete and order an MRI

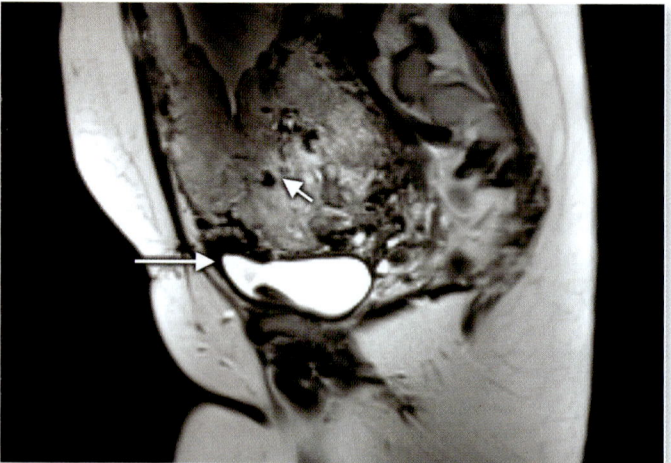

Figure 43.3: T2-weighted image shows a hyperintense heterogeneous placenta with multiple T2 hypointense bands (short arrow). There is interruption of the myometrial junctional zone adjacent to the bladder, which is suspicious for placenta accrete or in this case, a placenta percreta (long arrow).

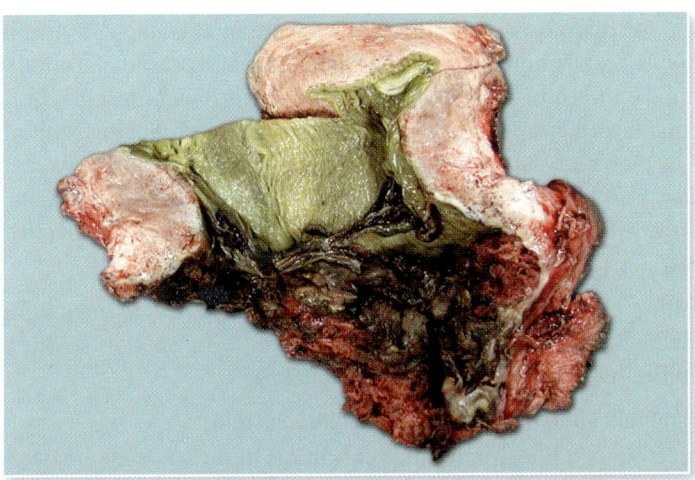

Figure 43.4: The image above shows abnormal attachment of the placenta into the lower uterus, which was proven to demonstrate microscopic penetration of chorionic villi that involved the uterine serosal lining

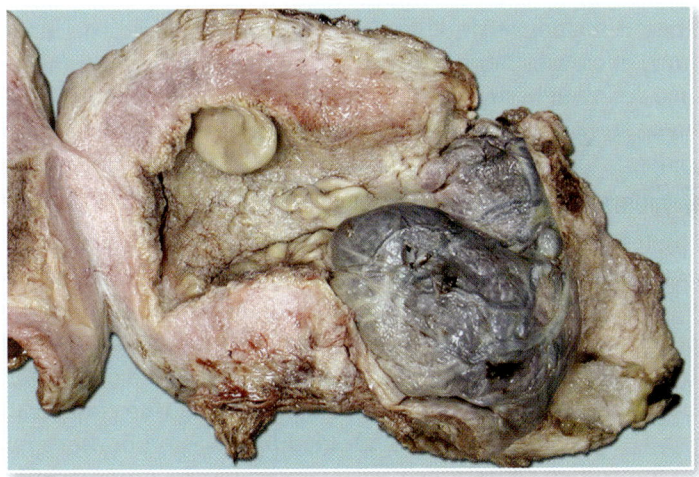

Figure 43.5: Abnormal placental attachment is identified into the lower uterus, and visual extension of the placenta appears to extend to the outer serosal lining

CLINICAL QUESTIONS

1. What is the best modality to diagnose placenta accreta?
Ans. Pelvic ultrasound characteristics that are associated with a placenta accreta are placental lacunae, loss of the retroplacental clear space, an irregular bladder wall and color Doppler abnormalities.[1] Both ultrasound and MRI have a high rate of sensitivity and specificity.

MRI is used for diagnosis when ultrasound is inconclusive. MRI findings may include heterogeneous signal intensity within the placenta or increased placental vascularity, dark, intraplacental bands on T2 weighted image, a bulging lower uterine segment, interruption of the normal layered appearance of the myometrium, direct invasion of adjacent pelvic structures by placental tissue, and tenting of the urinary bladder. In a recent meta-analysis ultrasound was found to have 83% sensitivity and 95% specificity for diagnosis of placenta accreta, while MRI had an 82% sensitivity and 88% specificity, respectively.[2,3]

2. What are the risk factors for placenta accreta?

Ans. Women with a prior cesarean delivery and placenta previa have a high incidence of placenta accreta/percreta.[4] The risk is also increased in patients with previous uterine surgery, an IVF pregnancy, and older maternal age.

3. What are common complications from placenta accreta?

Ans. Placenta accreta is a life-threatening condition that can cause heavy vaginal bleeding after delivery, commonly leading to disseminated intravascular coagulopathy (DIC), adult respiratory distress syndrome and kidney failure. Another possible complication is premature delivery and premature rupture of membranes (PROM).[5]

4. When should a patient with placenta accreta or percreta be delivered?

Ans. Women were less likely to have complications, if they were diagnosed antenatally. This allows for the formulation of a multiprofessional team for surgical discussion and planning which in-turn decreases hemorrhage and the need for blood transfusion.[6,7] Delivery with planned cesarean hysterectomy is recommended between 34 weeks and 37 weeks. Amniocentesis for fetal lung maturity prior to planned delivery does not seem to have any benefit.

5. What is the optimal treatment for placenta accreta?

Ans. Cesarean hysterectomy is the recommended treatment for placenta accreta. Cesarean hysterectomy carries a risk of about 50% to require a blood transfusion and admission to the intensive care unit. This increases the risk of obstetrical hemorrhage and blood transfusion.[7,8] One series reported an average of 5 units packed red blood cells per cesarean hysterectomy. These women are also at an increased risk for genitourinary tract complications, such as ureteral and bladder injuries, febrile complications and bowel dysfunction. For placenta percreta with bladder invasion or other morbid placental invasion, or for women who strongly wish to preserve their uterus for future pregnancy and who agree to close follow-up monitoring, conservative treatment with methotrexate is a valid option.[8]

■ TAKE-HOME MESSAGES

- Abnormal placentation can be classified as placenta accreta when the chorionic villi attach to the myometrium, placenta increta when the villi invade the myometrium, and placenta percreta when the villi invade through the myometrium.[1,2]
- The most common site of attachment of the placenta outside the uterus is the urinary bladder.[1,2]
- Placenta previa and history of a prior cesarean delivery or other procedures that can cause a uterine scar remain the most important predictors of placenta accreta.[1]

- In a recent meta-analysis ultrasound was found to have 83% sensitivity and 95% specificity for diagnosis of placenta accreta, while MRI had an 82% sensitivity and 88% specificity respectively.[2]
- MRI is used for diagnosis when ultrasound is inconclusive.[2] MRI findings may include heterogeneous signal intensity within the placenta or increased placental vascularity, dark, intraplacental bands on T2 weighted image, a bulging lower uterine segment, interruption of the normal layered appearance of the myometrium, direct invasion of adjacent pelvic structures by placental tissue, and tenting of the urinary bladder.[2,3]
- Conservative treatment for women with morbidly adherent placenta includes delivery of the fetus, closure of the uterus and returning the uterus to the pelvis. The patient is then treated with uterine artery embolization or with methotrexate therapy. Small study series have been reported with women who undergo conservative therapy with complete resolution of placental tissue while others required a hysterectomy at a later time.[5-7] Conservative treatment is a valid option for women with placenta percreta with bladder invasion or other morbid placental invasion, or for women who strongly wish to preserve their uterus for future pregnancy and who agree to close follow-up monitoring.[8-10]
- Cesarean hysterectomy is the recommended treatment for placenta accreta.[8] It carries a high risk of blood transfusion, admission to the intensive care unit, an increased risk for genitourinary tract complications, such as ureteral and bladder injuries, febrile complications and bowel dysfunction.[5,8,10]
- Women are less likely to have complications, if they are diagnosed antenatally. This allows for the formulation of a multiprofessional team for surgical discussion and planning which in turn decreases hemorrhage and the need for blood transfusion.[6]
- Delivery with planned cesarean hysterectomy is recommended between 34 weeks 37 weeks.[8,9] There does not appear to be any benefit to amniocentesis for fetal lung maturity prior to planned delivery.[9]

REFERENCES

1. Bowman ZS, Eller AG, Kennedy AM, et al. Accuracy of ultrasound for the prediction of placenta accreta. Am J Obstet Gyneol. 2014;211(2):177.e1-7.
2. Srisajjakul S, Prapaisilp P, Bangchokdee S. MRI of placental adhesive disorder. Br J Radiol. 2014;87(1042):20140294.
3. Meng X, Xie L, Song W. Comparing the diagnostic value of ultrasound and magnetic resonance imaging for placenta accrete: a systematic review and meta-analysis. Ultrasound Med Biol. 2013;39(11): 1956-65.
4. Bowman ZS, Manuck TA, Eller AG, et al. Risk factors for unscheduled delivery in patients with placenta accreta. Am J Obstet Gynecol. 2014;210(3):241.e1-6.
5. Perez-Delboy A, Wright JD. Surgical management of placenta accreta: to leave or remove the placenta? BJOG. 2014;121(2):163-9.
6. KE Fitzpatrick, S Sellers, P Spark, et al. The management and outcomes of placenta accreta, increta, and percreta in the UK: a population-based descriptive study. BJOG. 2014;121(1):62-70.
7. Clausen C, Lonn L, Langhoff-Roos J. Management of placenta percreta: a review of published cases. Acta Obstet Gynecol Scand. 2014; 93(2):138-43.
8. Sentilhes L, Goffinet F, Kayem G. Management of placenta accreta. Acta Obstet Gynecol Scand. 2013;92(10):1125-34.
9. Robinson BK, Grobman WA. Effectiveness of timing strategies for delivery of individuals with placenta percreta and accreta. Obstet Gynecol. 2010;116(4): 835-42.
10. Bailit JL, Grobman WA, Rice MM, et al. Morbidly adherent placenta treatments and outcomes. Obstet Gynecol. 2015;125(3): 683-9.

CHAPTER

Fetal Malpresentation

44

Melissa D Mendez

■ CLINICAL CASE

MJ is a 27-year-old G2P1 at 37 weeks and 1 day by LMP and 10 week ultrasound. She had a previous spontaneous vaginal delivery (SVD) that was uncomplicated. Her first baby is now 3 years old. Her current pregnancy has been uncomplicated. However, you have noted that she is persistent breech presentation. Yesterday, in clinic, you counseled your patient on the risks, benefits and indications of a version procedure. She elected to proceed with the version in order to have another vaginal delivery. You have her admitted to obstetric triage to utilize the ultrasound room to proceed with the version. You confirm the breech presentation with transabdominal ultrasound as shown in Figure 44.1.

Menarche: Age 13.

Menses: Every 32 days, lasting 6 days.

Pregnancy: One previous SVD full term, no complications. No complications with this current pregnancy except persistent breech presentation.

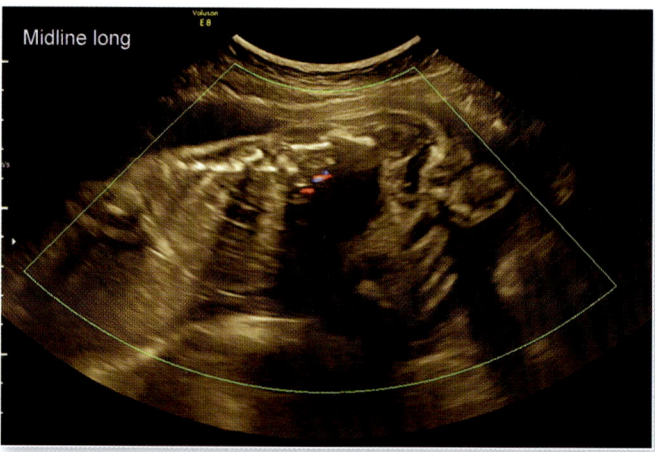

Figure 44.1: Transabdominal ultrasound demonstrating the lower uterine segment and cervical os and the breech presenting parts

Sexual history: In a monogamous relationship. No history of sexually transmitted diseases.

Contraception: None.

Review of Systems

- No chest pain or shortness of breath
- No diarrhea or constipation
- No urinary frequency, no hematuria or dysuria
- No headaches, visual changes or right upper quadrant pain

- *Past medical history*: Noncontributory
- *Past surgical history*: None
- *Vaccines*: Up-to-date
- *Current medications*: Prenatal vitamins
- *Allergies*: History of rash with penicillin
- *Social history*: She does not smoke; no drug use, and no alcohol
- *Family history*: Mother with history of heart attack at age 55. Father 60 years old with diabetes type II.

Physical Examination

- *Vital signs*: Temperature 37.0°C oral, BP 110/65, P 75, BMI 26
- *General*: Pleasant, well groomed, alert and oriented times three
- *Cardiac examination*: Regular rate and rhythm, no heart murmur
- *Chest examination*: Lungs clear to auscultation bilaterally
- *Abdomen*: Non-distended, non-tender. Fetal heart tones 130 sec baseline reassuring
- *Pelvic examination*: 1 cm dilated/thick/and high.

■ CLINICAL QUESTIONS

1. **What are the risk factors for having a fetus with malpresentation?**

Ans. Breech presentation is persistent at term in about 3–4% pregnancies.[1] Risk factors include multifetal gestation, fundal placenta, pelvic tumors and prior breech presentation. Uterine anomalies also increase the rate the malpresentation at term. Uterine anomalies may be caused by abnormal fusion or resorption of the Müllerian ducts and can occur in up to 10% of the population.[1] After the Term Breech Trial, ACOG recommended planned CS for delivery for persistent breech presentation.

2. **What are the indications for an external cephalic version?**

Ans. An external cephalic version is an obstetrical procedure that maneuvers the breech fetus into a cephalic presentation through the maternal gravid uterus. The fetus should be 36–37 weeks with a persistent malpresentation. The timing of an external cephalic version should be balanced against the risk for preterm labor.[3,4] The reported success rate is between 35% and 85%, with an average of 58%. There are higher success rates in women who are nonobese, multiparous, with abundant amniotic fluid index (AFI) and unengaged presenting part. A version is contraindicated in women in whom vaginal delivery is not an option, patients with uterine malformation, multifetal pregnancy, women who have ruptured membranes, placenta previa, and non-reassuring fetal status. A previous uterine scar is not a contraindication for cephalic version. A recent prospective cohort assessing 1,500 patients over 10 years found no difference in success rate between previous CS and no CS scar.[4]

3. **What are the risks associated with an external cephalic version?**

Ans. Patients should be counseled about the risks associated with a version. These include placental abruption, uterine rupture, fetal compromise, fetomaternal hemorrhage, and emergent CS rates in 0.5 %.[4] Even if successful, these pregnancies still have a higher rate of CS for dystocia, malpresentation, and non-reassuring fetal heart tracings.

4. **Are there any techniques that may increase the chances for a successful external cephalic version?**

Ans. For an external cephalic version, you may consider using the following tocolytics, epidural, and nitrous oxide. There may be a higher success rate for external cephalic version, if attempted with epidural anesthesia.[5-7] Tocolytics, such as betamimetics (turbultaline) and calcium-channel blockers (nifedipine) have shown no proven benefits for preterm labor or for the CS over placebo.[7,8]

5. **Do women want an external cephalic version?**

Ans. Studies have shown that women who undergo an external cephalic version do, hoping that it will be successful and allow them to obtain a vaginal delivery.[9] The majority of patients report satisfaction and would recommend the procedure to others.[10] Some women may also try alternative methods, such as moxibustion, acupuncture and yoga poses. None of these methods have been shown to increase the rates of a cephalic presentation.[11]

■ TAKE-HOME MESSAGES

- Breech presentation is persistent at term in about 3–4% pregnancies.[1]
- Risk factors include multifetal gestation, fundal placenta, uterine anomalies, pelvic tumors and prior breech delivery.[1]
- After the Term Breech Trial, ACOG recommended planned CS for delivery for persistent breech presentation, although subsequent studies demonstrated no difference in intelligence at 2 years of age.[1]
- Indications for version procedure are 35–37 weeks gestation, breech or transverse presentation, with no contraindications.[2]
- A version has a success rate in 35–85%, with an average of 58%.[3,4]
- Higher success rates are noted with attempted version in women who are nonobese, multiparous and have an abundant AFI and an unengaged presenting part.[4]
- Contraindications to an external cephalic version include ruptured membranes, need for immediate delivery, placenta previa, non-reassuring fetal status, uterine malformation, and multifetal gestation.[4] A previous uterine scar is not a contraindication for an external cephalic version.
- Risks associated with version include placental abruption, uterine rupture, fetal compromise and fetomaternal hemorrhage.[4]
- An attempted external cephalic version may result in an emergent CS rates 0.5% of the time.[4]
- Even if successful, these pregnancies still have a higher rate of CS for dystocia, malpresentation and non-reassuring fetal heart tone tracing.[4]
- For a version, you may consider using the tocolytics, epidural, nitrous oxide.[5-7]

REFERENCES

1. Chan YY, Jayaprakasan K, Tan A, et al. Reproductive outcomes in women with congenital uterine anomalies:a systematic review. Ultrasound Obstet Gynecol. 2011;38(4):371-82.
2. Burgos J, Cobos P, Rodríguez L, et al. Is external cephalic version at term contraindicated in previous caesarean section? A prospective comparative cohort study. BJOG. 2014;121(2):230-5.
3. Khaw KS, Lee SW, Ngan Kee WD, et al. Randomized trial of anaesthetic interventions in external cephalic version for breech presentation. Br J Anaesth. 2015;114(6):944-50.
4. Hutton EK, Hannah ME, Ross SJ et al. The early external cephalic version (ECV) 2 trial: an international multicenter randomized controlled trial of timing of ECV for breech pregnancies. BJOG. 2011;118(5):564-77.
5. Weiniger CF. Analgesia/anesthesia for external cephalic version. Curr Opin Anesthesiol. 2013;26(3):278-87.
6. Cluver C, Gyte GM, Sinclair M, et al. Interventions for helping to turn term breech babies to head first presentation when using external cephalic version. Cochrane Database Syst Rev. 2015; 9;2:CD000184. doi: 10.1002/14651858.CD000184.pub4.
7. Wilcox CB, Nassar N, Roberts CL. Effectiveness of nifedipine tocolysis to facilitate external cephalic version: a systematic review. BJOG. 2011;118(4):423-8.
8. Theron GB, Kader R. Obstetric outcome after successful external cephalic version for breech presentation at term. Int J Gynaecol Obstet. 2014;127(3):298-9.
9. de Hundt M, Velzel J, de Groot CJ, et al. Mode of delivery after successful external cephalic version: a systematic review and metaanalysis. Obstet Gynecol. 2014;123(6):1327-34.
10. Bogner G, Hammer BE, Schausberger C. Patient satisfaction with childbirth after external cephalic version. Arch Gynecol Obstet. 2014;289(3):523-31.
11. Guittier M-J, Pichon M, Irion O, et al. Recourse to alternative medicine during pregnancy: motivations of women and impact of research findings. medicine Altern Complement Med. 2012;18(12):1147-53.

CHAPTER

Gestational Hypertensive Disorders

45

Melissa D Mendez, Sanja Kupesic Plavsic

■ CLINICAL CASE

MS is a 23-year-old G1P0 at 35 weeks by her LMP who presents to the clinic complaining of a headache. She describes the headache as severe, in the back of her head. Her headache resolved with Tylenol. She denies any visual problems or right upper quadrant pain. She has no contractions, no loss of fluid and she is able to feel the baby moving. Patient is alert and oriented at this time.

Menarche: Age 11.

Menses: 28/5.

LMP: 36 weeks ago.

Pregnancy: First pregnancy, no complications.

Sexual history: In a monogamous relationship with the father of the baby. She denies a history of sexually transmitted diseases.

Contraception: None.

Review of Systems

- No chest pain or shortness of breath
- No diarrhea or constipation
- No urinary frequency, no hematuria or dysuria

- *Past medical history:* Noncontributory
- *Past surgical history:* Noncontributory
- *Vaccines:* Up-to-date, including Tdap at 32 weeks gestation and the flu shot during the second trimester
- *Current medications:* Prenatal vitamins daily
- *Allergies:* No known drug allergies
- *Social history:* She does not smoke; no history of drug and/or alcohol use
- *Family history:* Noncontributory.

Physical Examination

- *Vital signs*: T37.2°C oral, BP 170/110, P 83, BMI 31
- *Cardiac examination*: Regular rate and rhythm, no heart murmur
- *Chest examination*: Lungs clear to auscultation bilaterally
- *Abdomen*: Non-distended, non-tender. Fetal heart tones cannot be auscultated
- *Extremities*: 2+ pitting edema, 2+ deep tendon reflexes
- *Sterile vaginal examination*: 2/50/–2
- *FHTs*: 120s positive accelerations, no decelerations, moderate variability
- *Tocometer*: Contractions every 20 minutes
- Ultrasound revealed intrauterine growth restriction. Doppler ultrasound was performed and findings are illustrated in Figures 45.1 to 45.5.
- After ultrasound was completed patient started complaining of epigastric and right upper quadrant pain and blurry vision. Blood pressure was obtained and nurse measured systolic blood pressure >200. The patient was immediately transferred to labor and delivery for induction of labor with oxytocin and anticipated delivery. The patient was found to have proteinuria with a protein to creatinine ratio of 0.85 and severe range blood pressures. She was given the diagnosis of pre-eclampsia with severe features.
- *Labor course*: Magnesium sulfate was given for seizure prophylaxis. The patient progressed to 5 cm dilatation at which point she requested an epidural. An amniotomy was performed after the epidural was placed and she progressed to 6 cm. Our patient did not progress past 6 cm despite adequate contractions assessed by internal intrauterine pressure catheter. She was taken to the operating room for a primary low-transverse cesarean section (LTCS) resulting in a delivery of 1,250 g male infant with Apgar scores 3,7; cord gases: 6.98 arterial and 6.95 venous. Patient received 24 hours of IV magnesium sulfate for postpartum seizure prophylaxis.

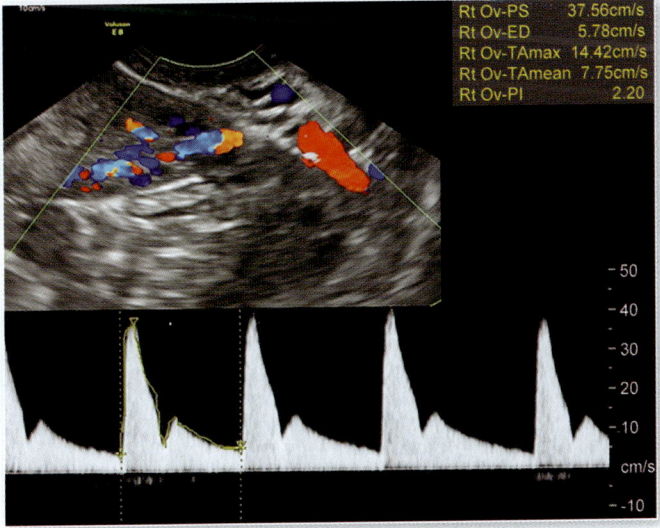

Figure 45.1: Uterine artery on the side of placenta revealed a prominent diastolic notch and elevated vascular resistance and pulsatility index (PI 2.20)

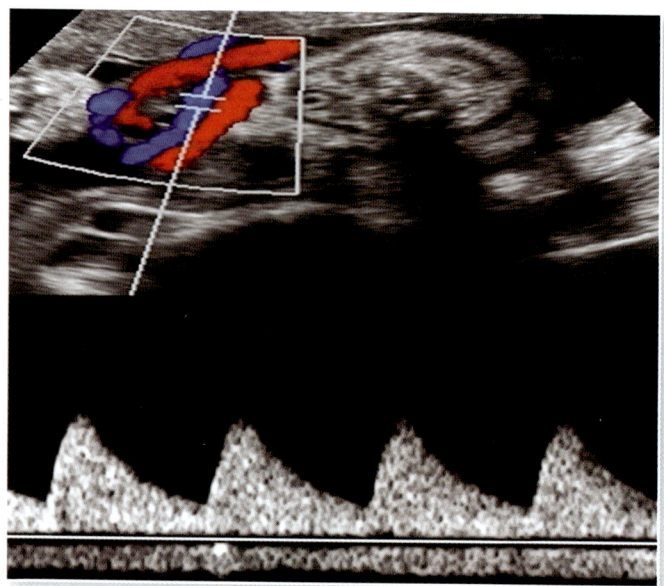

Figure 45.2: In normal pregnancy, the end-diastolic flow velocity in the umbilical artery increases in relation to the systolic velocity. This physiologic increase in diastolic blood flow reflects a reduction of peripheral vascular resistance due to increasing villous differentiation in the placenta. It is also caused by an increase in the vessels' caliber, increased cardiac output and compliance. Doppler waveform of the umbilical artery has a characteristic saw-tooth appearance of arterial flow in one direction and continuous umbilical venous blood flow in the other

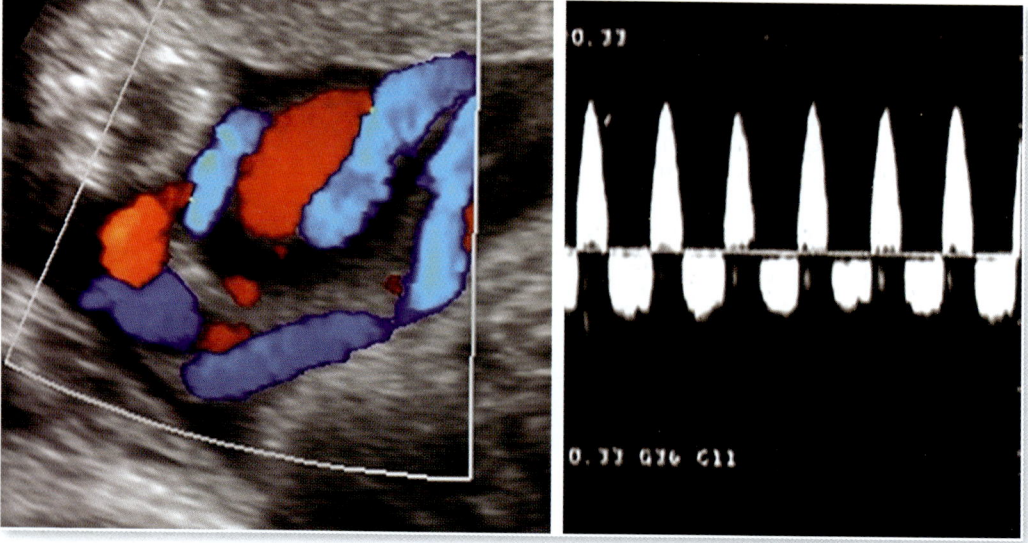

Figure 45.3: In our patient, umbilical artery Doppler shows absence and reversed diastolic velocity

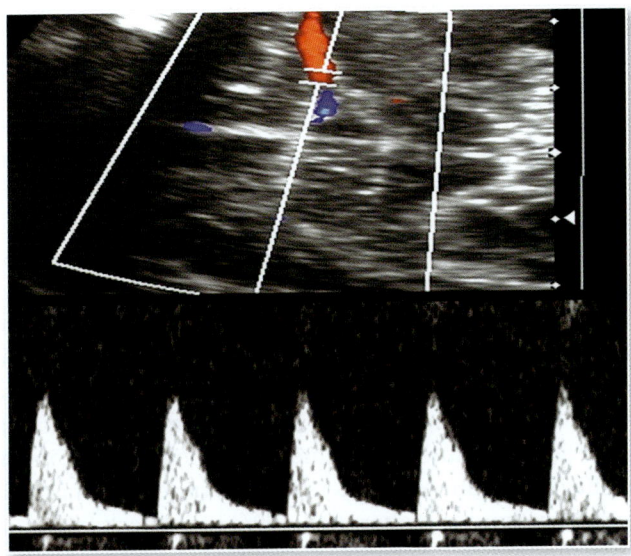

Figure 45.4: In normal pregnancy blood flow velocity signals obtained from the midpoint of the middle cerebral artery, approximately 1 cm from the circle of Willis are characterized by a sharp systolic upstroke followed by a steep postsystolic down stroke and a low end-diastolic component

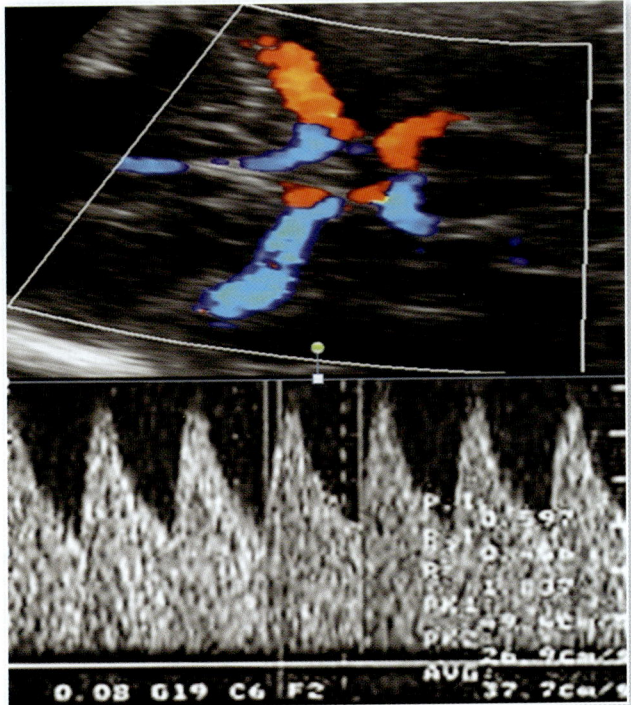

Figure 45.5: Increased diastolic flow velocities and decreased resistance index in the middle cerebral artery were noted in our patient. This phenomenon called brain-sparing effect is induced by hypoxemia, and involves a redistribution of the fetal blood in favor of the fetal brain

CLINICAL QUESTIONS

1. What are the definitions of hypertensive disorders of pregnancy?

Ans. There are four classifications of hypertensive disorders of pregnancy: (1) Chronic hypertension of any cause; (2) Chronic hypertension with superimposed pre-eclampsia; (3) Gestational hypertension occurring after 20 weeks gestation and consisting of elevated blood pressure 140/90 with no proteinuria and no severe features; (4) Pre-eclampsia without severe features, defined as blood pressure of greater than or equal to systolic 140 or diastolic 90 on two occasions and greater than 4 hours apart and proteinuria.[1] Proteinuria is defined as the excretion of 300 mg or more of protein on a 24-hour urine collection. Alternatively, proteinuria may be established by a urine protein to creatinine ratio of 0.3 or higher. Pre-eclampsia with severe features is defined as blood pressure greater or equal to systolic 160 or diastolic 110 on two occasions, at least four hours apart with proteinuria.[1] Severe features can include thrombocytopenia, impaired liver function tests, renal insufficiency, pulmonary edema or new onset cerebral or visual disturbances. Also, if the blood pressure is higher than 160/110 the task force recommends giving antihypertensive medications. Eclampsia is defined as new onset grand malseizures in a woman with pre-eclampsia.[1]

2. What are risk factors for developing pre-eclampsia?

Ans. Pre-eclampsia is usually seen in the extremes of ages: in the very young and very old gravidas. It can also be seen in pregestational diabetics, renal diseases, chronic hypertension and multiple gestations. Being overweight or obese also increases the risk of developing pre-eclampsia.[2]

3. How is preeclampsia treated?

Ans. Pre-eclampsia is primarily treated by delivery of the fetus. If the patient is greater than 37 weeks and pre-eclamptic, then you should deliver the patient. If the patient is 34–37 weeks and nonsevere, waiting until as close as possible to 37 weeks may increase maternal morbidity but may greatly reduce neonatal respiratory distress syndrome.[3] If the patient is preterm and stable, you can give antenatal corticosteroids and attempt to wait until at least 34 weeks. Delivery does not require a CS unless indicated for other reasons.[1,3]

Magnesium sulfate has been shown to decrease the risk of eclampsia as compared to phenytoin and probably reduces maternal death.[4] Magnesium sulfate is given as a 6 g IV bolus followed by 2 g/hour IV for seizure prophylaxis. Traditionally, magnesium sulfate is infused for 24 hours postpartum. There is some evidence that infusing for 6–12 hours in stable severe pre-eclampsia may have similar outcomes to infusing with 24 hours and be associated with less medication exposure and less side effects.[5,6] Postpartum women with blood pressures 150 mm Hg systolic or 100 mm Hg diastolic on two occasions taken four hours apart should be treated with antihypertensive medication.[7] Antihypertensive medications may include methyldopa, beta-blockers, slow-release nifedipine and diuretics as considered appropriate.[7]

4. Is there any way to predict or prevent pre-eclampsia?

Ans. Hypertensive disorders of pregnancy increase potentially life threatening conditions among maternal near-miss cases and maternal deaths during the intrapartum and postpartum period.[8] Later in life, these women may be at risk for chronic hypertension, cardiovascular heart disease and strokes.[9] Currently, there is no FDA approved labor imaging test that may accurately predict who will develop pre-eclampsia. Low-dose aspirin (81 mg) is indicated to prevent pre-eclampsia after 12 weeks gestation in women who are at high risk to develop pre-eclampsia.[10] According to the USPTF, women should be counseled on their increased risk for further hypertensive disorders and cardiovascular disease later in life.[11]

■ TAKE-HOME MESSAGES

- Pre-eclampsia without severe features is defined as blood pressure of greater than or equal to systolic 140 or diastolic 90 on two occasions and greater than 4 hours apart and proteinuria. Proteinuria is defined as the excretion of 300 mg or more of protein on a 24-hour urine collection. Alternatively, proteinuria may be established by a urine protein to creatinine ratio of 0.3 or higher.[1]
- Pre-eclampsia with severe features is defined as blood pressure greater or equal to systolic 160 or diastolic 110 mm Hg on two occasions, at least four hours apart with proteinuria. Severe features can include thrombocytopenia, impaired liver function tests, renal insufficiency, pulmonary edema or new onset cerebral or visual disturbances.[1]
- Risk factors for developing pre-eclampsia are: extremes of ages, obesity, pregestational diabetics, renal diseases, chronic hypertension and multiple gestations.[2]
- Preeclampsia is primarily treated by delivery of the fetus. The gestational age and the severity of the disease will determine when and how to deliver. This should be tailored to the individual patient.[3]
- Magnesium sulfate has been shown to decrease the risk of eclampsia as compared to phenytoin and probably reduces maternal death.[4]
- Postpartum women with blood pressures 150 mm Hg systolic or 100 mm Hg diastolic on two occasions taken four hours apart should be treated with antihypertensive medication which may include methyldopa, beta blockers, nifedipine and diuretics as appropriate.[7]
- Low-dose aspirin (81 mg) is indicated to prevent pre-eclampsia after 12 weeks gestation in women who are at high risk to develop pre-eclampsia.[10]
- Women with a history of pre-eclampsia are at increased risk for further hypertensive disorders and cardiovascular disease later in life.[11]
- Color Doppler velocimetry (measurement of vascular resistance, peak systolic velocity and assessment of notch) from the uterine, umbilical artery and middle cerebral artery can determine hemodynamic repercussion caused by gestational hypertensive disease.[12-15]

■ REFERENCES

1. American College of Obstetrics and Gynecology. The Task Force Report on Hypertension in Pregnancy. 2013;122(5):1122-31.
2. Paré E, Parry S, McElrath TF, Pucci D, Newton A, Lim KH. Clinical risk factors for pre-eclampsia in the 21st century. Obstet Gynecol. 2014;124(4):763-70.
3. Broekhuijsen K, van Baaren GJ, van Pampus MG, Ganzevoort W, Sikkema JM, Woiski MD, et al. Immediate delivery versus expectant monitoring for hypertensive disorders of pregnancy between 34–37 weeks of gestation (HYPITAT-II): an open-label, randomized controlled trial. Lancet. 2015;385(9986):2492-501.
4. Duley L, Gulmezoqlu AM, Henderson-Smart DJ, Chou D. Magnesium sulfate and other anticonvulsants for women with pre-eclampsia. Cochrane Database Syst Rev. 2010;(11):CD000025.
5. Maia SB, Katz L, Neto CN, Caiado BV, Azevedo AP, Amorim MM. Abbreviated (12-hour) versus traditional (24- hour) postpartum magnesium sulfate therapy in severe preeclampsia. Int J Gynaecol Obstet. 2014;126(3):260-4.
6. Darngawn L, Regi JR, Bansai R, Jeyaseeian L. A shortened postpartum magnesium sulfate prophylaxis in pre-eclamptic women at low risk of ecplamsia. Int J Gynaecol Obstet. 2012;116(3):237-9.
7. Brown CM, Garovic VD. Drug treatment of hypertension in pregnancy. Drugs. 2014;74(3):283-96.

8. Abalos E, Cuesta C, Carroli G, Qureshi Z, Widmer M, Vogel JP, et al. WHO Multicountry Survey on maternal and Newborn Health Research Network. Pre-eclampsia, eclampsia and adverse maternal and perinatal outcomes: a secondary analysis of the World Health Organization Multicountry Survey on Maternal and Newborn Health. BJOG. 2014;121 Suppl 1:14-24.
9. Bellamy L, Casas J, Hingorani AD, Williams DJ. Pre-eclampsia and risk of cardiovascular disease and cancer in later life: systematic review and meta-analysis. BMJ. 2007; online doi 10.1136/bmj.39335.385301.BE.
10. LeFevre ML and US Preventative Services Task Force. Low dose aspirin use for the prevention of morbidity and mortality from pre-eclampsia: US Preventive Services Task Force recommendation statement. Ann Intern Med. 2014;161(11):819-26.
11. Andersgaard AB, Acharya G, Mathiesen EB, Johnson SH, Straume B, Øian P. Recurrence and long-term maternal health risks of hypertensive disorders of pregnancy: A population-based study. Am J Obstet Gynecol. 2012;206(2):143.e1-143.e8.
12. Sibai B, Dekker G, Kupferminc M. Pre-eclampsia. Lancet. 2005;365:785-99.
13. Martin AM, Bindra R, Curcio P, et al. Screening for pre-eclampsia and fetal growth restriction by uterine artery Doppler at 11-14 weeks of gestation. Ultrasound Obstet Gynecol. 2001;18:583-6.
14. Gomez O, Martinez JM, Figueras F, et al. Uterine artery Doppler at 11–14 weeks of gestation to screen for hypertensive disorders and associated complications in an unselected population. Ultrasound Obstet Gynecol. 2005;26:490-4.
15. Papageorghiou AT, Yu CKH, Bindra R, et al. Multicentre screening for pre-eclampsia and fetal growth restriction by transvaginal uterine artery Doppler at 23 weeks of gestation. Ultrasound Obstet Gynecol. 2001;18:441-9.

CHAPTER 46

Operative Delivery

Melissa D Mendez, Sushila Arya

■ CLINICAL CASE

LF is a 27-year-old G1P0 with uncomplicated prenatal care at 39 weeks and 5 days gestational age by her LMP and a 14-week ultrasound. She had prenatal testing which showed no chromosomal abnormalities and a female fetus. She was admitted to labor and delivery for active labor at 6 cm cervical dilation. She requested and received an epidural for pain control. She progressed to complete dilatation and plus 1 station 4 hours later, and began to push. On reviewing fetal heart tracing, category II with deep repetitive variable decelerations is noticed. The patient has been pushing for two hours, and she is now plus 2 station. The fetus is in occiput anterior position and the patient exerts reasonable maternal effort.

Menarche: Age 9.

Menses: 28/5.

LMP: 41 weeks ago.

Pregnancy: As above.

Sexual history: In a monogamous relationship with her husband of 5 years. No history of sexually transmitted diseases.

Contraception: Previous use of Mirena IUD.

Review of Systems

- No chest pain or shortness of breath
- No diarrhea or constipation
- No urinary frequency, no hematuria or dysuria
- *Past medical history*: Noncontributory
- *Past surgical history*: Left radial fracture from a skating accident
- *Vaccines*: Up-to-date
- *Current medications*: Prenatal vitamins
- *Allergies*: No known drug allergies
- *Social history*: She does not smoke, no drug use, no alcohol use
- *Family history*: Grandmother with history of diabetes.

Physical Examination

- *Vital signs*: Temperature 36.9°C oral, BP 118/65, P 75, BMI 26
- *Cardiac examination*: Regular rate and rhythm, no heart murmur
- *Chest examination*: Lungs clear to auscultation bilaterally
- *Abdomen*: Nondistended, non-tender. Fetal heart tones auscultated at 130s beats per minute
- *Pelvic examination*: As above
- Patient was counseled about her options to achieve quick delivery for the category II tracing, completely dilated cervix, 2+ fetal station and pushing for 2 hours. Instrumental delivery (vacuum assisted, provider preference and experience) was recommended and explained to the patient. She consented for vacuum-assisted delivery after understanding the risks, benefits and alternatives. Neonatology team was called in for delivery. Bladder was drained; anesthesia is adequate; fetal position and station confirmed, and vacuum (Kiwi) was applied at the flexion point.

■ CLINICAL QUESTIONS

1. What are the indications for an operative delivery?

Ans. In the United States, about 3% of all deliveries are done via vaginal operative delivery.[1] Indications for operative delivery include non-reassuring heart rate status which could be defined as prolonged bradycardia, repetitive late decelerations, decreased variability, or thick meconium.[2] In addition, the cervix must be fully dilated, membranes ruptured and the fetal head engaged. The maternal pelvis should feel adequate for vaginal delivery (Figs 46.1 and 46.2).[2]

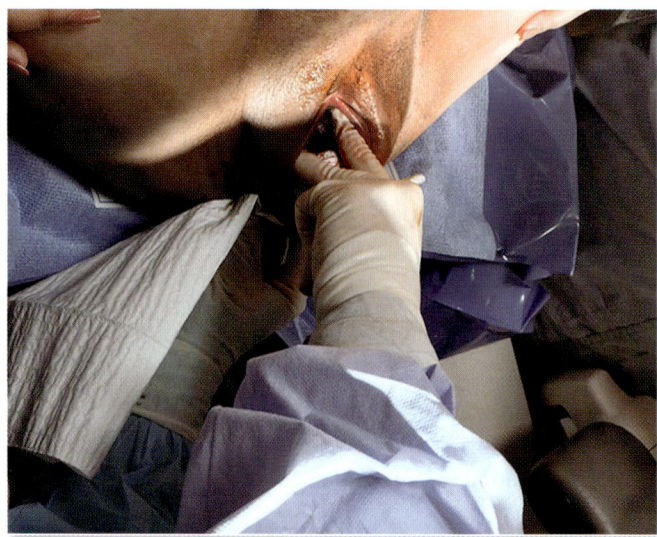

Figure 46.1: Vacuum application at the flexion point. Vacuum was built to safety zone (green mark), and gentle constant traction was applied with contractions concomitant with maternal pushing efforts

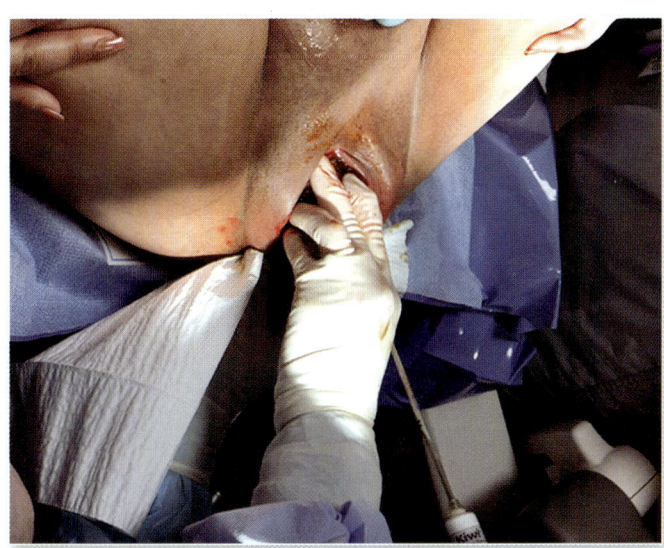

Figure 46.2: With two sets of pulls the fetal head was delivered. Vaccum was released and baby was delivered with gentle traction and maternal pushing without difficulty. Total vacuum application time was two minutes

2. What are potential complications of operative deliveries?

Ans. Operative deliveries are associated with a higher rate of postpartum hemorrhage, fetal scalp lacerations, fetal scalp hematomas and sepsis. The use of forceps and a longer active second stage of labor are associated with increased maternal morbidity, such as third and fourth degree lacerations.[3,4] Neonatal injuries could include bruising, lacerations, cephalohematoma or retinal hemorrhage.[5] Suboptimal placement was found in one study to be as high as 28% for both vacuum and forceps placement, especially for malposition of the fetal head. This may also contribute to neonatal trauma and maternal hemorrhage rates. Improper instrumentation also increased the rate of cesarean delivery.[4]

3. Is there a role for episiotomy at the time of operative delivery?

Ans. Anal sphincter tear rates were not statistically different with use of episiotomy compared with no episiotomy at the time of operative delivery. Short-term complications of perineal injury include pain, infection and hemorrhage.[5] Long-term complications include pelvic pain, dyspareunia and incontinence of urine, flatus or feces. The rate of anal sphincter tearing with an operative delivery is about twice that without an operative delivery, regardless of the use of episiotomy.[6]

4. Should antibiotics be given for operative vaginal delivery?

Ans. A recent Cochrane review examined this question.[7] They found one study which showed no statistical significance in rates of endomyometritis for women undergoing an operative delivery with either forceps or vacuum. At this time, antibiotic prophylaxis for operative vaginal delivery is not recommended.[7]

TAKE-HOME MESSAGES

- Operative vaginal delivery is a delivery in which the operator uses forceps or a vacuum to extract the fetus from the vagina. It is estimated that in the United States, about 3% of all deliveries are done via vaginal operative delivery.[1]
- Indications for operative delivery include non-reassuring heart rate status which could be defined as prolonged bradycardia, repetitive late decelerations, decreased variability or thick meconium.[2] The cervix must be fully dilated, membranes ruptured and the fetal head engaged. The maternal pelvis should feel adequate for vaginal delivery.[2]
- Contraindications for operative vaginal delivery include extreme fetal prematurity, fetal bleeding diathesis, unengaged head, unknown fetal position, brow or face presentation, and suspected fetal pelvic disproportion.[8, 9]
- Operative deliveries are associated with a higher rate of postpartum hemorrhage, fetal scalp lacerations, fetal scalp hematomas, and sepsis.[3]
- Operative deliveries are associated with a higher rate of third and fourth degree lacerations, and long-term effects of perineal lacerations, especially if wound breakdown occurs, could include pelvic pain, dyspareunia, and incontinence of urine, flatus or feces.[3, 6]

REFERENCES

1. Martin JA, Hamilton BE, Ventura SJ, et al. Births: final data for 2010. Natl Vital Stat Rep. 2012;61(1):1-72.
2. American College of Obstetricians and Gynecologists. ACOG Practice Bulletin No. 154: Operative vaginal delivery. Obstet Gynecol. 2015;126(5):e56-65.
3. Ducarme G, Hamel JF, Bouet PE, et al. Maternal and neonatal morbidity after attempted operative vaginal delivery according to fetal head station. Obstet Gynecol. 2015;126(3):521-9.
4. Ramphul M, Kennelly MM, Burke G, Murphy DJ. Risk factor and morbidity associated with suboptimal instrument placement at instrumental delivery: observational study nested within the instrumental delivery and ultrasound randomized controlled trial ISRCTN 72230496. BJOG 2015;122(4):558-63.
5. Macleod M, Strachan B, Bahl R, et al. A prospective cohort study of maternal and neonatal morbidity in relation to use of episiotomy at operative vaginal delivery. BJOG. 2008;115(13):1688-94.
6. Lewicky-Gaupp C, Leader-Cramer A, Johnson LL, et al. Wound complications after obstetric anal sphincter injuries. Obstet Gynecol. 2015;125(5):1088-93.
7. Liabsuetrakal T, Choobun T, Peeyananjarassri K, Islam QM. Antibiotic prophylaxis for operative vaginal delivery. Cochran Database Syst Rev. 2014 Oct 13;10:CD004455. doi: 10.1002/14651858.CD004455.pub3.
8. Committee on Practice Bulletins—Obstetrics. ACOG Practice Bulletin No. 154 Summary: Operative Vaginal Delivery. Obstet Gynecol. 2015;126(5):1118.
9. Gei AF, Belfort MA. Forceps-assisted vaginal delivery. Obstet Gynecol Clin North Am. 1999;26:345.

CHAPTER

Cesarean Section

47

Mary Traci Groening

■ CLINICAL CASE

RB is a 26-year-old G2P1 at 39 weeks 3 days gestation by LMP consistent with a 10-week ultrasound who presented to labor and delivery triage complaining of regular contractions every 6 minutes for three hours. She denies loss of fluid and vaginal bleeding. She had good prenatal care with a well-known nurse midwife clinic. She denies any problems with her current pregnancy, including gestational diabetes, preterm labor, or high blood pressure. Of note, she did desire a trial of labor, as her first delivery was a primary low transverse cesarean delivery for non-reassuring fetal status during labor. She was admitted to labor and delivery in active labor at 5 cm, and progressed to 8 cm without further dilation despite adequate oxytocin augmentation. The patient underwent a repeat cesarean section for arrest of active phase at 8 cm, failed trial of labor. Figures 47.1 to 47.13 illustrate the course of the procedure.

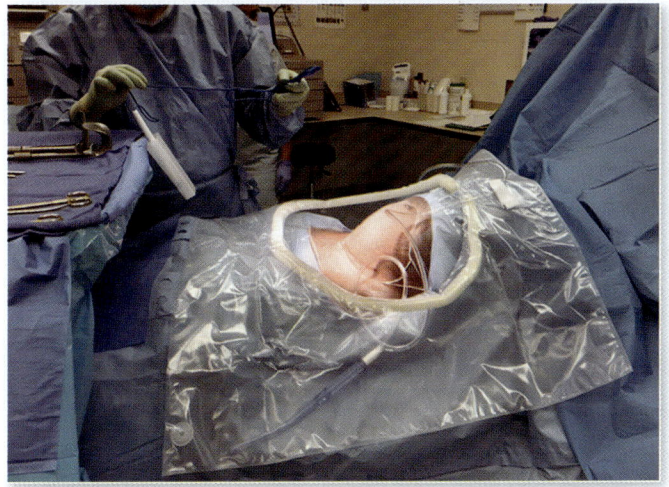

Figure 47.1: Patient positioning and draping for cesarean section

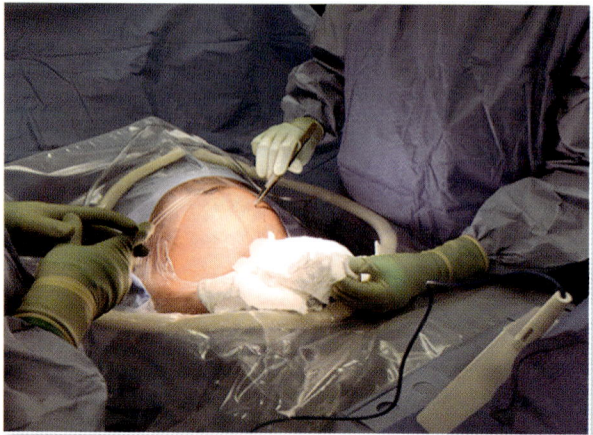

Figure 47.2: Testing the effectiveness of the spinal or epidural anesthesia (epidural used in this patient)

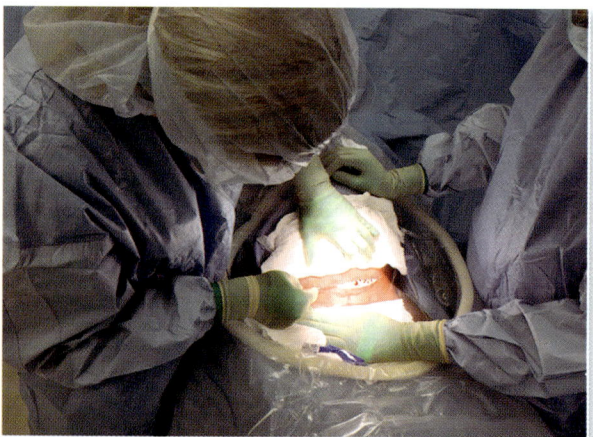

Figure 47.3: Pfannenstiel incision performed on this patient

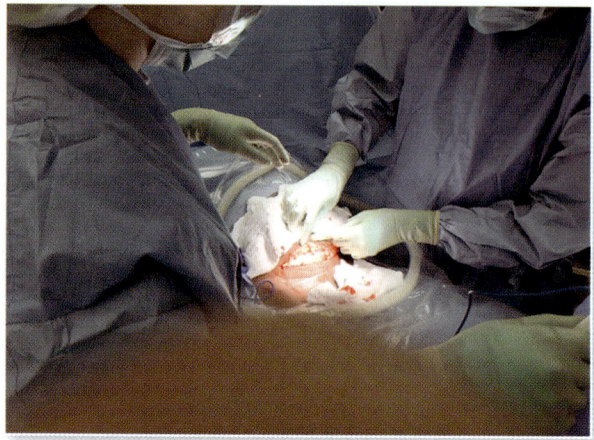

Figure 47.4: Examining incision and cauterizing bleeding

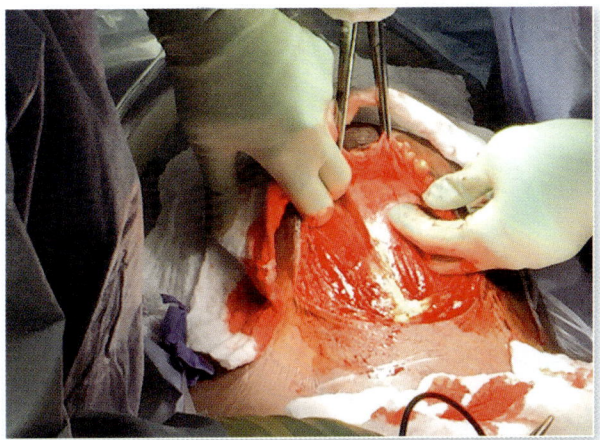

Figure 47.5: Blunt dissection of underlying rectus muscles from fascia

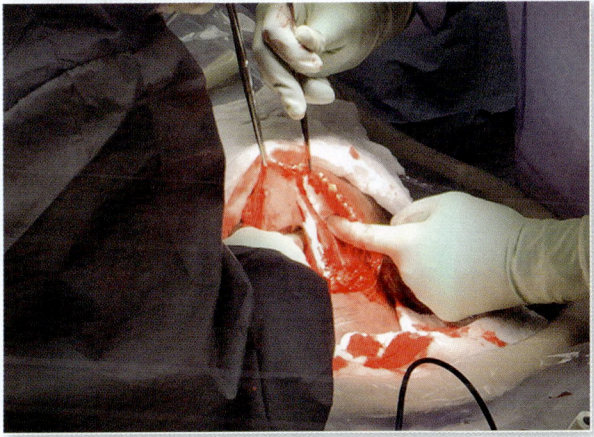

Figure 47.6: Kocher clamps used during blunt dissection

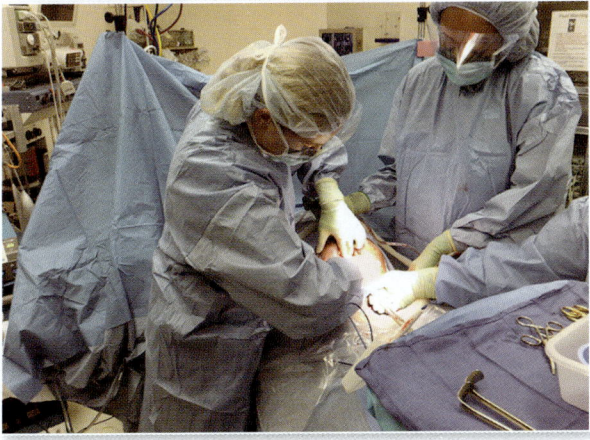

Figure 47.7: After entry into the peritoneal cavity, hysterotomy was made and extended using cephalad–caudad blunt motion

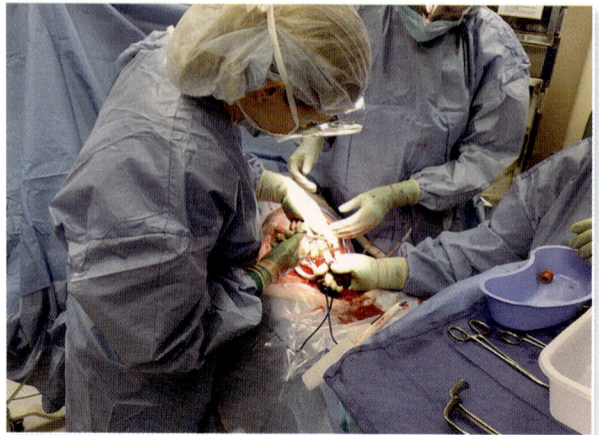

Figure 47.8: Delivery of fetal head

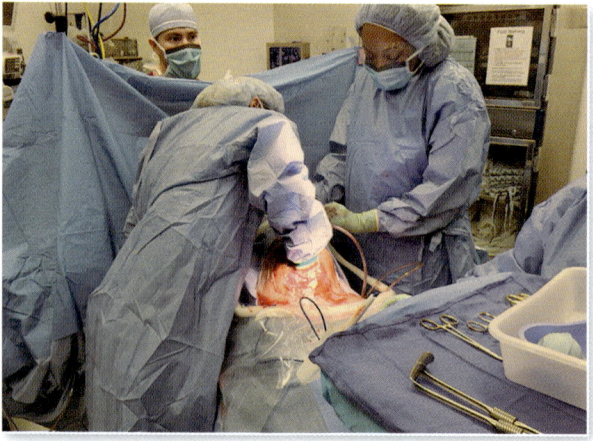

Figure 47.9: Delayed cord clamping after delivery of neonate

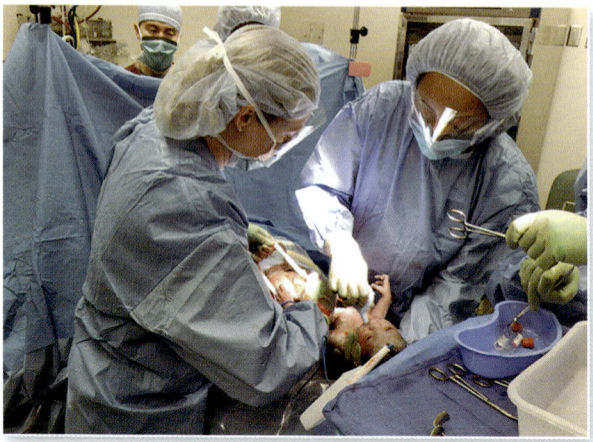

Figure 47.10: After cord is clamped and cut, neonate is handed to waiting pediatrics team. Cord blood is collected

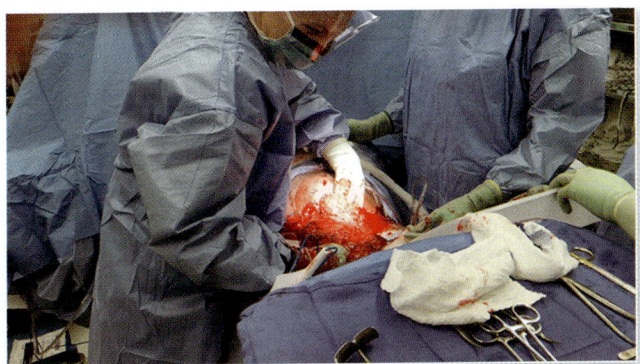

Figure 47.11: Spontaneous removal of placenta with fundal massage

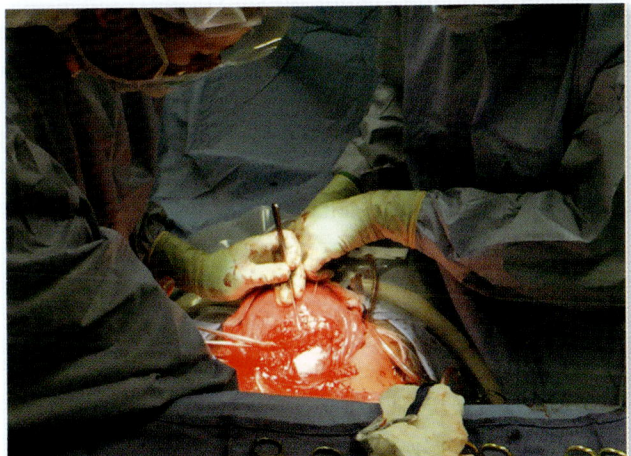

Figure 47.12: Hysterotomy repair in 2 layers: first layer locked/running suture and second layer imbricating unlocked/running (both with 3–0 vicryl on a CT-1 needle)

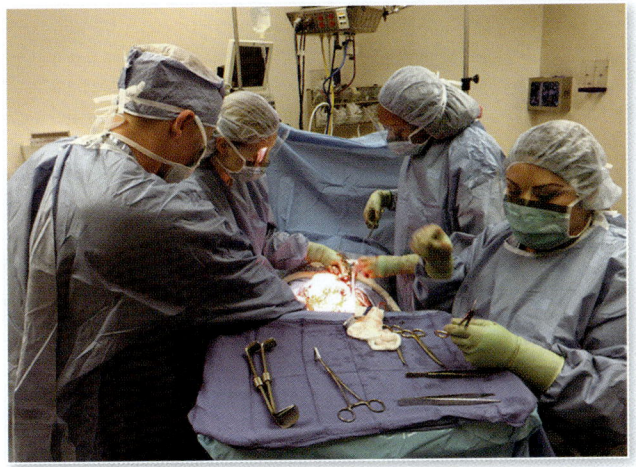

Figure 47.13: The operating room team: scrub technician far right, first assistant on patient's left, primary surgeon on patient's right (if surgeon is right handed), second assistant on far left

CLINICAL QUESTIONS

1. What are the increased risks to a patient who undergoes a cesarean delivery compared to vaginal delivery?

Ans. The risk factors include postpartum bleeding, genital tract injury, wound infection, systemic infection, wound disruption, wound hematoma and death.[1,2] In addition, morbidity and mortality may be related to one of the following causes: uterine rupture, anesthetic complications, shock, cardiac arrest, acute renal failure, assisted venous thromboembolic event, hemorrhage requiring hysterectomy or transfusion.[3-7]

2. What antibiotics are usually given preoperatively to reduce infection?

Ans. Antimicrobial prophylaxis is recommended for all CS unless the patient is already receiving appropriate antibiotics (e.g., for chorioamnionitis) and that prophylaxis should be administered within 60 minutes before the start of the cesarean delivery. A single dose of a targeted antibiotic, such as a first-generation cephalosporin, is the first-line antibiotic of choice, unless significant drug allergies are present. For women with a history of a significant penicillin or cephalosporin allergy (anaphylaxis, angioedema, respiratory distress or urticaria) a single-dose combination of clindamycin with an aminoglycoside is a reasonable alternative choice for cesarean delivery prophylaxis.[7]

3. What uterotonic medications can be given to reduce postpartum hemorrhage?

Ans.
- Oxytocin infusion (10–40 IU in 1 liter crystalloid over 4–8 hours)
- Misoprostol (200–800 µg rectal or sublingual)[8]

TAKE-HOME MESSAGES

- Cesarean delivery accounts for 1/3rd of all deliveries in the US and is the most common major surgery performed (1.3 million women per year).[9,10]
- Cesarean delivery is the most common residency surgical procedure performed.[11]
- Cesarean delivery has increased morbidity and mortality than vaginal delivery for infection, bleeding, wound complications and death.[12]
- Women are typically positioned to the left to avoid vena cava compression and improve blood flow to the uterus and the placenta. A Cochrane review in 2013 found no apparent benefit to a 20-degree left lateral table tilt compared to a supine position. The data were too weak to produce any recommendations.[8]
- There is insufficient data to recommend chlorhexidine vs. iodine for skin preparation.[5]
- Antibiotic prophylaxis prior to skin incision is recommended to decrease risk of wound infection and endometritis.[8]
- Most practitioners use the traditional Pfannenstiel incision. Recent data suggest lower rates of complication with the Joel–Cohen incision, a straight lateral incision about two centimeters above the Pfannenstiel location.[8]
- The bladder flap helped minimize infection before antibiotics but no longer serves a useful purpose. CS without a bladder flap appears not to add additional risks, but significantly shortens operative time.[8]
- Blunt extension of the uterine incision in the cranial–caudad direction is recommended to decrease lateral extensions, blood loss, and operative time.[8]
- Spontaneous delivery of the placenta is recommended to allow dilated sinuses to contract and reduce blood loss, endometritis, and wound infection.[8]
- Exteriorizing the uterus for repair may be surgeon's preference, as febrile complications and surgical time were similar between uterine exteriorization and intraabdominal repair.[8]

- Double-layer hysterotomy repair may help reduce uterine rupture during a future trial of labor.[8]
- There are conflicting studies regarding closure of the visceral and parietal peritoneum to reduce adhesions.[8]
- Routine adhesion barrier use is not recommended.[13,14]
- The subcutaneous tissue should be re-approximated if greater than 2 cm to reduce wound disruption, hematomas, seromas, and infection. Routine use of a drain is not recommended.[7]
- Subcuticular skin suturing is recommended over staples to reduce pain, wound complications, and increase cosmetics. Operative time may be increased by 10 minutes.[7,15]

REFERENCES

1. Hofmeyr GJ, Barrett JF, Crowther CA. Planned caesarean section for women with a twin pregnancy. Cochrane Database of Systematic Reviews 2011, Issue 12. Art. No.: CD006553. DOI: 10.1002/14651858.CD006553.pub2.
2. Liu S, Liston RM, Joseph KS, Heaman M, Sauve R, Kramer MS. Maternal mortality and severe morbidity associated with low-risk planned cesarean delivery versus planned vaginal delivery at term. Maternal Health Study Group of the Canadian Perinatal Surveillance System. CMAJ 2007;176:455-60.
3. Deneux-Tharaux C, Carmona E, Bouvier-Colle MH, Breart G. Postpartum maternal mortality and cesarean delivery. Obstet Gynecol. 2006;108:541-8.
4. Abenhaim HA, Azoulay L, Kramer MS, Leduc L. Incidence and risk factors of amniotic fluid embolisms: a population-based study on 3 million births in the United States. Am J Obstet Gynecol 2008;199:49.e1-49.e8.
5. Silver RM, Landon MB, Rouse DJ, Leveno KJ, Spong CY, Thom EA, et al. Maternal morbidity associated with multiple repeat cesarean deliveries. National Institute of Child Health and Human Development Maternal-Fetal Medicine Units Network. Obstet Gynecol. 2006;107:1226-32.
6. Hannah ME, Whyte H, Hannah WJ, Hewson S, Amankwah K, Cheng M, et al. Maternal outcomes at 2 years after planned cesarean section versus planned vaginal birth for breech presentation at term: the international randomized Term Breech Trial. Term Breech Trial Collaborative Group. Am J Obstet Gynecol. 2004;191:917-27.
7. Gregory KD, Jackson S, Korst L, Fridman M. Cesarean versus vaginal delivery: whose risks? Whose benefits? Am J Perinatol. 2012;29:7-18.
8. Dahlke JD, Mendez-Figueroa H, Rouse DJ et al. Evidence-based surgery for cesarean delivery: an updated systematic review. Am J Obstet Gynecol. 2013;209(4):294-306.
9. Centers for Disease Control and Prevention. Nation Center for Health Statistics: vital statistics. Available at: http://www.cdc.gov/nchs/vitalstats.htm. Accessed Oct. 1, 2012.
10. Hall MJ, DeFrances CJ, Williams SN, Golosinskiy A, Schwartzman A. National Hospital Discharge Survey: 2007 summary. Natl Heal Stat Report. 2010;29:1-20:24.
11. Ciottii M, Johnston MJ. Minimum Thresholds for Obstetrics and Gynecology Procedures. Available at: https://www.acgme.org/acgmeweb/Portals/0/PFAssets/ProgramResources/220_Ob_Gyn%20Minimum_Numbers_Announcment.pdf.
12. Safe Prevention of the Primary Cesarean Delivery. Obstetric Care Consensus. Number. 1, March 2014.
13. Edwards RK, Ingersoll M, Gerkin RD, et al. Carboxymethylcellulose adhesion barrier placement at primary cesarean delivery and outcomes at repeat cesarean delivery. Obstet Gynecol. 2014;123(5):923-8.
14. Gaspar-Oishi M, Aeby T. Cesarean delivery times and adhesion severity associated with prior placement of a sodium hyaluronate-carboxycellulose barrier. Obstet Gynecol. 2014;124(4):679-83.
15. American College of Obstetricians and Gynecologists. ACOG Practice Bulletin No. 120: Use of prophylactic antibiotics in labor and delivery. Obstet Gynecol. 2011;117(6): 1472-83.

CHAPTER

Caudal Regression Syndrome

48

Ulrich Honemeyer, Sanja Kupesic Plavsic

MG is a 29-year-old primigravida presenting at 23 weeks 2 days for fetal anatomy scan. Her history is significant for preexisting diabetes mellitus type 2. The patient is on metformin and low carbohydrate diet since 4 years. Six weeks ago insulin therapy was introduced due to poor blood sugar control.

Menarche: Age 10.

Menses: 30–60/5–6 days, irregular.

LMP: 25 weeks ago.

Sexual history: Two male partners over her lifetime. For five years she is in a monogamous relationship with her husband.

Review of Systems

- No headaches, no problems with vision
- No history of blood clots DVT or PE
- No heart palpitations, no shortness of breath
- Normal urination, regular bowel movement, no nausea and vomiting
- *Past medical history*: No hospitalizations
- Vaccines are up to date (hepatitis B vaccine series, and MMR booster; flu shot past winter)
- *Past surgical history*: None
- *Meds*: None
- *Allergies*: None known drug allergies
- *Social history*: Receptionist, denies smoking, drugs and alcohol
- *Family history*: Mother: age 52, with no medical problems. Father: age 60, with history of diabetes and high blood pressure. No family history of congenital anomalies.

Physical Examination

- *Vital signs*: T 36.8°C oral; BP 125/85; P 86; BMI 22
- *Blood type/Rh*: A (+)

- Rubella titer, hepatitis test, syphilis test, HIV test, CBC and urine culture performed in first trimester were within normal limits. Quad screening performed at 18 weeks gestation was also within normal limits. Normal physical and pelvic examinations. Fetal anatomy examination was performed and findings are presented in Figures 48.1 to 48.6.

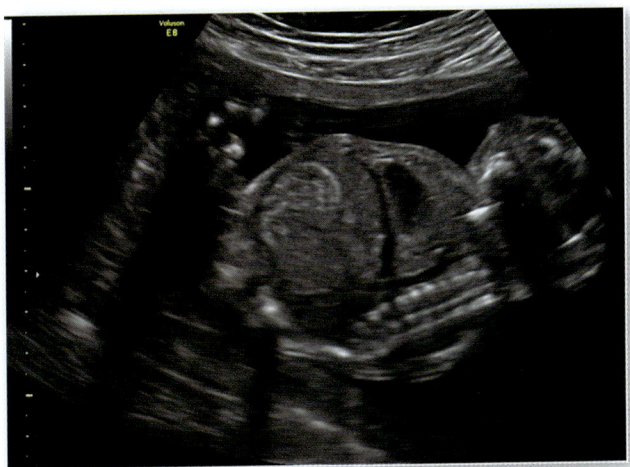

Figure 48.1: B-mode ultrasound demonstrates abnormal shape of the fetal chest and absence of the lumbar and sacral spine

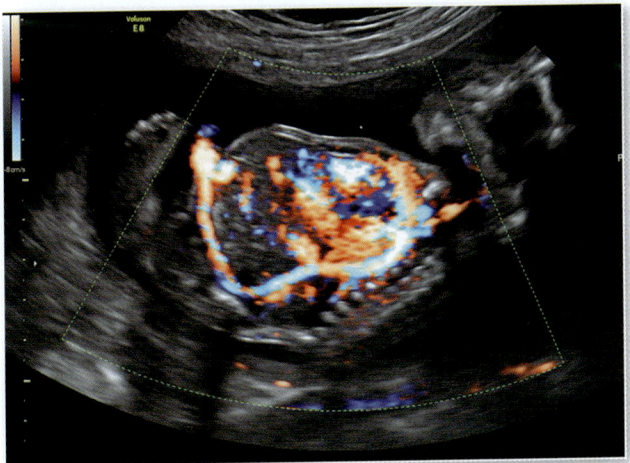

Figure 48.2: The same fetus assessed by high definition (HD) flow Doppler technique demonstrating blood vessels of the whole fetal circulation. Renal flow is not appreciated and kidneys could not be visualized. There is a normal amount of amniotic fluid

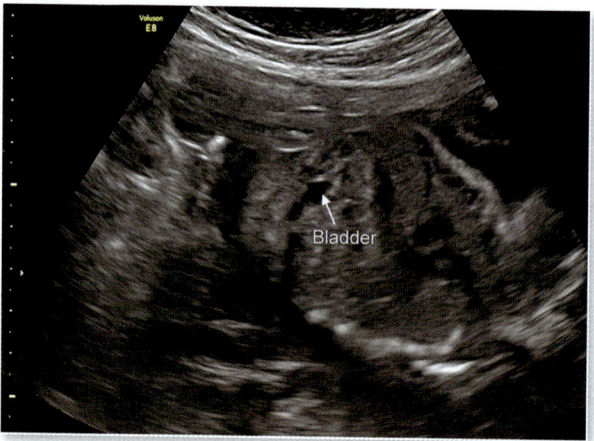

Figure 48.3: Urinary bladder contains a small volume of urine

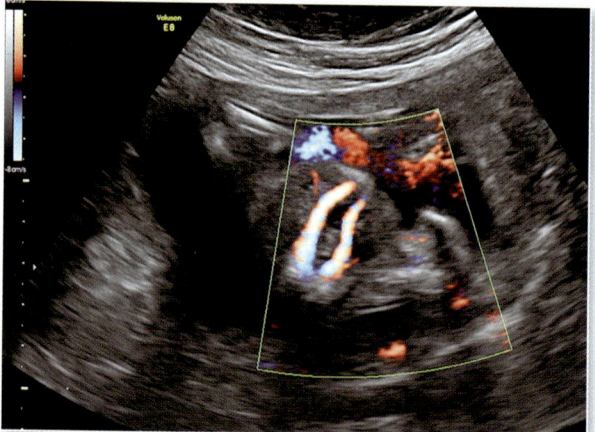

Figure 48.4: HD flow Doppler reveals bilateral umbilical arteries running around the urinary bladder

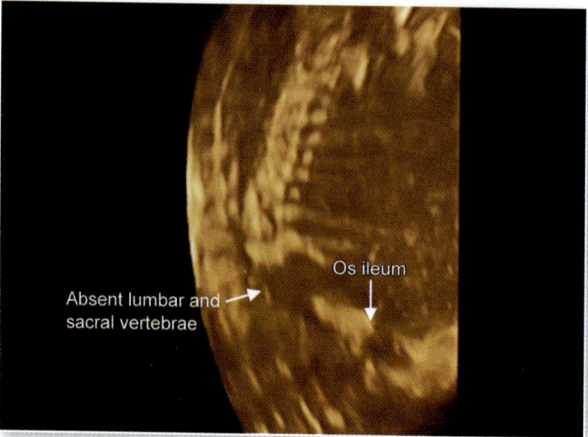

Figure 48.5: Three-dimensional ultrasound demonstrates absence of lumbar and sacral vertebrae and small hip bones

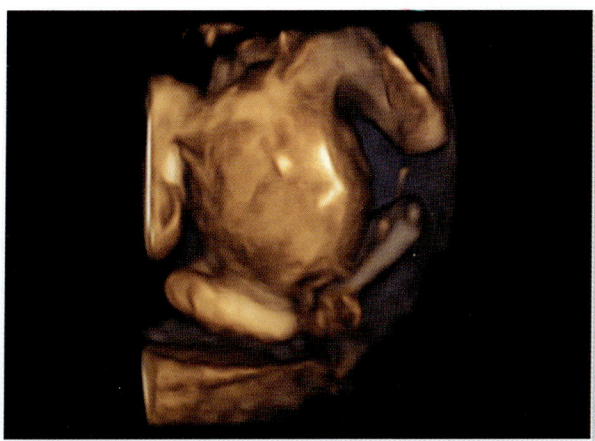

Figure 48.6: Three-dimensional ultrasound demonstrates fixed "lotus seat" position with two hypoplastic lower limbs and absent left fibula

■ CLINICAL QUESTIONS

1. What is quad screen blood test and when it is performed?

Ans. Quad screen blood test includes alpha feto-protein (AFP), human chorionic gonadotropin (hCG), estriol and inhibin A. A quad test is performed in the second trimester.

2. Discuss the ultrasound findings and the differential diagnoses.

Ans. Biometry was corresponding to the calculated gestational age by LMP (23 weeks 2 days). B mode ultrasound demonstrates abnormal shape of the fetal chest and absence of the lumbar and sacral spine (See Figs 48.1 and 48.2).[1,2] The bladder contains a small volume of urine. Kidneys could not be visualized and renal flow is not appreciated on HD flow Doppler (See Figs 48.1 to 48.4). Three-dimensional ultrasound demonstrates absence of lumbar and sacral vertebrae and small hip bones (Fig. 48.5). Hypoplastic lower limbs and absent left fibula are suggestive of abnormal development of the caudal region of the spine (Fig. 48.6). Lower extremities are noted in the fixed flexed position.[3] Surface rendering demonstrates normal facial features (Fig. 48.7).

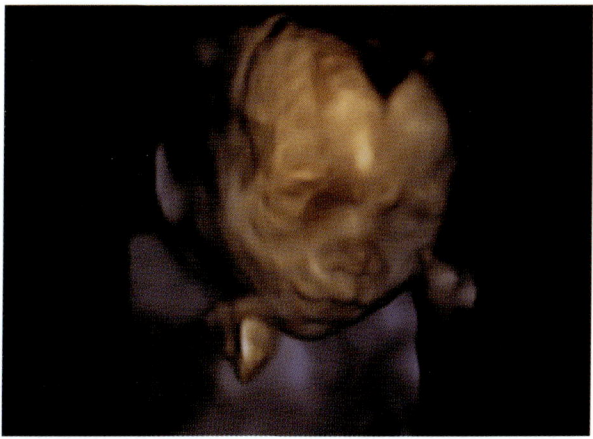

Figure 48.7: Surface rendering of the fetal face. There is no evidence of facial abnormalities

Sonographic findings are suggestive of caudal regression syndrome (CRS). Differential diagnosis includes sirenomelia and VACTERL association.[4] Table 48.1 illustrates the differences between caudal regression syndrome and sirenomelia. VACTERL is an acronym including the following abnormalities: V: verterbral abnormalities; A: anal atresia; C: cardiac defects; T: tracheal anomalies including tracheoesophageal fistula; E: esophageal atresia, R: renal abnormalities and L: limb abnormalities.

Table 48.1 Sonographic findings in caudal regression syndrome and sirenomelia[5,6]

Sonographic findings	Caudal regression syndrome	Sirenomelia
Lower extremities	Bilateral hypoplasia	Single or fused
Renal anomalies	Unilateral renal agenesis Horseshoe kidney Ureteral duplication	Renal agenesis or dysgenesis
Anus	Normal or imperforate	Absent
Amniotic fluid	Normal or increased	Oligohydramnios
Umbilical artery	Two umbilical arteries	Single umbilical artery

3. Why AFP was within normal limits?

Ans. Sacral agenesis is a close defect. Therefore, AFP was within normal limits.

TAKE-HOME MESSAGES

- The prevalence of CRS is estimated to 1–5 per 100,000 newborns.[7,8]
- CRS occurs with increased incidence in mothers with insulin dependent diabetes. It is estimated that approximately 16% of CRS occur in women with diabetes.[9] Other factors associated with CRS are alcohol, retinoic acid, hypoxia and amino acid imbalances.[9] In some cases CRS is associated with genetic mutations: VANGL1 gene located on the short (p) arm of chromosome 1 (1p13) and HLXB9.
- A diagnosis of CRS is made by ultrasound and magnetic resonance imaging (MRI).[1-8]
- Treatment of CRS requires coordinated efforts of an interprofessional team consisting of pediatricians, neurologists, neurosurgeons, urologists, nephrologists, orthopedists, orthopedic surgeons, cardiologists, etc.[1-10] Multiple surgeries may be necessary to treat complex spinal, limb, urological and cardiac abnormalities associated with this syndrome.

REFERENCES

1. Aslan H, Yanik H, Celikaslan N, et al. Prenatal diagnosis of caudal regression syndrome: a case report. BMC Pregnancy Childbirth 2001;1(1):8.
2. Unsinn KM, Geley T, Freund MC, Gassner I. US of the spinal cord in newborns: spectrum of normal findings, variants, congenital anomalies, and acquired diseases. Radiographics. 2000;20(4):923-38.
3. Moritoki Y, Kojima Y, Kamisawa H, et al. Neuropathic bladder caused by caudal regression syndrome without any other neurogenic symptoms. Case Rep Med. http://www.ncbi.nlm.nih.gov/pubmed/22761628. Date published June 12, 2012.
4. Boulas MM. Recognition of caudal regression syndrome. Adv Neonatal Care. 2009;9(2):61-9.
5. Das BB, Rajegowda BK, Bainbridge R, Giampietro PF. Caudal regression syndrome versus sirenomelia: a case report. J Perinatol. 2002;22(2):168-70.
6. Zaw W, Stone DG. Caudal regression syndrome in twin pregnancy with type II diabetes. J Perinatol 2002;22(2):171-4.
7. Levene MI. Disorders of the spinal cord, cranial and peripheral nerves. In: Fetal and Neonatal Neurology and Neurosurgery, 4th ed. Levene MI, Chervenak FA. Philadelphia, PA: Churchill Livingstone Elsevier. 2009; p. 781.
8. Jones KL. Ed. Smith's Recognizable Patterns of Human Malformation. 6th ed. Philadelphia, PA: Elsevier Saunders 2006, pp730.
9. Caudal Regression Syndrome. National Organization of Rare Disorders. https://rarediseases.org/rare-diseases/caudal-regression-syndrome/. Date published 2013.
10. Torre M, Buffa P, Jasonni V, Cama A. Long-term urologic outcome in patients with caudal regression syndrome, compared with meningomyelocele and spinal cord lipoma. J Pediatr Surg. 2008;43(3):530-3.

CHAPTER 49

Fetal Hydronephrosis

Ulrich Honemeyer, Sanja Kupesic Plavsic

■ CLINICAL CASE

CC is a 35-year-old P2G1, presenting at 22 weeks gestation for fetal anatomy scan. Her history is noncontributory.

Menarche: Age 12.

Menses: 28–30/5 days, regular.

LMP: 22 weeks ago.

Sexual history: In monogamous relationship with her husband.

Review of Systems

- No headaches, no problems with vision
- No history of blood, clots DVT, or PE
- No heart palpitations, no shortness of breath
- Normal urination, regular bowel movement, no nausea and vomiting
- *Past medical/surgical history*: No hospitalizations
- Vaccines are up-to-date (hepatitis B vaccine series, and MMR booster; flu shot past winter)
- *Medications*: Folic acid over the counter
- *Allergies*: None
- *Social history*: Fashion designer; denies smoking, drugs and alcohol
- *Family history*: No family history of congenital anomalies. Mother: age 62, with no medical problems. Father: age 63, with history of diabetes and high blood pressure.

Physical Examination

- *Vital signs*: T36.9°C oral BP 120/80; P 78; BMI 20. Blood type/Rh: A (+)
- Rubella titer, hepatitis test, syphilis test, HIV test, CBC and urine culture performed in first trimester were within normal limits. Quad screening performed at 18 weeks gestation was also within normal limits

Section 2: Obstetrics

- Normal physical and pelvic examinations
- Fetal anatomy examination was performed and relevant findings are presented in Figures 49.1 to 49.4.

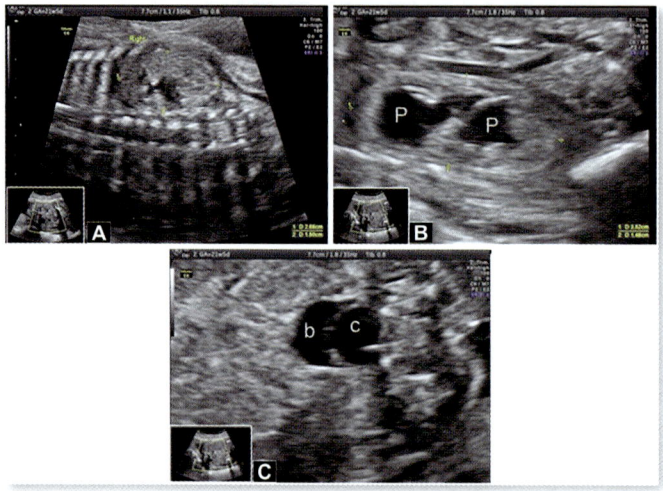

Figures 49.1A to C: Double right kidney with two pelvi-calyceal systems (P) at 22 weeks gestation (A and B). Image C illustrates bladder (b) with uretrocele (c)

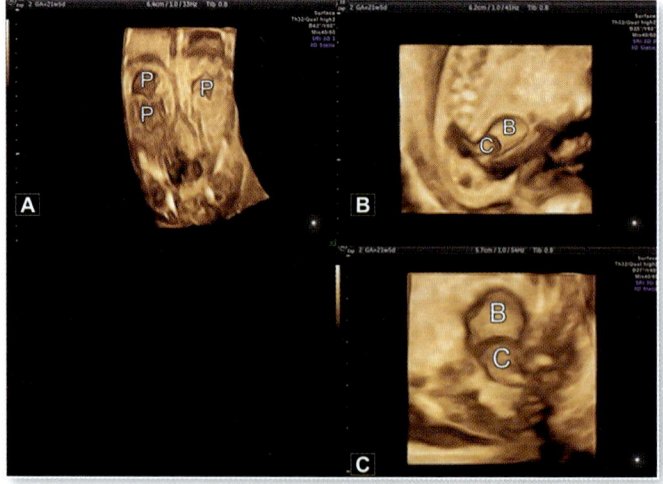

Figures 49.2A to C: Three-dimensional US image (surface rendering) of double kidney and ureterocele at 22 weeks gestation. (A) Both kidneys and pelvi-calyceal systems (P); (B and C) Surface rendering of bladder (B) and ureterocele (C)

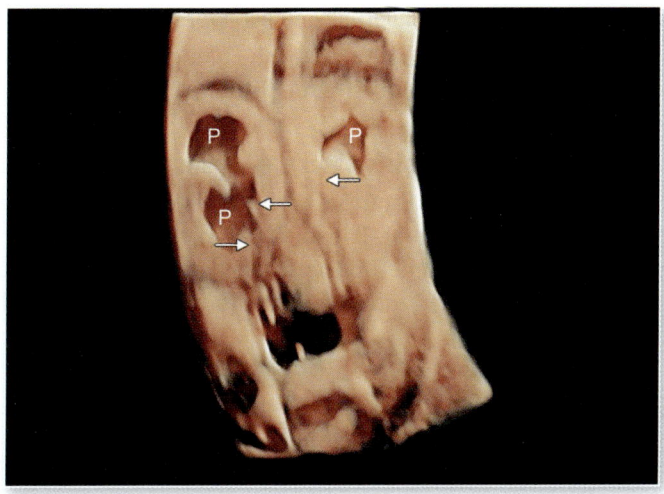

Figure 49.3: Surface mode HD life rendering of the double right kidney, right double ureter (two arrows) and ureterocele at 22 weeks gestation

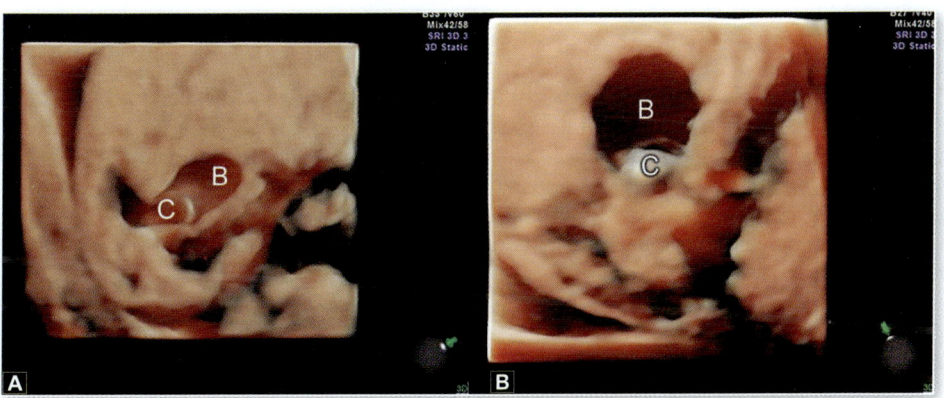

Figures 49.4A and B: Surface mode HD life rendering of the bladder (B) and ureterocele (C) of the same patient in lateral (A) and AP view (B)

■ CLINICAL QUESTIONS

1. What is the most likely diagnosis?

Ans. Figures 49.1 to 49.4 illustrate dilatation of the renal collecting system. Sonographic findings are consistent with fetal hydronephrosis.

2. What is the most common etiology of this finding?

Ans. Nearly 2/3rd of fetal hydronephrosis are attributed to ureteropelvic junction (UPJ) obstruction. The remaining third is secondary to vesicoureteral reflux, megaureter or posterior urethral valves.[1]

3. At what gestational age can ultrasonography detect fetal hydronephrosis?

Ans. Ultrasonography can detect fetal kidneys and the bladder by 12 weeks' gestation. At 20 weeks' gestation fetal urinary system is better visualized and hydronephrosis is easier to detect.[2]

4. Which ultrasonographic parameters are assessed in patients with fetal hydronephrosis?

Ans. Ultrasonographic urogenital evaluation of the fetus should determine whether the abnormality is unilateral or bilateral. The following parameters should also be assessed and reported: fetal gender, renal anteroposterior (AP) pelvic diameter, bladder distension, bladder sagittal length, volume of amniotic fluid and associated pathologic conditions/US findings.[2]

■ TAKE-HOME MESSAGES

- In almost 50% of cases fetal hydronephrosis is transient and resolves by the third trimester. The presence of oligohydramnios and additional renal or extrarenal anomalies suggest significant pathology.[1]
- The most commonly used scoring system for fetal hydronephrosis uses renal pelvic diameter (RPD) measurement. Mild hydronephrosis is defined as RPD of 4–10 mm, and more severe hydronephrosis as RPD >10 mm.[3,4]
- In fetuses with increased RPD, ultrasonographic imaging should asses the presence of caliectasis, parenchymal echogenicity, parenchymal thinning, presence of ureteromegaly, enlarged bladder size and wall thickness, and if present, the anomalies of kidney and urinary tract.[3,5]
- Fetuses with hydronephrosis are at increased risk for Down syndrome and congenital anomalies of the kidney and urinary tract and require comprehensive prenatal evaluation.[6]
- Repeat antenatal ultrasound examinations are indicated to help guide management decisions. Fetuses with second trimester hydronephrosis should undergo repeat testing in the third trimester to assess progression. Repeat ultrasound examinations are usually performed every two to three weeks in fetuses with bilateral involvement (or an affected solitary kidney), and at 32–34 weeks gestation in those with unilateral involvement.[1,3,5,6]
- Sonographic signs for diagnosis of lower urinary tract obstruction are oligohydramnios and thick walled or dilated bladder.[1] Bilateral hydroureteronephrosis, dilated posterior urethra, perinephric urinoma and progressive calyceal or ureteric dilatation correlate with postnatal pathology and the need for surgery.[3] Abnormally large or small kidneys, parenchymal thinning, cysts, increased echogenicity and oligohydramnios are suggestive of renal dysplasia and impaired renal function.[5] Oligohydramnios refers to a reduced amount of amniotic fluid, which results in pulmonary maldevelopment and somatic compression, and is associated with increased neonatal morbidity and mortality.
- Prenatal diagnosis of severe hydronephrosis (renal pelvic diameter >20 mm) correlates with high incidence (90%) of moderate and severe postnatal hydronephrosis. Prenatal diagnosis of moderate hydronephrosis (renal pelvic diameter 10–20 mm) is associated with moderate postnatal hydronephrosis in 20%, and improvement in 80% of the newborn infants. Data from the literature indicate that delaying the postnatal renal ultrasound in infants with prenatal diagnosis of mild hydronephrosis (renal pelvic diameter <10 mm) reduces the number of postnatal studies and significantly decreases hospitals' inpatient workload.[7]
- The efficacy and utility of continuous antibiotic prophylaxis in children with congenital antenatal hydronephrosis is uncertain. The literature has both supportive and contradictory evidence.[8]
- Diagnostic and therapeutic interventions for fetuses with suspected lower urinary tract obstruction and oligohydramnios should be performed only at specialized centers.[9]

- A ureterocele is a cystic dilatation of the terminal ureter within the bladder and/or the urethra. It may present as an incidental finding on antenatal ultrasonography, or may present as hydroureteronephrosis during antenatal ultrasonography when the ureterocele causes obstruction of the distal portion of the affected ureter.[10] The most common classification system for ureterocele is based upon whether the ureterocele is located entirely within the bladder (e.g. intravesical) or if a portion extends beyond the bladder neck or urethra (e.g. ectopic). In our case, the intravesical ureterocele is presented with hydroureteronephrosis.

REFERENCES

1. Passerotti CC, Kalish LA, Chow J, et al. The predictive value of the first postnatal ultrasound in children with antenatal hydronephrosis. J Pediatr Urol. 2011;7(2):128-36.
2. Liu DB. Antenatal hydronephrosis. Medscape website. http://emedicine.medscape.com/article/1016305-overview. Last updated March 27, 2015.
3. Johnson CE, Elder JS, Judge NE, et al. The accuracy of antenatal ultrasonography in identifying renal abnormalities. Am J Dis Child. 1992;146(10):1181-4.
4. Freedman AL, Johnson MP, Gonzalez R. Fetal therapy for obstructive uropathy: past, present, future? Pediatr Nephrol. 2000;14(2):167-76.
5. Corteville JE, Gray DL, Crane JP. Congenital hydronephrosis: correlation of fetal ultrasonographic findings with infant outcome. Am J Obstet Gynecol. 1991;165(2):384-8.
6. Sidhu G, Beyene J, Rosenblum ND, et al. Outcome of isolated antenatal hydronephrosis: a systematic review and meta-analysis. Pediatr Nephrol. 2006;21(2):218-24.
7. Maayan-Metzger A, Lotan D, Jacobson JM, Raviv-Zilka L, et al. The yield of early postnatal ultrasound scan in neonates with documented antenatal hydronephrosis. Am J Perinatol. 2011;28(8):613-8.
8. Herz D, Merguerian P, McQuiston L. Continuous antibiotic prophylaxis reduces the risk of febrile UTI in children with asymptomatic antenatal hydronephrosis with either ureteral dilation, high-grade vesicoureteral reflux, or ureterovesical junction obstruction. J Pediatr Urol. 2014;10(4):650-4.
9. Sinha A, Bagga A, Krishna A, et al. Revised guidelines on management of antenatal hydronephrosis. Indian J Nephrol. 2013;23(2):83-97.
10. Cavaliere A, Ermito S, Mammaro A, et al. Ultrasound scanning in fetal renal pelvis dilatation: not only hydronephrosis. J Prenat Med. 2009;3(4):60-1.

CHAPTER 50

Asymptomatic Adnexal Mass in Pregnancy

Sanja Kupesic Plavsic

■ CLINICAL CASE

AL is a 27-year old G1P2 who is scheduled for fetal anatomy scan at 20 weeks' gestation. She is asymptomatic and so far has an uncomplicated pregnancy course.

Menarche: Age 14.

Menses: 30/5 days, regular.

LMP: 20 weeks ago.

Pregnancies: One uncomplicated pregnancy, vaginal term delivery (3,500 g/54 cm, Apgar 9/10).

Sexual history: Three male partners over her lifetime. *Chlamydia* test and Pap smear performed in first trimester were normal.

Review of Systems

- No headaches, no problems with vision
- No history of blood clots DVT or PE
- No heart palpitations, no shortness of breath
- No abdominal/pelvic pain
- No nausea, vomiting, constipation and/or diarrhea
- Normal urination; no symptoms of UTI

- *Past medical history*: None—no hospitalizations
- *Past surgical history*: None
- Vaccines: Up- to-date
- *Medilines*: None
- *Allergies*: Non known drug allergies
- *Social history*: AL is a housewife. She is vegetarian, does not smoke, does not drink alcoholic drinks, and reports no history of substance abuse
- *Family history*: Mother: age 50, with no medical problems. Father: age 55, with no medical problems. No family history of uterine, breast, ovarian or colon cancer.

Physical Examination

- *Vital signs*: T 36.8°C oral, BP 125/80; P 65; BMI 22
- Normal heart, lungs, thyroid and neck
- *Abdominal examination and pelvic examinations*: Normal
- *Fetal anatomy scan reveals*: A single live IUP measuring 19 weeks 6 days (consistent with dates). Anatomy is well visualized, and there are no apparent fetal anomalies. Cervix was measured transvaginally at 4.0 cm without funneling, indicating low risk of preterm labor. In the left adnexa there is a complex mass measuring 4.5 × 4.0 × 3.6 cm (Fig. 50.1). Right ovary is within the normal sonographic limits. There is no free fluid in the cul-de-sac.

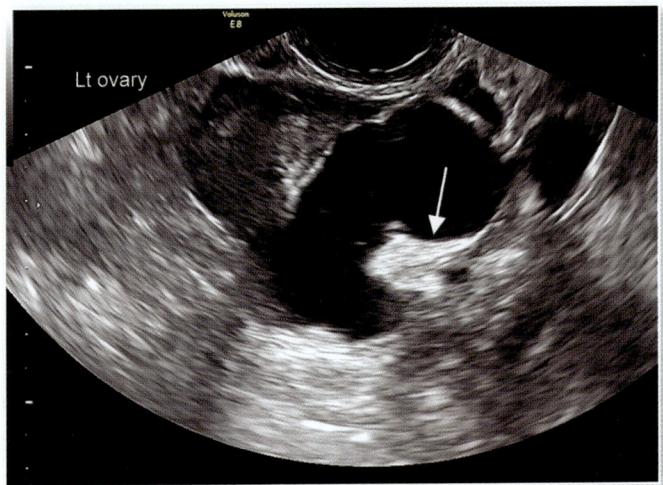

Figure 50.1: In the left adnexa, there is a complex mass measuring 4.5 × 4.0 × 3.6 cm. Rokitansky nodule (pointed by an arrow) is a sonographic finding suggestive of a dermoid cyst

■ CLINICAL QUESTIONS

1. How should the patient be counseled?

Ans. The patient should be informed about the presence of a left adnexal mass. Sonographic and Doppler findings are typical for an uncomplicated ovarian dermoid. Further radiologic evaluation is not required. Because dermoid cysts are liable to torsion, the patient should be counseled to avoid rotational movements to prevent the risk of torsion. In case of low abdominal and/or pelvic pain, the patient should immediately refer to the hospital.

2. Is surgical intervention in this patient indicated and can it be postponed?

Ans. Sonographic and Doppler findings indicate a dermoid cyst. Color Doppler demonstrates moderate impedance blood flow signals obtained from the central part of the lesion, which virtually excludes adnexal torsion, and is reassuring of a benign etiology (Fig. 50.2). Thick media is typical for preexisting vessels of benign tumors and contribute to moderate-to-high vascular resistance. This patient is asymptomatic and dermoid cyst is an incidental finding. At this time surgery is not indicated, and the patient should be re-scanned in 1–2 months (to check for growth and morphology changes of the lesion).

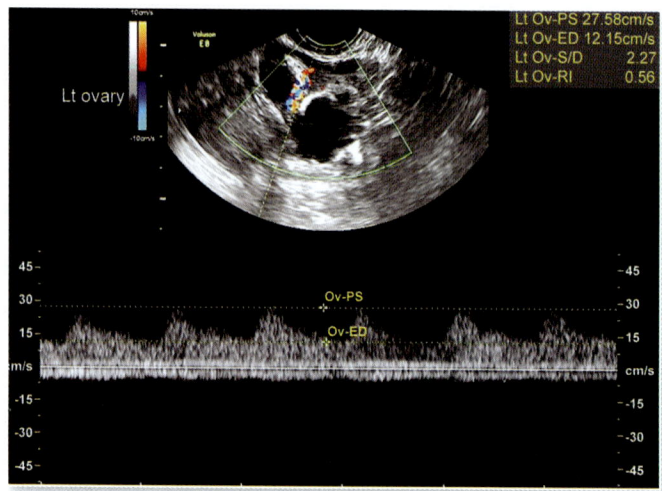

Figure 50.2: Color Doppler image of the same adnexal mass. Moderate vascular impedance blood flow signals (RI 0.56, PI 0.70) are obtained from the central part of the lesion

3. **How can the likelihood of malignancy be determined and what is the best next step for this patient?**

Ans. Dermoid cysts have characteristic sonographic features of hair and sebum, and the diagnosis is reasonably certain without surgical exploration. Biochemical tumor markers in pregnancy are of limited value. The levels of CA-125, alpha-fetoprotein, lactate dehydrogenase, human chorionic gonadotropin and inhibin A are elevated during pregnancy and fluctuate with gestational age. The resistance and pulsatility indices measure resistance within blood vessels. In this patient, color Doppler is reassuring of a benign ovarian lesion, based on moderate vascular resistance blood flow signals. Neovascularization seen in malignant tumors has typically low vascular resistance due to the abnormal distribution and scant muscular layer of the vessels.

■ TAKE-HOME MESSAGES

- Expectant management of ovarian dermoid cysts is feasible in pregnant patients in whom the diagnosis was made incidentally on ultrasound scan.[1,2]
- Most adnexal masses in pregnancy are benign cystic lesions (usually functional ovarian cysts) smaller than 5 cm in diameter. It is estimated that about 70% of all ovarian cysts in pregnancy which are incidentally diagnosed by ultrasound in first trimester spontaneously resolve.[1-3]
- The majority of the cysts which persist throughout pregnancy measuring 5 cm or greater are dermoid cysts.[2,4]
- Dermoid cysts have characteristic sonographic features of hair and sebum, and the diagnosis is reasonably certain without surgical exploration.[1,5,6]
- Biochemical tumor markers in pregnancy are of limited value. The levels of CA-125, alpha-fetoprotein, lactate dehydrogenase, human chorionic gonadotropin and inhibin A are elevated during gestation and fluctuate with gestational age.[7]

- In patients with large and bilateral dermoid cysts surgery should be considered, because the size may cause difficulty in second and third trimesters of pregnancy.[2,8]
- Surgical intervention is warranted when acute complications, such as adnexal torsion, hemorrhage, rupture or infection occur.[7-9]
- It is estimated that between 8% and 10% of adnexal masses that persist during pregnancy are malignant.[10]

REFERENCES

1. Zanetta G, Mariani E, Lissoni A, et al. A prospective study of the role of ultrasound in the management of adnexal masses in pregnancy. BJOG. 2003;110(6):578-83.
2. Runowicz C, Brewer MB. Adnexal masses in pregnancy. UpToDate. http://www.uptodate.com/contents/adnexal-mass-in-pregnancy. Accessed February 6, 2015.
3. Sherard GB 3rd, Hodson CA, Williams HJ, et al. Adnexal masses and pregnancy: a 12-year experience. Am J Obstet Gynecol. 2003;189(2):358-62.
4. Caspi B, Levi R, Appelman Z, et al. Conservative management of ovarian cystic teratoma during pregnancy and labor. Am J Obstet Gynecol. 2000;182(3):503-5.
5. Bernhard LM, Klebba PK, Gray DL, Mutch DG. Predictors of persistence of adnexal masses in pregnancy. Obstet Gynecol. 1999;93(4):585-9.
6. Kupesic S, Plavsic B. Adnexal torsion: color Doppler and three-dimensional ultrasound. Abdom Imaging. 2010; 35(5):602-6.
7. Yakasai IA, Bappa LA. Diagnosis and management of adnexal masses. J Surg Tech Case Rep. 2012;4(2):79-85.
8. Agarwal N, Kriplani A, Bhatla N, et al. Management and outcome of pregnancies complicated with adnexal masses. Arch Gynecol Obstet. 2003;267(3):148-52.
9. Schmeler KM, Mayo-Smith WW, Peipert JF, et al. Adnexal masses in pregnancy: surgery compared with observation. Obstet Gynecol. 2005;105:1098-103.
10. Leiserowitz GS, Xing G, Cress R, et al. Adnexal masses in pregnancy: how often are they malignant? Gynecol Oncol. 2006; 101(2):315-21.

CHAPTER 51

Adnexal Mass and Pelvic Pain in Pregnancy

Sanja Kupesic Plavsic, Ulrich Honemeyer

■ CLINICAL CASE

SM is a 36-year-old G1 who is presenting to ER with low abdominal and pelvic pain. She complains of abdominal bloating and cramping pain (severity 9/10) in her right lower pelvic area which began 2 hours ago. She feels nauseous, and has vomited three times. She does not complain of vaginal bleeding. Seven weeks ago she underwent ovulation induction with clomiphene citrate and gonadotropins, followed by an intrauterine insemination (IUI). Ten days ago normal intrauterine pregnancy was confirmed by ultrasound.

Menarche: Age 13.

Menses: 28/4 days, regular, spots the first couple of days, then heavy for two days.

LMP: 8 weeks ago.

Pregnancies: None.

Sexual history: Three male partners over her lifetime. For 5 years, she is in a monogamous relationship with her husband. First two years, she used condoms for birth control. Last three years, she attempted to get pregnant. After infertility work-up, she underwent two rounds of IUI. *Chlamydia* test and Pap smear were performed 6 months ago and were normal.

Review of Systems

- No headaches, no problems with vision
- No history of blood clots DVT or PE
- No heart palpitations, no shortness of breath
- Positive for right lower abdominal/pelvic pain
- No constipation and/or diarrhea. Positive for nausea and vomiting (3x)
- Decreased urination

- *Past medical history*: None (no hospitalizations)
- *Past surgical history*: None
- *Vaccines*: Up-to-date (hepatitis B vaccine series, and MMR booster; flu shot past winter)
- *Medications*: None
- *Allergies*: None known drug allergies

- *Social history*: High school teacher, denies smoking, denies drugs; occasionally has a drink once per week
- *Family history*: Mother: age 62, with no medical problems, retired. Father: age 70, with history of diabetes and high blood pressure. No family history of uterine, breast, ovarian or colon cancer.

Physical Examination

- *Vital signs*: BP 115/75; P 85; BMI 24
- Normal heart, lungs, thyroid and neck
- *Abdominal examination*: Tenderness over LLQ and evidence of rebound tenderness
- *Pelvic examination*: Cervix with no lesions, no cervical motion tenderness. Uterus is enlarged, anteverted. Right adnexa enlarged and very tender to palpation, left adnexa enlarged, difficult to assess the size of adnexal masses because of the tenderness
- Pelvic ultrasound was performed and sonographic findings are illustrated in Figures 51.1 to 51.4.

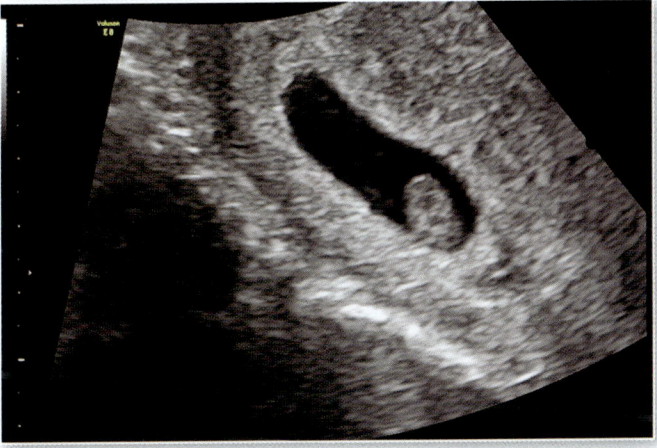

Figure 51.1: Intrauterine gestational sac with embryonic pole

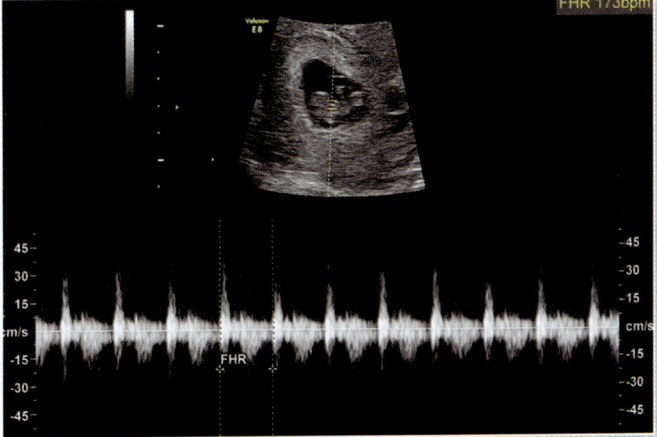

Figure 51.2: Regular embryonic heart action (frequency of 178 bpm) is obtained

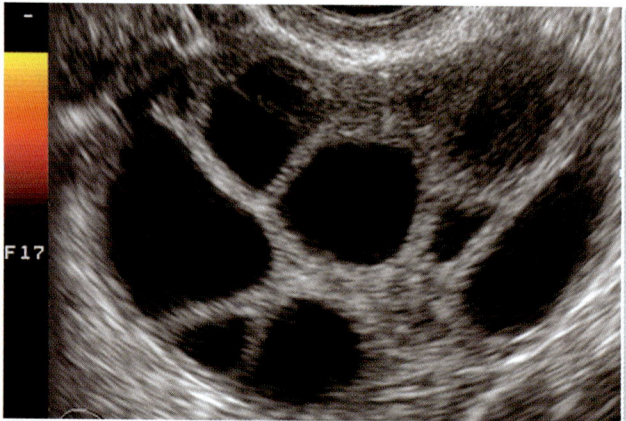

Figure 51.3: Power Doppler US image of the torsed right hyperstimulated ovary. Note absence of intraovarian blood flow signals. Doppler findings are suggestive of complete adnexal torsion

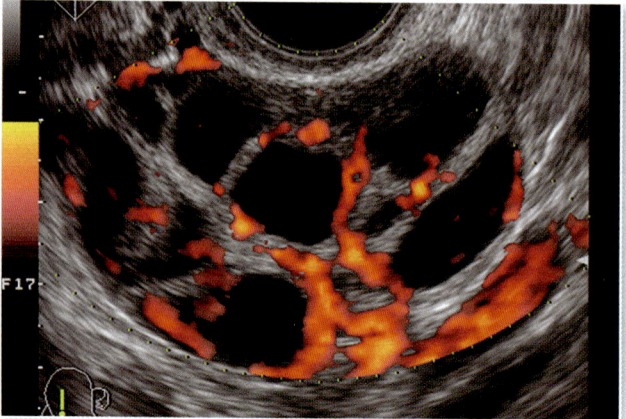

Figure 51.4: Power Doppler image of the contralateral hyperstimulated ovary. Note prominent intraovarian flow. From Kupesic S (ed). Color Doppler, 3D and 4D Ultrasound in Gynecology, Infertility and Obstetrics. Figure 9.11. p. 121; New Delhi: Jaypee Brothers Medical Publisher; 2011.

■ CLINICAL QUESTIONS

1. How should the adnexal mass be assessed?

Ans. Investigations include beta-hCG (to assess the dynamics of beta-hCG), white blood cell counts (WBC), CRP, hematocrit, hemoglobin, electrolytes, and pelvic ultrasound.

Results of our patient's laboratory and imaging findings are as following:
- Beta-hCG: 98,410 mIU/mL
- Laboratory findings reveal normal WBC, CRP, and electrolytes, and no evidence of hemoconcentration

- Pelvic ultrasound depicts intrauterine gestational sac with embryonic pole and regular heart action (Figs 51.1 and 51.2). Sonographic findings are consistent with 8 weeks gestation. The ovaries are enlarged and measure 10 × 12 cm (right) and 11 × 12 cm (left) with numerous fluid-filled cysts. There is free fluid in the cul-de-sac. There are no sonographic signs of ectopic pregnancy
- Power Doppler US does not obtain intraovarian blood flow signals from the right ovary (Fig. 51.3), while normal intraovarian perfusion is detected from the contralateral ovary (Fig. 51.4). Sonographic and Doppler findings are suggestive of the right ovarian/adnexal torsion.

2. **When is surgical intervention indicated and can it be postponed?**

Ans. Sonographic and Doppler findings indicate complete torsion of the right hyperstimulated ovary for which urgent surgical intervention is required.

3. **What is the best surgical route? Laparoscopy or laparotomy?**

Ans. Laparoscopy procedure is recommended to treat patients suffering from ovarian torsion in pregnancy due to shorter hospital stay, fewer postoperative complications and ovarian preservation.

■ TAKE-HOME MESSAGES

- Ultrasound is a method of choice for the assessment of pelvic masses in pregnancy.[1,2]
- Color and pulsed Doppler ultrasound is useful for detection of adnexal torsion.[3,4]
- Surgical intervention is warranted when acute complications (such as adnexal torsion, ovarian rupture, bleeding and/or infection) develop.[1,5]
- Ovarian torsion is suspected in the presence of ovarian enlargement, worsening unilateral pain, nausea, and vomiting. Color Doppler is particularly useful for diagnosis of ovarian torsion. Untwisting of torquated adnexa followed by observation of improved color at laparoscopy (Figures 51.5 to 51.8) is safe and effective.[4]
- Surgical intervention of adnexal masses in pregnancy is needed when malignancy is suspected and when the size of the tumor is likely to cause difficulty.[6,7]

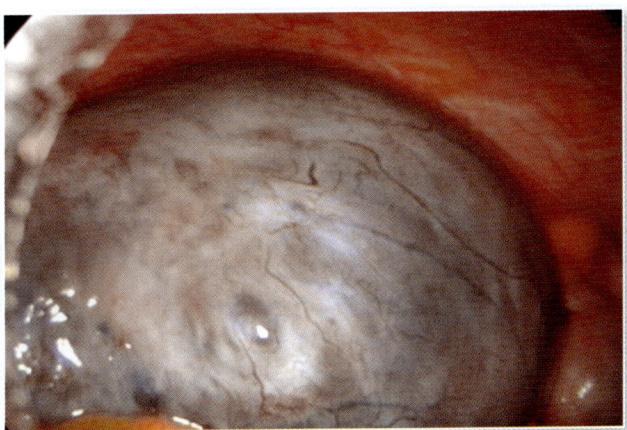

Figure 51.5: Laparoscopic image of the torsed hyperstimulated ovary. Note typical bluish color

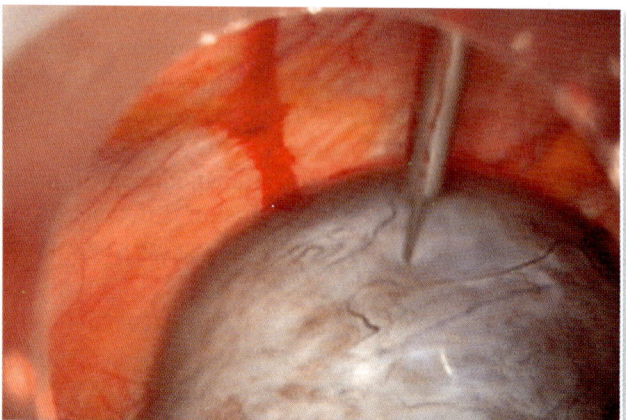

Figure 51.6: Multiple luteinized cysts were punctured

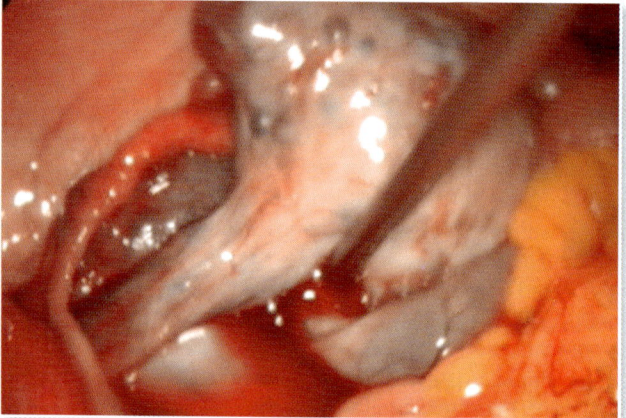

Figure 51.7: Intraoperative unwinding of the right adnexa was performed

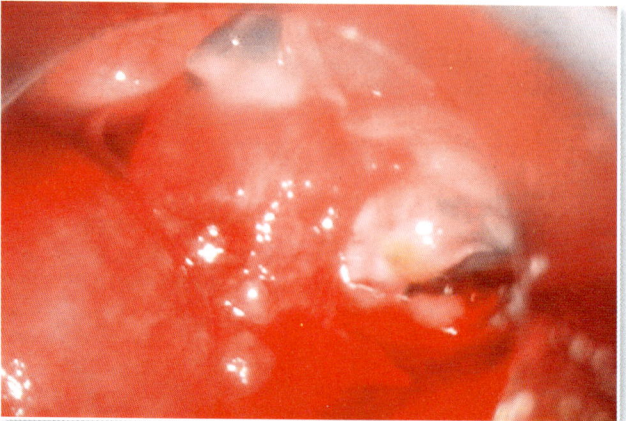

Figure 51.8: Reestablished circulation of the right ovary was noted 10–15 minutes following detorsion of what initially appeared to be a nonviable ovary. No postoperative complications were noted and the ovary was proved functional by ultrasonography

- Patients undergoing ovarian surgery prior to 8 weeks gestation in whom the corpus luteum is removed require progesterone supplementation (50–100 mg vaginally every 8–12 hours or 50 mg (1 mL) intramuscularly).[6] After 10 weeks of gestation, the placenta is the primary provider of progesterone, so progesterone supplementation is no longer indicated.[6,7]
- During the first and second trimesters, laparoscopy is safe as laparotomy.[8] Data from the literature indicate that laparoscopy procedure is recommended to treat patients suffering from ovarian torsion in pregnancy due to shorter hospital stay, fewer postoperative complications and ovarian preservation.[9]
- When ovarian malignancy is suspected, a vertical incision should be performed.[6,10] If the mass has features suggesting malignancy, ipsilateral salpingo-oophorectomy should be performed. The mass should be sent for frozen section and all suspicious lesions should be biopsied.[6,10]

REFERENCES

1. Giuntoli RL 2nd, Vang RS, Bristow RE. Evaluation and management of adnexal masses during pregnancy. Clin Obstet Gynecol. 2006;49(3):492-505.
2. Chiang G, Levine D. Imaging of adnexal masses in pregnancy. J Ultrasound Med. 2004;23(6):805-19.
3. Yen CF, Lin SL, Murk W, et al. Risk analysis of torsion and malignancy for adnexal masses during pregnancy. Fertil Steril. 2009; 91(5):1895-902.
4. Kupesic S, Plavsic B. Adnexal torsion: color Doppler and three-dimensional ultrasound. Abdom Imaging. 2010;35(5):602-6.
5. Yakasai IA, Bappa LA. Diagnosis and management of adnexal masses in pregnancy. J Surg Tech Case Rep. 2012;4(2):79-85.
6. Leiserowitz GS, Xing G, Cress R, et al. Adnexal masses in pregnancy: how often are they malignant? Gynecol Oncol. 2006; 101(2):315-21.
7. American College of Obstetricians and Gynecologists. ACOG Practice Bulletin. Management of adnexal masses. Obstet Gynecol. 2007;110(1):201-14.
8. Schmeler KM, Mayo-Smith WW, Peipert JF, et al. Adnexal masses in pregnancy: surgery compared with observation. Obstet Gynecol. 2005;105:1098-103.
9. Lo LM, Chang SD, Horng SG, et al. Laparoscopy versus laparotomy for surgical intervention of ovarian torsion. J Obstet Gynaecol Res. 2008;34(6):1020-5.
10. Palmer J, Vatish M, Tidy J. Epithelial ovarian cancer in pregnancy: a review of the literature. BJOG. 2009;116(4):480-91.

CHAPTER

Appendicitis in Pregnancy

52

Safa Farrag, Humera Chaudhary, Sanja Kupesic Plavsic

■ CLINICAL CASE

LR is a 25-year G2P1who is presenting at 20 weeks' gestation with a severe right lower quadrant (RLQ) abdominal and pelvic pain. The pain started few hours ago, and is progressively worsening. It started around the umbilicus then migrated to the right lower quadrant; 8/10 in severity; movement makes it worse; staying still makes it slightly better. The pain is associated with nausea, loss of appetite, abdominal bloating and vomiting (LR vomited twice during the past hour). She had chills but did not check her temperature. She has never had this type of pain before. Her last clinic visit was seven days ago. Her vital signs and labs were within normal limits at that time.

Menarche: Age 14.

Menses: 28/4 days, regular.

LMP: 22 weeks ago.

Pregnancies: 1 uncomplicated pregnancy 4 years ago. The course of current pregnancy was also normal.

Deliveries: 1 normal vaginal term delivery.

Sexual history: Five partners in her lifetime; she is with the last partner for 3 years.

Contraception: She was using oral contraception pills after the delivery of her first child till three months prior to the current pregnancy; no condom use.

Review of Systems

- No vaginal bleeding or discharge
- No diarrhea or constipation; complains of nausea and vomiting
- No urinary symptoms
- No headache. No chest pain or cough
- No lower extremity edema

- *Past medical history*: Treated for gonorrhea 1 year ago; hospitalized for normal vaginal delivery

- *Past surgical history*: None
- *Vaccines*: Up to date (hepatitis B vaccine series, MMR booster and flu shot)
- *Current medications*: Tylenol 350 mg once at home when her pain started
- *Allergies*: No known drug allergies
- *Social history*: She is an accountant, no history of smoking, ETOH or drug abuse
- *Family history*: Mother (51 years), diagnosed with diabetes. Father (54 years) is healthy.

Physical Examination

- The patient is in moderate distress due to the pain
- *Vital signs*: T 38.5°C oral, BP 105/85, P 99
- *Cardiac examination*: S1, S2 present, grade 2 ejection systolic murmur at the heart base
- *Chest examination*: Clear lungs.
- *Skin*: No jaundice
- *Abdominal examination*: Soft, tender right lower quadrant, with mild rebound tenderness; gravid uterus palpated 1 cm above the umbilicus, fetal movement preserved
- *Pelvic examination*: Vaginal examination elicits more pain and discomfort than abdominal examination. Cervix is closed, no discharge. Uterine size corresponds to the gestational age. Adnexal masses could not be appreciated.

Laboratory Tests

White blood cells: 17,000 cells/mm^3; with left shift. Otherwise normal.

■ CLINICAL QUESTIONS

1. What is the differential diagnosis of the RLQ pain in pregnancy?

Ans.
- Ectopic pregnancy has to be ruled out first with any positive pregnancy test and an abdominal pain. Our patient is at 20 weeks gestation and ectopic pregnancy is an unlikely diagnosis
  - *Appendicitis*: Pain usually occurs close to McBurney's point in the majority of pregnant patients; however, with uterine enlargement, the location of appendix migrates a few centimeters in the cranial direction
  - *Differential diagnosis includes*: Pre-eclampsia, HELLP, and acute fatty liver of pregnancy
  - In later pregnancy uterine rupture (usually associated with vaginal bleeding and fetal decompensation) and placental abruption
  - Intra-amniotic infection should also be considered
  - *Pyelonephritis*: Associated with urinary symptoms
  - *Ovarian torsion*: Requires color Doppler ultrasound to be ruled out.

2. What is the next step in the work up?

Ans.
- *Abdominal ultrasound (US)*: May show the appendix as a tubular uncompressible structure in the RLQ. US can also rule out other causes of abdominal pain, such as ovarian torsion (Figs 52.1 to 52.3)
  - *Magnetic resonance imaging (MRI):* If US test was inconclusive; MRI is superior to CT due to the lack of exposure to the ionizing radiation.

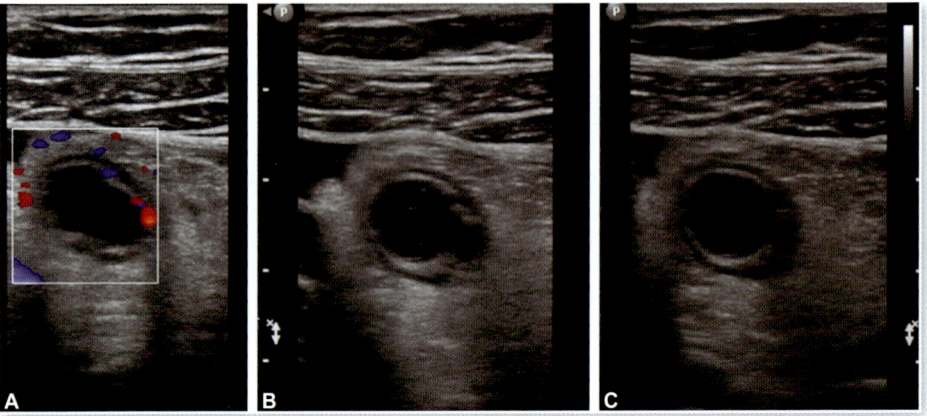

Figures 52.1A to C: Axial ultrasound images of the right lower quadrant show dilated fluid filled appendix that does not show compression. Figure A shows increased vascularity in appendiceal wall

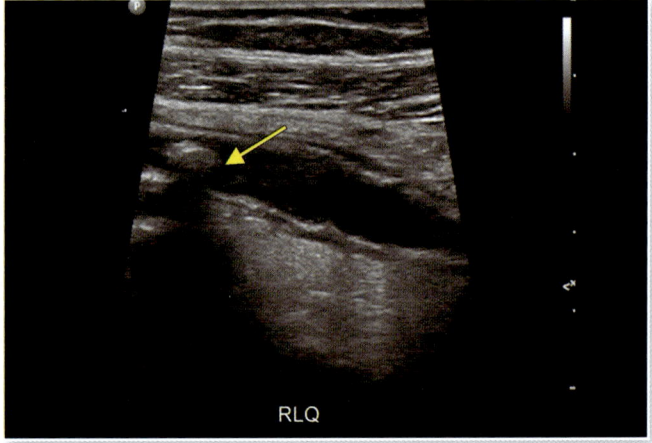

Figure 52.2: Sagittal ultrasound images through long axis of the appendix shows dilated fluid filled tubular blind ended structure containing an appendicolith at its base (arrow)

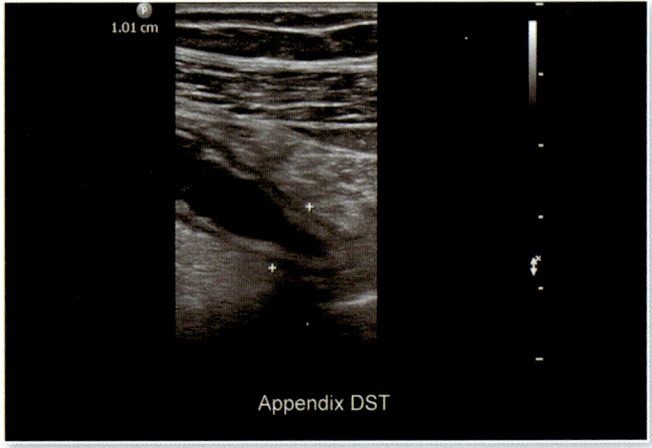

Figure 52.3: Dilated appendix measures 1 cm in diameter

3. What is the best treatment?

Ans. Prompt surgery, along with perioperative antibiotics is recommended for management of pregnant patients presenting with appendicitis. Laparoscopic appendectomy is safe and effective procedure, associated with good maternal and fetal outcome.

■ TAKE-HOME MESSAGES

- Acute appendicitis is the most common non-obstetric surgical emergency during pregnancy. The incidence of acute appendicitis during pregnancy is 1 in 800 to 1 in 1,500 pregnancies, with the lowest risk reported during the third trimester.[1,2]
- The site of the pain is usually the RLQ; however, it may migrate a few centimeters cephalad with the enlarging uterus, so pain may be localized in the mid or even the upper right side of the abdomen in the third trimester.[3]
- A detailed history and examination is vital to differentiate between the broad differential diagnoses. The clinical picture and laboratory findings may be atypical during pregnancy, so further imaging is required to confirm the diagnosis of appendicitis and to reduce the false positive rate.[4]
- Delayed management can result in life-threatening maternal and fetal complications, including appendicular perforation, premature delivery, miscarriage, and fetal loss. The prognosis is determined by the interval between the onset of presentation and the time of surgical intervention.[5]
- Abdominal ultrasonography is the most frequently utilized imaging test used in the evaluation of pregnant women with acute abdominal pain and concern for appendicitis.[6]
- MRI appears to be an excellent modality for excluding acute appendicitis in pregnant women when clinical and US examination are inconclusive, and to improve diagnostic accuracy to reduce the rate of negative appendectomies.[7,8]
- Treatment of appendicitis is appendectomy, with perioperative antibiotic treatment with second-generation cephalosporin to cover gram-negative and gram-positive aerobes, and clindamycin or metronidazole for anaerobes. Surgery should not be delayed for more than 24 hours after symptom onset to avoid appendicular perforation.[9]
- There is no strong evidence weather open or laparoscopic appendectomy is the preferred modality to treat appendicitis during pregnancy in regard to fetal or maternal safety. Laparoscopy surgery has been shown to offer some advantages over open laparotomy: Decreased postoperative pain, reduced hospital, and wound morbidity.[10] However, there is a low grade evidence that laparoscopic appendectomy might be associated with higher rates of fetal loss.[11]

■ REFERENCES

1. Abbasi N, Patenaude V, Abenhaim HA. Management and outcomes of acute appendicitis in pregnancy-population-based study of over 7000 cases. BJOG. 2014;121(12):1509-14.
2. Zingone F, Sultan AA, Humes DJ, West J. Risk of acute appendicitis in and around pregnancy a population-based cohort study from England. Ann Surg. 2015;261(2):332-7.
3. House JB, Bourne CL, Seymour HM, Brewer KL. Location of the appendix in the gravid patient. J Emerg Med. 2014;46(5):741-4.
4. Flexer SM, Tabib N, Peter MB. Suspected appendicitis in pregnancy. Surgeon. 2014;12(2):82-6.
5. Miloudi N, Brahem M, Ben Abid S, et al. Acute appendicitis in pregnancy: specific features of diagnosis and treatment. J Visc Surg. 2012;149(4):e275-9.
6. Drake FT, Kotagal M, Simmons LE, et al. Single institution and statewide performance of ultrasound in diagnosing appendicitis in pregnancy. J Matern Fetal Neonatal Med. 2015;28(6):727-33.
7. Theilen LH, Mellnick VM, Longman RE, et al. Utility of magnetic resonance imaging for suspected appendicitis in pregnant women. Am J Obstet Gynecol. 2015;212(3):345.e1-6.
8. Aggenbach L, Zeeman G, Cantineau AEP, et al. Impact of appendicitis during pregnancy: No delay in accurate diagnosis and treatment. Int J Surg. 2015;15:849.
9. Bickell NA, Aufses AH Jr, Rojas M, Bodian C. How time affects the risk of rupture in appendicitis. J Am Coll Surg. 2006;202(3):401-6.
10. Friedman JD, Ramsey PS, Ramin KD, Berry C. Pneumoamnion and pregnancy loss after second-trimester laparoscopic surgery. Obstet Gynecol. 2002;99(3):512-3.
11. Humphrey GMW, Al Samaraee A, Mills SJ, Kalbassi MJ. Laparoscopic appendicectomy in pregnancy: A systematic review of the published evidence. Int J Surg. 2014;12(11):1235241.

Congenital Heart Disease in Pregnancy

CHAPTER 53

Safa Farrag, Wael El-Mallah, Sanja Kupesic Plavsic

■ CLINICAL CASE

LR is a 25-year-old Hispanic G1P0 who is coming to the clinic as a new patient, with no prior clinic visits at 25 weeks gestation. She has recently moved from Mexico and was told that she has a heart murmur, but has never had any cardiac evaluation. Today she is complaining of fatigue and shortness of breath for the past four weeks. Symptoms occur while doing her regular physical activities like house cleaning. She feels well at rest. Her physical activities are minimally reduced, and she is still able to function, but she is concerned that her condition might get worse.

Menarche: Age 13.

Menses: 28/5 days, regular.

LMP: 25 weeks ago.

Pregnancies: None.

Deliveries: None.

Sexual history: Monogamous relationship with the husband.

Contraception: None.

Review of Systems

- No syncope. No chest pain or cough
- No nausea or vomiting
- No lower extremity edema
- No vaginal bleeding or uterine contractions
- No diarrhea or constipation
- No urinary problems
- *Past medical history:* Non-significant
- *Past surgical history:* Tonsillectomy at 12 years of age
- *Vaccines*: Up to date except for the flu shot
- *Current medications:* Over the counter folic acid in the first trimester
- *Allergies*: No known drug allergies
- *Social history:* LR is a housewife, no history of smoking, ETOH, and drug abuse
- *Family history:* Mother–50 years, had a valve replacement. Father–58 years, has hypertension.

Physical Examination

- The patient is in no distress
- *Vital signs:* T 36.4°C oral, BP 110/85, P 90, BMI 25
- *Cardiac examination:* S1, S2 present, right second intercostal space murmur, 3/6, no palpable thrill; murmur is radiating to the neck and over both carotid arteries; no diastolic murmur, no S4.
- *Chest examination:* Clear lungs
- *Abdominal examination:* Soft, tender right upper quadrant, no rebound tenderness; no Murphy sign. Gravid uterus palpated 3 cm above the umbilicus, fetal movements preserved
- *Pelvic examination:* No bleeding, cervix is closed
- *Skin:* No jaundice.

CLINICAL QUESTIONS

1. What does the above mentioned murmur suggest?

Ans. The right second intercostal space murmur suggests an outflow obstruction at the aortic valve area that is most likely due to aortic stenosis.

2. What is the most common cause of an isolated aortic stenosis murmur?

Ans. Bicuspid aortic valve is the most common cause of an isolated aortic stenosis murmur.

3. What are the best imaging tests to confirm the diagnosis?

Ans. A transthoracic echocardiography is the best imaging option to assess the aortic valve opening, gradient of flow across the valve, and ejection fraction. Further evaluation of the aortic arch and thoracic aorta can be done by MRI or transesophageal echocardiography (Figs 53.1 to 53.3).

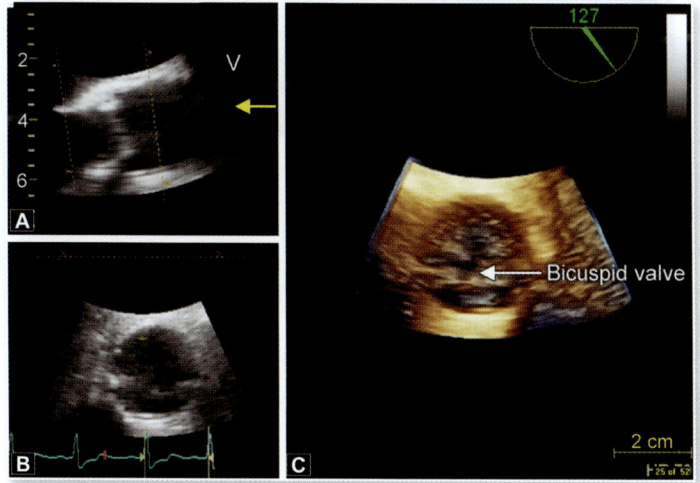

Figures 53.1A to C: Transesophageal echocardiogram depicting: (A) 2D image of a bicuspid stenotic aortic valve in longitudinal view; (B) 2D image of a bicuspid stenotic aortic valve short axis view; (C) 3D image of bicuspid stenotic aortic valve in short axis view

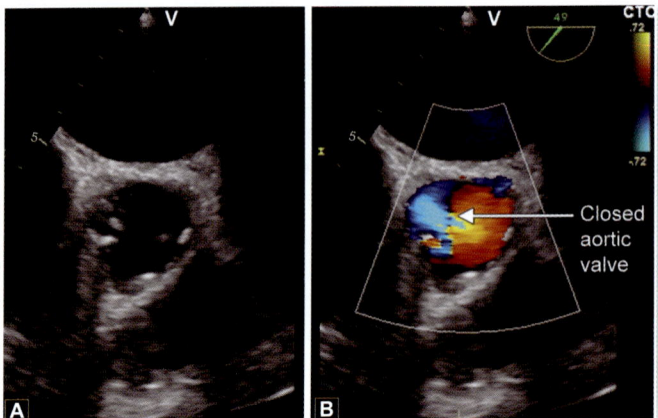

Figures 53.2A and B: (A) 2D image of a transesophageal echocardiogram depicting the closed bicuspid aortic valve without colors; (B) 2D image of a transesophageal echocardiogram depicting the closed bicuspid aortic valve with colors showing trivial aortic regurgitation

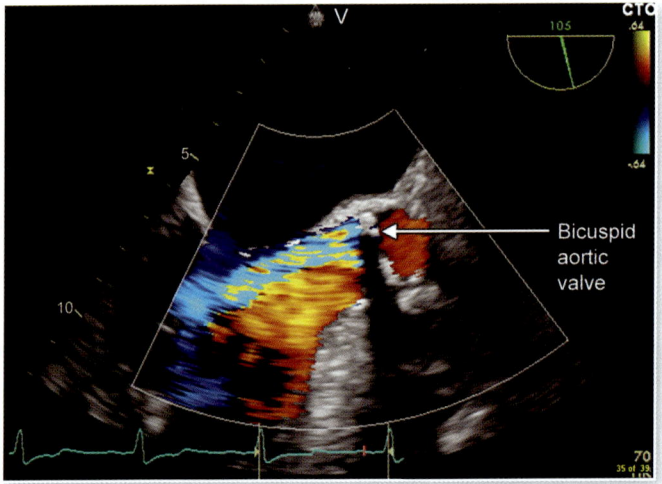

Figure 53.3: 2D image of a transesophageal echocardiogram depicting the bicuspid aortic valve in long axis view

4. **What is the best management of this patient with mild symptoms, mild stenosis by echo, and mildly reduced ejection fraction (55%)?**

Ans. Conservative treatment with bed rest, beta-blockers, and oxygen.

■ TAKE-HOME MESSAGES

- Cardiac disease complicates approximately 4% of all pregnancies in the United States. Congenital cardiac lesions are 3 times more common than acquired.[1] Bicuspid aortic valve is the most common congenital heart disease affecting 2% of the population.[2]

- According to the 2008 American College of Cardiology/American Heart Association (ACC/AHA) guidelines it is recommended to use echocardiographic screening for bicuspid aortic valve in first-degree relatives of a patient with known bicuspid aortic valve.[3]
- Aortic stenosis is a common complication of a bicuspid aortic valve. Symptoms can range from mild dyspnea, fatigue, palpitation, or anginal pain on strenuous or rapid prolonged exertion to symptoms at rest (based New York Heart Association (NYHA) classification).[4]
- Other complications of bicuspid aortic valve include aortic incompetence, especially in the setting of prolapsing cusps, endocarditis, or after balloon valvuloplasty. Complications also include aortopathy, aortic dissection, and endocarditis which can lead to valve perforation or destruction.[5] Aortic dissection during pregnancy is potentially lethal to both mother and fetus.[6]
- Echocardiogram is used to evaluate the size of aortic valve opening, gradient of flow across the valve and ejection fraction. MRI is recommended for imaging of the aortic arch, descending and abdominal aorta. Transesophageal echocardiography is another option for thoracic aortic imaging. Measurements of aortic size may vary depending on the technique used.[1,7]
- Severe aortic stenosis is determined when the valve area is <1 cm^2, the mean gradient >40 mmHg, aortic velocity >4.0 m/sec, and ejection fraction <55%. Pregnant women with mild to severe aortic stenosis and no or minimal symptoms can be treated conservatively with bed rest, oxygen and beta-blockers.[8]
- Pregnant women with severe symptoms of aortic stenosis can be treated with balloon valvotomy. Surgery should be avoided during pregnancy because of the risk to the fetus and the mother.[9]
- Aortic valve replacement is indicated in patients with severe symptoms of heart failure NYHA class III or IV with bicuspid AS, following failed or non-applicable valvotomy, patients with refractory heart failure NYHA class III or IV HF and bicuspid AR, and for aortic dissection.[10]

REFERENCES

1. Gandhi M, Martin SR. Cardiac Disease in Pregnancy. Obstet Gynecol Clin North Am. 2015;42(2):315-33.
2. Yuan SM. Bicuspid aortic valve in pregnancy. Taiwan J Obst Gynecol. 2014;53(4):47680.
3. Warnes CA, Williams RG, Bashore TM, et al. ACC/AHA 2008 Guidelines for the Management of Adults with Congenital Heart Disease: a report of the American College of Cardiology/American Heart Association Task Force on Practice Guidelines (writing committee to develop guidelines on the management of adults with congenital heart disease). Circulation 2008; 118 (23):e714-833.
4. Donnelly RT, Pinto NM, Kocolas I, Yetman AT. The immediate and long-term impact of pregnancy on aortic growth rate and mortality in women with Marfan syndrome. J Am Coll Cardiol. 2012;60(3):224-9.
5. Siu SC, Silversides CK. Bicuspid Aortic Valve Disease. J Am Coll Cardiol. 2010;55(25):2789-800.
6. Yang Z, Yang S, Wang F, Wang C. Acute aortic dissection in pregnant women. Gen Thorac Cardiovasc Surg. 2014,DOI 10.1007/s11748-014-0460-4.
7. Hiratzka LF, Bakris GL, Beckman JA, et al. 2010 ACCF/AHA/AATS/ACR/ASA/SCA/SCAI/SIR/STS/SVM guidelines for the diagnosis and management of patients with Thoracic Aortic Disease: a report of the American College of Cardiology Foundation/American Heart Association Task Force on Practice Guidelines, American Association for Thoracic Surgery, American College of Radiology, American Stroke Association, Society of Cardiovascular Anesthesiologists, Society for Cardiovascular Angiography and Interventions, Society of Interventional Radiology, Society of Thoracic Surgeons, and Society for Vascular Medicine. Circulation 2010;121(13):e266.
8. Bonow RO, Carabello BA, Chatterjee K, et al. 2008 Focused update incorporated into the ACC/AHA 2006 guidelines for the management of patients with valvular heart disease: a report of the American College of Cardiology/American Heart Association Task Force on Practice Guidelines (Writing Committee to Revise the 1998 Guidelines for the Management of Patients with Valvular Heart Disease): endorsed by the Society of Cardiovascular Anesthesiologists, Society for Cardiovascular Angiography and Interventions, and Society of Thoracic Surgeons. Circulation. 2008;118:e523.
9. Roos-Hesselink JW, Ruys TP, Stein JI, et al. Outcome of pregnancy in patients with structural or ischaemic heart disease: results of a registry of the European Society of Cardiology. Eur Heart J. 2013;34(9):657-65.
10. Task Force Members, Celia Oakley, Chairperson, Anne Child, et al. Expert consensus document on management of cardiovascular diseases during pregnancy, The Task Force on the Management of Cardiovascular Diseases During Pregnancy of the European Society of Cardiology. Eur Heart J. 2003;24(8):761-81.

Deep Venous Thrombosis in Pregnancy

CHAPTER 54

Safa Farrag, Humera Chaudhary, Sanja Kupesic Plavsic

■ CLINICAL CASE

GA is a 37-year-old G3P2, who was admitted to ER at 31 weeks gestation with twin pregnancy, complaining of left lower extremity pain. The pain started about 2 days ago. It is progressively worsening, 8/10 in severity, associated with mild swelling, redness and tenderness over the leg. She has no fever or chills, and has never experienced this pain before. Her last clinic visit was 2 weeks ago, when her weight, vital signs, and labs were within normal limits.

Menarche: Age 14.

Menses: 28/5 days, regular.

LMP: 33 weeks ago.

Pregnancy: 2 uncomplicated pregnancies 5 and 3 years ago. The course of current pregnancy was normal.

Delivery: Two normal vaginal term deliveries.

Sexual history: In monogamous relationship with her husband.

Contraception: She was using diaphragm and condoms prior to the current pregnancy.

Review of Systems

- No chest pain or shortness of breath
- No headache, no fever
- No vaginal bleeding or uterine colic
- No diarrhea or constipation
- No hematuria or dysuria

- *Past medical history*: Bilateral lower extremities varicose veins; BMI 34 prior to pregnancy
- *Past surgical history*: Cholecystectomy following the first pregnancy
- *Vaccines*: Up to date (hepatitis B vaccine series, MMR booster and flu shot)
- *Current medications*: None
- *Allergies*: No known drug allergy
- *Social history*: She is a hair stylist, smokes 1 pack of cigarettes per day for the past 10 years; cut down to 10 cigarettes per day during pregnancy; social ETOH, no drug abuse
- *Family history*: Mother—60 years, has diabetes and hypertension. Father—61 years, has hypertension.

Physical Examination

- The patient is in moderate distress due to the pain
- *Vital signs*: T 36.9°C oral, BP 105/85, P 90, BMI 35
- *Cardiac examination*: Normal.
- *Chest examination*: Clear lungs
- *Abdominal examination*: Soft, non-tender.
- *Pelvic examination*: No vaginal bleeding, cervix is closed
- *Extremities*: Left leg—swelling, erythema, tenderness, with increased left leg circumference >2 cm than the right side. Predominant bilateral varicose vein stage 2 and 3
- Gray scale and color Doppler ultrasound findings are presented in Figures 54.1 to 54.3.

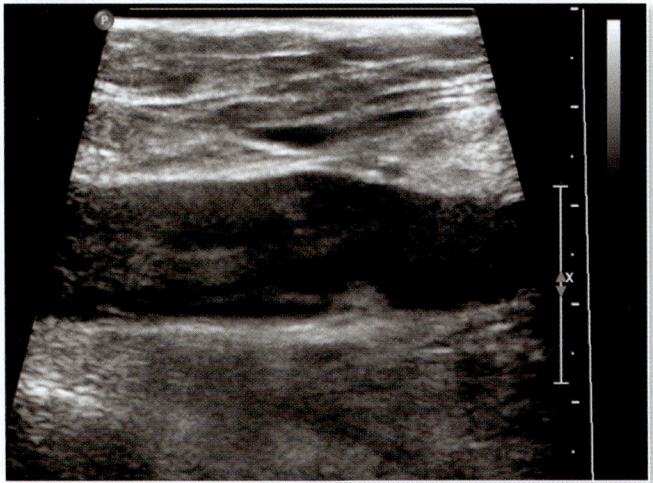

Figure 54.1: Gray scale ultrasound image shows distended left common femoral vein filled with internal echoes representing acute thrombus

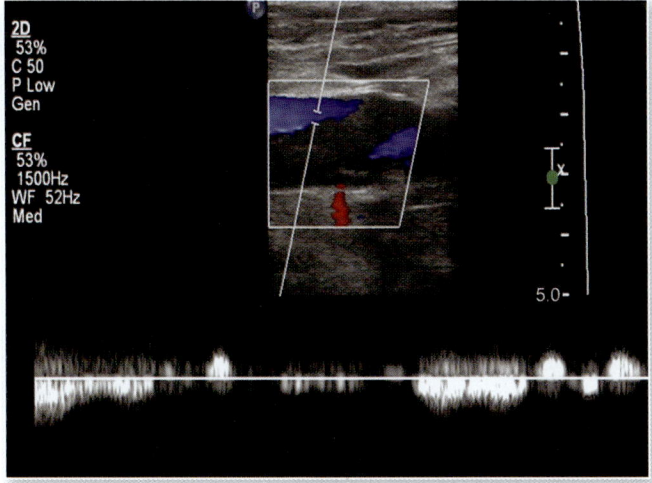

Figure 54.2: Color Doppler shows no flow in left common femoral vein at the site of thrombus

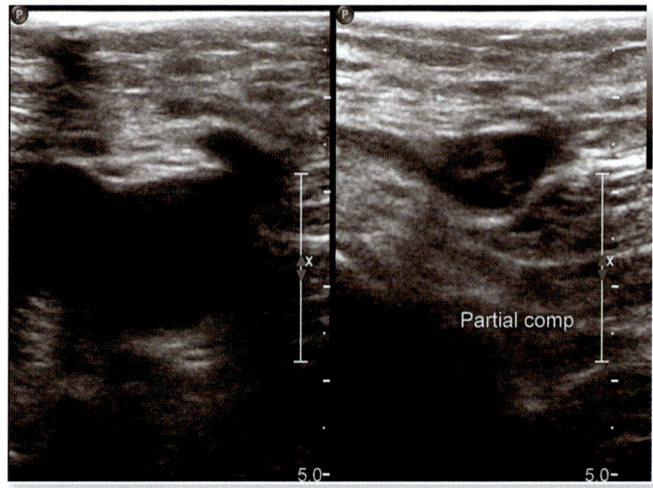

Figure 54.3: Gray scale ultrasound images show partial compression of left common femoral vein due to thrombosis

■ CLINICAL QUESTIONS

1. What is the best next step for the diagnosis?

Ans. Vein compression ultrasonography (CUS) preferably with Doppler (duplex ultrasound). D-Dimer and Wells score for DVT prediction are not used in pregnant women.

2. What are the most common thromboembolic events during pregnancy?

Ans. Besides DVT, pulmonary embolism (PE) is one of the most common thromboembolic events in pregnancy which should be suspected with any respiratory symptoms. Cerebral vein thrombosis should be suspected in pregnant patients with headache, altered mental status, and/or increased intracranial tension.

3. What are the most common risk factors for DVT in pregnant patients?

Ans. Age >30, smoking, history of DVT, twin/multiple pregnancy, assisted reproduction, varicose veins, systemic lupus erythematosus, BMI >30, parity >3, history of CS, antepartum or postpartum hemorrhage.

■ TAKE-HOME MESSAGES

- PE is the seventh leading cause of maternal mortality, responsible for 9% of maternal deaths. The incidence of venous thromboembolism (VTE) increases about 4-fold during pregnancy and at least 14-fold during the puerperium.[1,2]
- Compression of the left iliac vein by the overlying right iliac artery is thought to contribute to the predilection of left-sided DVT during pregnancy.[3]
- Pregnancy-associated changes in venous capacitance and compression of large veins by the gravid uterus promote stasis and increase of several coagulation factors, including factors VII, VIII, IX, X, XII, and fibrinogen, along with a decrease in protein S anticoagulant response to activated protein C decreases contribute to increased risk of thromboembolic incidents.[2,4]

- The best diagnostic tool for DVT is CUS with Doppler (non-invasive, readily available, and does not involve radiation).[5]
- Any patient presenting with respiratory symptoms should initially get a chest X-ray to rule out other pathology. For the diagnosis of pulmonary embolism, the patient will need CUS, especially in the presence of lower extremity symptoms. The decision whether to get computed-tomographic angiography (CTA) or ventilation-perfusion (V/Q) is challenging due to the risk of ionizing radiation to the mother and fetus associated with both, however, if the CXR is abnormal then a CTA is preferred, while if it is negative then a V/Q may be the alternative choice.[5,6]
- Warfarin should be avoided in the antepartum period due to teratogenicity.[7]
- Low molecular weight heparin (LMWH) is preferable to unfractionated heparin in the setting of pregnancy due to its lower rate of heparin-induced thrombocytopenia (HIT), allergic reactions and osteoporosis.[8]
- Anticoagulant therapy generally continues for at least six weeks postpartum. Patients with persistent risk factors for VTE may require a longer duration of therapy.[9]
- LMWH is the drug of choice for thromboprophylaxis during pregnancy, and should be considered in women with personal history of VTE and known thrombophilia.[8,10]

REFERENCES

1. Chang J, Elam-Evans LD, Berg CJ, et al. Pregnancy-related mortality surveillance—United States, 1991-1999. MMWR Surveill Summ. 2003;52(2):1-8.
2. Lussana F, Coppens M, Cattaneo M, Middeldorp S. Pregnancy-related venous thromboembolism: risk and the effect of thromboprophylaxis. Thromb Res. 2012;129(6):673-80.
3. Bourjeily G, Paidas M, Khalil H, Rosene-Montella K, Rodger M. Pulmonary embolism in pregnancy. Lancet. 2010;375(9713):500-12.
4. Marik PE, Plante LA. Venous thromboembolic disease and pregnancy. N Engl J Med. 2008;359(19):2025-33.
5. Gray G, Nelson-Piercy C. Thromboembolic disorders in obstetrics. Best Pract Res Clin Obstet Gynaecol. 2012;26(1):53-64.
6. Cahill AG, Stout MJ, Macones GA, Bhalla S. Diagnosing pulmonary embolism in pregnancy using computed-tomographic angiography or ventilation-perfusion. Obstet Gynecol. 2009;114(1):124-9.
7. Marshall AL. Diagnosis, treatment, and prevention of venous thromboembolism in pregnancy. Postgrad Med. 2014;126(7):25-34.
8. Guimicheva B, Czuprynska J, Arya R. The prevention of pregnancy-related venous thromboembolism. Br J Haematol. 2015;168(2):163-74.
9. Kamel H, Navi BB, Sriram N, Hovsepian DA, et al. Risk of a thrombotic event after the 6-week postpartum period. N Engl J Med. 2014;370(14):1307-15.
10. Lussana F, Coppens M, Cattaneo M, Middeldorp S. Pregnancy-related venous thromboembolism: risk and the effect of thromboprophylaxis. Thromb Res. 2012;129(6): 673-80.

CHAPTER 55

Gallstones in Pregnancy

Safa Farrag, Humera Chaudhary, Padilla Osvaldo, Sanja Kupesic Plavsic

■ CLINICAL CASE

MH is a 29-year-old Caucasian G3P2, who came to ER complaining of the RUQ colicky pain at 24 weeks gestation. The pain is not radiating, 8/10 in severity, and started two hours after she ate her lunch. There is no nausea or vomiting, fever or chills associated with this pain. She has never had this pain before. Her clinic visit was last week, and her vital signs and laboratory findings were within normal limits at that time.

Menarche: Age 15.

Menses: 30/5 days, regular.

LMP: 26 weeks ago.

Pregnancies: Two uncomplicated pregnancies 5 and 3 years ago. The course of current pregnancy was also normal.

Deliveries: Two normal vaginal term deliveries.

Sexual history: In monogamous relationship with her husband.

Contraception: She was using oral contraceptive pills after the delivery of her second child till three months prior to the current pregnancy.

Review of Systems

- No headache, no fever
- No chest pain or cough
- No nausea or vomiting
- No lower extremity edema
- No vaginal bleeding or uterine colic
- No diarrhea or constipation

- No urinary problems
- *Past medical history*: None, except for two hospitalizations for normal vaginal deliveries
- *Past surgical history*: Appendectomy 12 years ago
- *Vaccines*: Up to date (hepatitis B vaccine series, MMR booster, and flu shot).
- *Current medications*: Tylenol 350 mg once at home when her pain started
- *Allergies*: No known drug allergies
- *Social history*: MH is a housewife, no history of smoking, ETOH, and drug abuse
- *Family history*: Mother—61 years, diagnosed with hypertension and diabetes; history of cholecystectomy at the age of 35. Father died of prostate cancer at the age of 68. No brothers or sisters.

Physical Examination

- The patient is in moderate distress due to RUQ abdominal pain
- *Vital signs*: T 36.5°C oral, BP 105/85, Pulse 90, BMI 30
- *Cardiac examination*: S1, S2 present, grade 2 ejection systolic murmur at the heart base
- *Chest examination*: Clear lungs.
- *Skin*: No jaundice
- *Abdominal examination*: Soft, tender right upper quadrant, no rebound tenderness; no Murphy sign. Gravid uterus palpated 3 cm above the umbilicus, fetal movements preserved
- *Pelvic examination*: No vaginal bleeding, cervix is closed
- Figures 55.1 and 55.2 illustrate abdominal ultrasound findings.

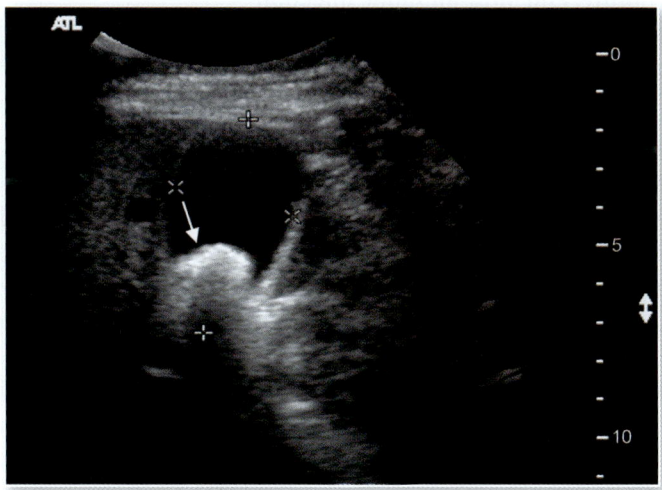

Figure 55.1: A 2 × 3 cm gallstone visualized close to the neck of the gallbladder. There is no evidence of gallbladder wall thickening

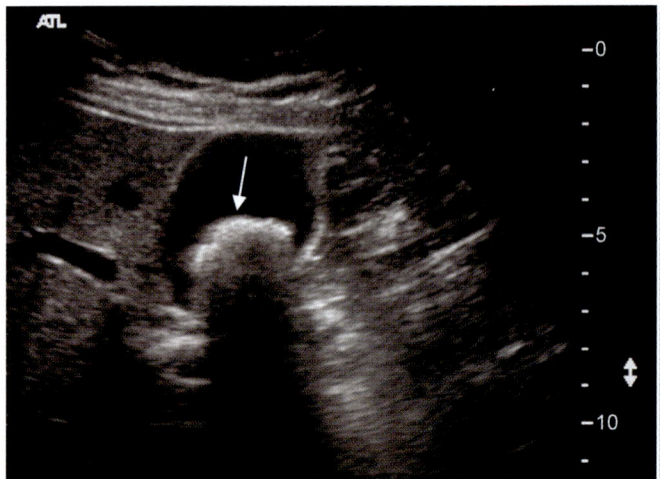

Figure 55.2: "Shadowing" phenomenon: note the absence of echoes posterior to the calculus

■ CLINICAL QUESTIONS

1. **What is the differential diagnosis of the RUQ pain in pregnancy?**

   Ans. • *Gallstones*: Uncomplicated or complicated (cholecystitis, cholangitis and biliary pancreatitis)
   • Pregnancy related RUQ pain in pre-eclampsia, HELLP, acute fatty liver of pregnancy, uterine rupture, and intra-amniotic infection
   • Nonpregnancy related RUQ pain like hepatitis, peptic ulcer disease or right lower lobe pneumonia.

2. **What is the initial work up of this patient?**

   Ans. • *Initial laboratory check*: CBC, LFT, and lipase
   • In uncomplicated gallstones, all the labs are expected to be normal
   • Leukocytosis is detected in patients with cholecystitis and cholangitis, intra-amniotic infection and/or pneumonia. Thrombocytopenia is evident in patients with HELLP, along with high BP and elevated LFT. Furthermore, RUQ pain with elevated LFT is seen in patients with acute fatty liver and HELLP. Elevated lipase levels are noticed in patients with biliary pancreatitis
   • *Abdominal ultrasound*: Demonstrates gallstones and biliary sludge (Figs 55.1 and 55.2); however, if a gallstone is in the common bile duct or ampulla of Vater causing cholangitis or pancreatitis, the endoscopic ultrasound (EUS) is more accurate for diagnostic and therapeutic approach.

3. **What is the best initial treatment?**

   Ans. Treatment consists of supportive care including pain control with acetaminophen for mild pain vs IV opioids for severe pain, and intravenous fluid. Pain usually subsides within 1–2 hours. Antibiotics are indicated in patients with cholecystitis and/or cholangitis.

4. When is cholecystectomy indicated?

Ans.
- Cholecystectomy is indicated if the pain is recurrent and causing distress, in patients with cholecystitis not responding to conservative management, or pancreatitis requiring endoscopic retrograde cholangiopancreatogram (ERCP)
- For patients near term, cholecystectomy should be postponed to about 6 weeks after delivery
- Because our patient did not respond to conservative treatment, cholecystectomy was performed. Figures 55.3 and 55.4 describe pathology and histology findings.

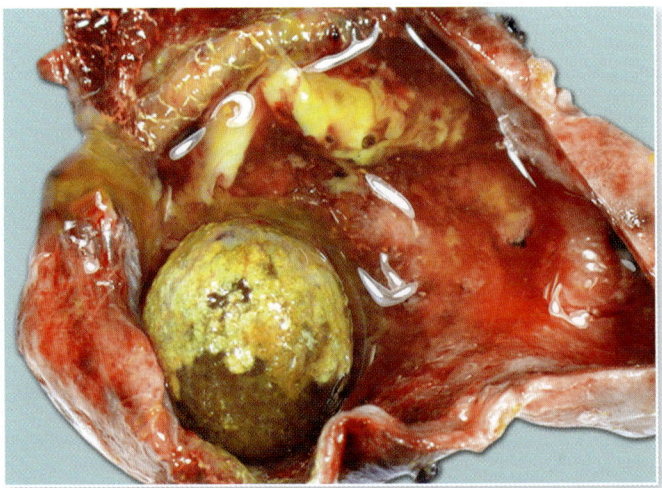

Figure 55.3: Gallbladder is opened to reveal erythematous mucosal and serosal surfaces, compatible with acute cholecystitis. In addition, there is yellow purulent material, which is consistent with aggregates of neutrophils (abscess formation). Finally, a green-yellow gallbladder stone is identified

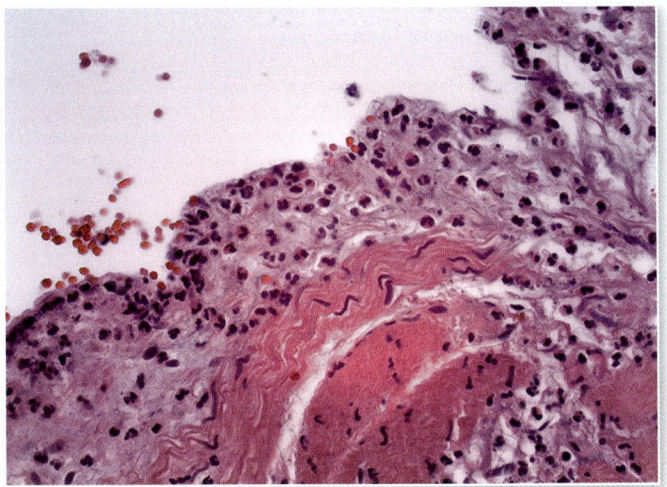

Figure 55.4: The specimen demonstrates the gallbladder mucosa infiltrated with numerous multilobed granulocytes, consistent with acute cholecystitis

■ TAKE-HOME MESSAGES

- Pregnancy is a risk factor for gallstone disease. The major independent risk factor for gallstones is pre-pregnancy obesity.[1,2]
- The spectrum of gallstone disease ranges from biliary colic to life-threatening pancreatitis, so the management should be tailored to the patient according to her clinical presentation.[3]
- Majority of pregnant patients will have uncomplicated cholelithiasis, however some of them may develop complicated gallstone disease (CGD) as acute cholecystitis, choledocholithiasis and gallstone pancreatitis.[4]
- Bilirubin and transaminases are not affected by normal pregnancy, while amylase and lipase levels have been reported to increase slightly.[5] Significantly elevated transaminase levels are associated with complicated gallstones or acute fatty liver or HELLP.[6]
- Gallstones and sludge are easily visualized by ultrasound, with sensitivity and specificity approaching 100%.[3,7] Abdominal ultrasound is routinely performed, and despite being a sensitive test for cholelithiasis, it is insensitive for the detection of common bile duct (CBD) stones.[8]
- The advantage of using the endoscopic ultrasound (EUS) is its ability to perform intervention such as sphincterotomy and stone extraction.[9]
- For recurrent biliary colic primary surgical management during pregnancy is reasonable because recurrence is common with conservative therapy, and surgical therapy appears to be safe for the mother and the fetus.[10]

■ REFERENCES

1. Igbinosa O, Poddar S, Pitchumoni C. Pregnancy associated pancreatitis revisited. Clin Res Hepatol Gastroenterol. 2013;37(2):177-81.
2. Veerappan A, Gawron JA, Soper NJ, Keswani NJ. Delaying cholecystectomy for complicated gallstone disease in pregnancy is associated with recurrent postpartum symptoms. J Gastrointest Surg. 2013;17(11):1953-9.
3. Date RS, Kaushal M, Ramesh A. A review of the management of gallstone disease and its complications in pregnancy. Am J Surg. 2008;196(4):599-608.
4. Ko CW. Risk factors for gallstone-related hospitalization during pregnancy and the postpartum. Am J Gastroenterol. 2006; 101(10): 2263–8.
5. Larsson A, Palm M, Hansson LO, Axelsson O. Reference values for clinical chemistry tests during normal pregnancy. BJOG, 2008;115(7):874-81.
6. Goel A, Ramakrishna B, Zachariah U, et al. How accurate are the Swansea criteria to diagnose acute fatty liver of pregnancy in predicting hepatic microvesicular steatosis? Gut, 2011;60(1):138-9.
7. Gilo NB, Amini D, Landy HJ. Appendicitis and cholecystitis in pregnancy. Clin Obstet Gynecol. 2009;52(4):586-96.
8. Al-Hashem H, Muralidharan V, Cohen H, Jamidar PA. Biliary disease in pregnancy with an emphasis on the role of ERCP. J Clin Gastroenterol. 2009; 43(1): 58-62.
9. Artifon EL, Kumar A, Eloubeidi MA, Chu A, Halwan B, Sakai P, et al. Prospective randomized trial of EUS versus ERCP-guided common bile duct stone removal: an interim report. Gastrointest Endosc. 2009;69(2):238-43.
10. Othman MO, Stone E, Hashimi M, Parasher G. Conservative management of cholelithiasis and its complications in pregnancy is associated with recurrent symptoms and more emergency department visits. Gastrointest Endosc. 2012;76(3):564-9.

CHAPTER 56

Liver Disease in Pregnancy

Safa Farrag, Humera Chaudhary, Sanja Kupesic Plavsic

■ CLINICAL CASE

MR is a 25-year-old Hispanic G2P1, who comes to ER with severe itching at 32 weeks gestation. Her symptoms started 7 days ago. The itching is all over her body, but seems to be more pronounced on the palms and soles. The symptoms worsen during night time preventing her from sleeping. She has no abdominal pain, no nausea or vomiting. She had similar symptoms during her first pregnancy that resolved with medications. Her last clinic visit was a month ago. At that time, her blood pressure, laboratory tests and US were within expected normal limits.

Menarche: Age 13.

Menses: 28/5, regular.

LMP: 34 weeks ago.

Pregnancies: Previous pregnancy 4 years ago, with full term normal vaginal delivery of a healthy baby.

Sexual history: In monogamous relationship with husband for the past 5 years.

Contraception: IUD was removed 2 months prior to the current pregnancy.

Review of Systems

- No headaches, no fever
- No nausea or vomiting
- No abdominal pain
- No diarrhea or constipation
- No urinary symptoms
- *Vaccines*: Up to date (hepatitis B vaccine series, MMR booster, annual flu shot)
- *Past medical history:* Similar pruritus during her first pregnancy, she cannot recall the treatment provided at that time
- No history of hepatitis, or known liver disease

- *Past surgical history:* Tonsillectomy
- *Medications:* None
- *Allergies:* No known drug allergies
- *Social history:* Ms/MR just moved to the US from Chile. She is employed as accountant. Used to drink alcohol heavily prior to the first pregnancy, but stopped 5 years ago; no history of smoking, and illegal drug abuse
- *Family history:* Mother—age 66, with hypertension. Father—age 68, with diabetes mellitus.

Physical Examination

- *Vital signs:* T 36°C oral, BP 110/75, Pulse 85
- *Cardiac examination:* No murmurs or gallops
- *Chest examination:* Clear lungs
- *Skin:* Multiple excoriations on both upper and lower extremities and abdomen; no jaundice
- *Abdomen:* Soft, non-tender; no hepatosplenomegaly; bowel sounds present
- Gravid uterus, size appropriate for gestational age, fetal movements present
- *Pelvic examination:* No vaginal bleeding, cervix is closed
- *Initial laboratory results:* AST 157IU/L, ALT 250IU/L, bilirubin 2.9 mg/dL, alkaline phosphatase 250 IU/L. Total bile acid was 35 Umol/L (N <10 Umol/L), gamma-glutamyl transpeptidase (GGTP) and lipase are normal, CBC and coagulation profile are normal, negative hepatitis serology, no proteinuria. Normal abdominal ultrasound findings (Figs 56.1 and 56.2).

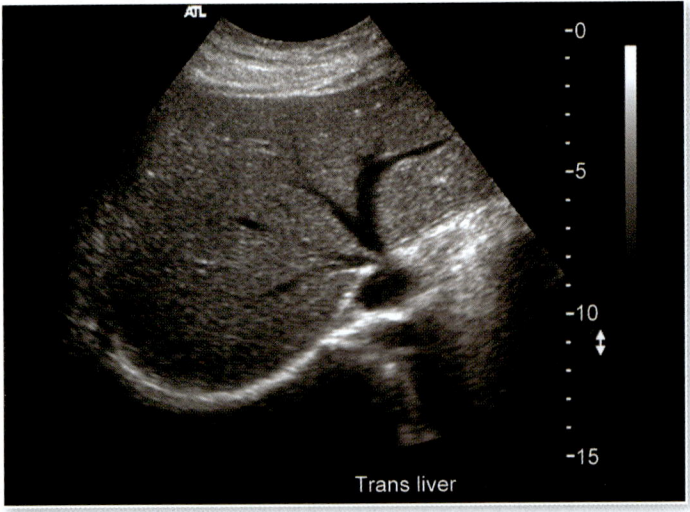

Figure 56.1: Ultrasound reveals normal liver. No biliary dilatation is present

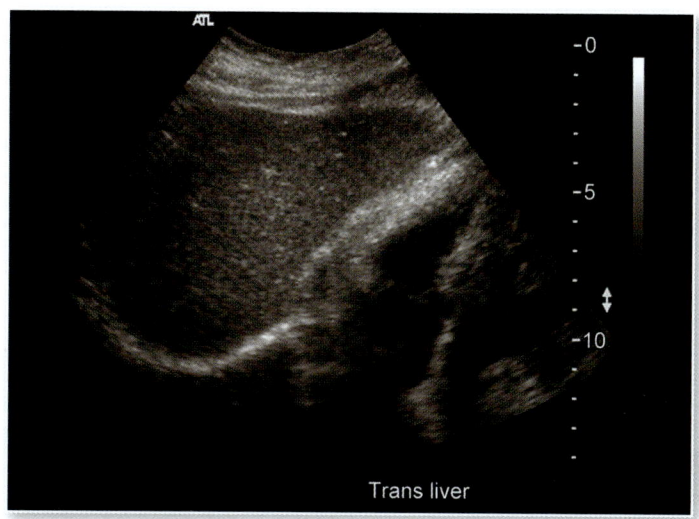

Figure 56.2: Normal liver on abdominal ultrasound with no evidence of biliary dilatation

CLINICAL QUESTIONS

1. What is the most likely diagnosis?
Ans. The most likely diagnosis is intrahepatic cholestasis, because of the following:
- The presence of pruritus during the third trimester, elevated ALT>AST, and mildly elevated bilirubin along with high total bile acid. Positive history of intrahepatic cholestasis in previous pregnancy and lab findings explain the symptoms and confirm the diagnosis
- Lack of nausea and vomiting, and the fact that she is in the third trimester
- Hyperemesis gravidarum is ruled out as a cause of elevated LFTs
- Lack of abdominal pain, high blood pressure and proteinuria (rule out pre-eclampsia), lack of thrombocytopenia (rules out HELLP as a cause of elevated LFTs)
- Lack of coagulopathy, high blood pressure, leukocytosis, and lack of nausea/vomiting during the third trimester rule out acute fatty liver of pregnancy.

2. What is the best initial treatment?
Ans. Ursodeoxycholic acid (UDCA) will help to improve pruritus and normalize serum bile acid.

3. Why delivery may be indicated for patients with intrahepatic cholestasis?
Ans. Due to the risk of fetal complications including prematurity, meconium staining of amniotic fluid, respiratory distress, fetal distress, and demise.

4. What are the indications for delivery prior to 36 weeks?
Ans.
- Intense intolerable pruritus despite medical treatment, and
- History of stillbirth due to intrahepatic cholestasis in previous pregnancy.

TAKE-HOME MESSAGES

- There are multiple liver diseases associated with pregnancy. The most important and common ones are: hyperemesis gravidarum, intrahepatic cholestasis of pregnancy, pre-eclampsia/eclampsia, HELLP syndrome (hemolysis, elevated liver enzymes and low platelets), and acute fatty liver of pregnancy (AFLP).[1]
- Around 25% of pregnant patients report pruritus, which is usually benign. However, in combination with abnormal liver function tests, a diagnosis of intrahepatic cholestasis of pregnancy (ICP) should be considered.[2] ICP is the most common pregnancy associated liver disease, which typically presents in late second and third trimesters of pregnancy, with main complaints of pruritus (typically of the palms and soles), abnormal liver function tests and elevated serum bile acid levels.[3]
- Affected women have an increase in hepatic sequelae including gallstone disease, hepatitis C, fibrosis, and cholangitis.[4] Some patients with ICP may have an underlying liver disease.[5]
- ICP harbors an increased risk for stillbirth (intrauterine death), which increases with higher bile acid levels. In a large prospective cohort study of women with ICP and total bile acid concentrations ≥40 mmol/L, a significant increased risks of adverse perinatal outcomes (including stillbirth) were detected.[6]
- Ursodeoxycholic acid (UDCA) is the first line treatment for ICP. Use of UDCA improves pruritus, lowers bile acids, and liver function tests. [7,8]
- Severe pruritus not responding to medical treatment and a previous history of stillbirth due to intrahepatic cholestasis require early termination of pregnancy. According to the most recent data from the literature patients with total serum bile acid concentrations ≥100 mmol/L should be offered a delivery prior to 36 weeks of gestation.[9]
- A decision-analytic model found delivery at 36 weeks of gestation without amniocentesis for fetal lung maturity testing or corticosteroid administration to be the optimal strategy to reduce maternal and neonatal morbidity and mortality.[10]

REFERENCES

1. Than NN, Neuberger J. Liver abnormalities in pregnancy. Best Practice Res Clin Gastroenterol. 2014;27(4):565-75.
2. Walker I, Chappell LC, Williamson C. Abnormal liver function tests in pregnancy. BMJ: 2013;347:f6055.
3. Williamson C, Geenes V. Intrahepatic cholestasis of pregnancy. Obstet Gynecol. 2014;124(1):120-33.
4. Marschall HU, Wikström Shemer E, Ludvigsson JF, Stephansson O. Intrahepatic cholestasis of pregnancy and associated hepatobiliary disease: a population-based cohort study. Hepatology. 2013;58(4):1385-91.
5. Turunen K, Mölsä A, Helander K, et al. Health history after intrahepatic cholestasis of pregnancy. Acta Obstet Gynecol Scand 2012;91(6):679.
6. Geenes V, Chappell LC, Seed PT, et al. Association of severe intrahepatic cholestasis of pregnancy with adverse pregnancy outcomes: a prospective population-based case-control study. Hepatology. 2014;59(4):1482-91.
7. Chris A, Kassam M. Intrahepatic cholestasis of pregnancy: diagnosis and management; a survey of Royal Australian and New Zealand College of Obstetrics and Gynaecology fellows. Aust N Z J Obst Gynaecol. 2014;54(3):263-7.
8. Bacq Y, Sentilhes L, Reyes HB, et al. Efficacy of ursodeoxycholic acid in treating intrahepatic cholestasis of pregnancy: a meta-analysis. Gastroenterology. 2012;143(6):1492-501.
9. Lo JO, Shaffer BL, Allen AJ, et al. Intrahepatic cholestasis of pregnancy and timing of delivery. J Matern Fetal Neonatal Med. 2014;28(18):2254-8.
10. Brouwers L, Koster MP, Page-Christiaens GC, et al. Intrahepatic cholestasis of pregnancy: maternal and fetal outcomes associated with elevated bile acid levels. Am J Obstet Gynecol. 2015;212(1):100.e1-7.

CHAPTER 57

Kidney Stones in Pregnancy

Safa Farrag, Humera Chaudhary, Sanja Kupesic Plavsic

CLINICAL CASE

GA is a 25 years old G2P1 who is admitted to ER at 28 weeks gestation, complaining of a right flank pain. The pain is 8/10 in severity, started about one hour ago and radiates to the right groin. It is associated with nausea and vomiting. She has no fevers or chills, and never had this pain before. Her last clinic visit was 2 weeks ago, when her weight, vital signs, and labs were within normal limits.

Menarche: Age 12.

Menses: 30/5 days, regular.

LMP: 30 weeks ago.

Pregnancy: One uncomplicated pregnancy 4 years ago. The course of current pregnancy was normal.

Delivery: One normal vaginal term delivery.

Sexual history: In monogamous relationship with her husband.

Contraception: She was using oral contraceptive pills till two months prior to the current pregnancy.

Review of Systems

- No headache, no fever
- No chest pain or cough
- No lower extremity edema
- No vaginal bleeding or uterine contractions
- No diarrhea or constipation
- No dysuria
- *Past medical history*: None
- *Past surgical history*: Appendectomy

- *Vaccines*: up to date (hepatitis B vaccine series, MMR booster and flu shot)
- *Current medications*: Tylenol 350 mg once 30 minutes ago
- *Allergies*: No known drug allergy
- *Social history*: She is a teacher, does not smoke, no ETOH and drug abuse
- *Family history*: Mother—55 years, with diabetes. Father—58 years, with hypertension.

Physical Examination

- The patient is in moderate distress due to the pain
- *Vital signs*: T 36.5°C oral, BP 105/85, P 90, BMI 29
- *Cardiac examination*: S1, S2 present, grade 2 ejection systolic murmur at the heart base
- *Chest examination*: Clear lungs.
- *Skin*: No jaundice
- *Abdominal examination*: Soft; tender right flank and right lower quadrant, no rebound tenderness; moderate CVA tenderness
- Gravid uterus level 4 cm above the umbilicus; fetal movements preserved
- *Pelvic examination*: No vaginal bleeding, cervix is closed
- *Lab*: UA: 10–20 RBC/HPF (10–20 red blood cells per high power field), no WBC, no bacteria, negative nitrate and negative leukocyte esterase. CBC and CMP within normal limits.

CLINICAL QUESTIONS

1. What is the best next step for the diagnosis of this patient?

Ans. Patient's symptoms are suggestive of nephrolithiasis. Abdominal ultrasound is the gold standard imaging study for renal colic during pregnancy (Figs 57.1 and 57.2).

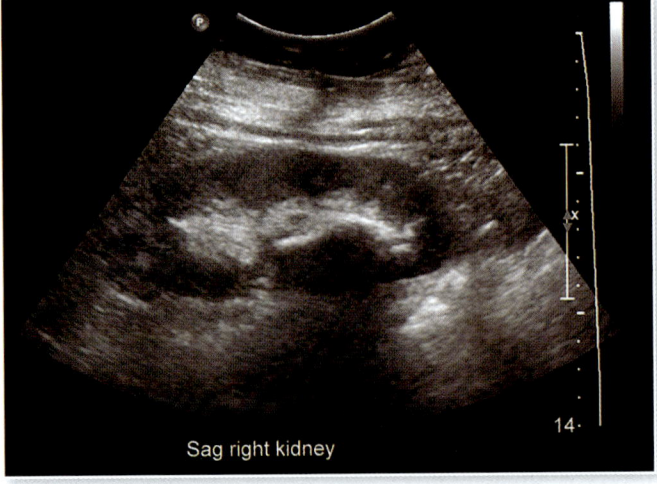

Figure 57.1: Ultrasound image of the right kidney. Note hyperechogenic calculi

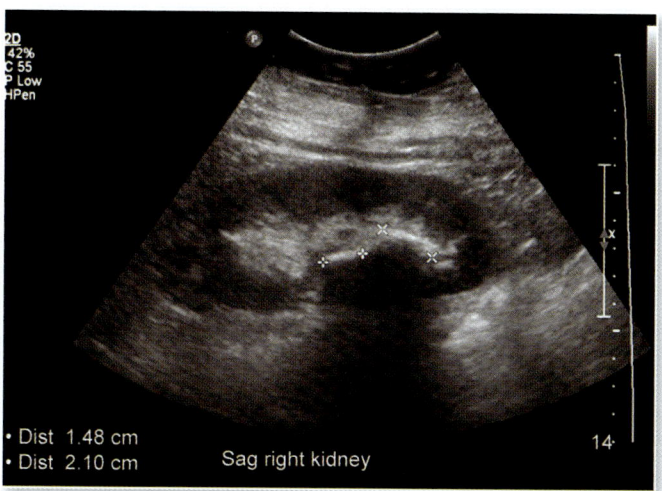

Figure 57.2: The same patient. Two nonobstructing calculi measuring 1.5 and 2.1 cm are noted in mid and lower pole calices of right kidney

2. What is the best management of nephrolithiasis during pregnancy?

Ans. Conservative management, including: aggressive hydration, pain control with narcotics, and anti-emetics for nausea, waiting for improvement of symptoms and stone passage.

3. What if conservative management fails?

Ans. If the patient continues to have pain, persistent nausea and vomiting, develops fever, renal function impairment, or complications such as pre-eclampsia, preterm labor, or if the stone is >1 cm, the intervention should consist of:
- Placement of the ureteral stent
- Placement of the nephrostomy tube, or
- Ureteroscopy with or without limited fluoroscopy.

4. What interventions for nephrolithiasis are contraindicated during pregnancy?

Ans.
- Shockwave lithotripsy, and
- Percutaneous nephrolithotomy.

■ TAKE-HOME MESSAGES

- Kidney stones (nephrolithiasis) are relatively rare during pregnancy. The incidence of the symptomatic cases is approximately 1 in 2,000 pregnancies. The most common presenting symptoms are colicky flank pain and hematuria.[1]
- Preterm premature rupture of membranes, preterm labor and pre-eclampsia are the most serious risks of symptomatic nephrolithiasis during pregnancy.[2]
- Renal ultrasonography is the initial imaging modality of choice for pregnant patients with renal colic.[3,4]

- MRI should be considered as a second-line test during pregnancy. It is not associated with radiation exposure, and is approved by the American College of Radiology during pregnancy. It is usually performed when US fails to establish a diagnosis and/or in patients with continued symptoms despite conservative management.[5]
- Most patients improve with conservative management, especially if the stone is of a passable size (<1 cm) and infection is absent. Conservative management includes: aggressive hydration, pain control with narcotics and antiemetics.[6,7]
- Intervention is indicated in patients with failed conservative treatment, persistence of symptoms, stone >1 cm, infection, renal impairment, only one functioning kidney and/or obstetric or non-obstetric complications. It consists of temporary drainage by ureteral stent or nephrostomy tube. Alternatively, ureteroscopy can be performed under US guidance, or using limited fluoroscopy with the pelvis covered, under spinal, general or local anesthesia.[6,8] Another option to reduce radiation exposure to the fetus while performing ureteroscopy utilizes an inverted C-arm fluoroscopic imaging unit.[9]
- Ureteroscopic stone removal appears to be similarly safe in pregnant and nonpregnant patients. A systematic review and meta-analysis of 14 reports assessing outcomes in 108 patients noted nine complications with this technique.[10]

REFERENCES

1. Masselli G, Derme M, Laghi F. Imaging of stone disease in pregnancy. Abdom Imaging. 2013;38(6):1409-14.
2. Swartz MA, Lydon-Rochelle MT, Simon D, et al. Admission for nephrolithiasis in pregnancy and risk of adverse birth outcomes. Obstet Gynecol. 2007;109(5):1099-104.
3. Mandeville JA, Gnessin E, Lingeman JE. Imaging evaluation in the patient with renal stone disease. Semin Nephrol. 2011;31(3):254-8.
4. Fulgham PF, Assimos DG, Pearle MS, Preminger GM. Clinical effectiveness protocols for imaging in the management of ureteral calculous disease: AUA technology assessment. J Urol. 2013;189(4):1203-13.
5. Kanal E, Barkovich AJ, Bell C, et al. ACR guidance document for safe MR practices: 2007. Am J Roentgenol. 2007;188(6):1447-74.
6. Semins MJ, Matlaga BR. Kidney stones during pregnancy. Nat Rev Urol. 2014;11(3):163-8.
7. Semins MJ, Matlaga BR. Kidney stones and pregnancy. Adv Chronic Kid Dis. 2012;20(3):260-4.
8. Deters LA, Belanger G, Shah O, Pais VM Jr. Ultrasound-guided ureteroscopy in pregnancy. Clin Nephrol. 2013;79(2):118-23.
9. Cocuzza M, Colombo JR Jr, Lopes RI. Use of inverted fluoroscope's C-arm during endoscopic treatment of urinary tract obstruction in pregnancy: a practicable solution to cut radiation. Urology. 2010;75(6):1505-8.
10. Semins MJ, Trock BJ, Matlaga BR. The safety of ureteroscopy during pregnancy: a systematic review and meta-analysis. J Urol. 2009;181(1):139-43.

CHAPTER 58

Thyroid Nodule in Pregnancy

Safa Farrag, Humera Chaudhary, Sanja Kupesic Plavsic

■ CLINICAL CASE

AR is a 36-year-old G3P2 who comes to the clinic for follow-up visit. She is 20 weeks pregnant and this is her first visit in this pregnancy. She recently moved from Mexico to the United States. She is concerned about a mass in her neck that she accidentally noticed a week ago. Before pregnancy, it was a small, pea size lesion more to the right of her neck, which has progressively increased in size to about 2 × 4 cm during the course of last month. The nodule is not tender, and is not associated with other swellings in the neck. She also complains of hoarseness and trouble swallowing.

Menarche: 14 years.

Menses: 30/4, regular.

LMP: 22 weeks ago.

Pregnancies: Previous pregnancies 3 and 5 years ago; full term uncomplicated vaginal deliveries.

Sexual history: In monogamous relationship with her husband for the past 8 years.

Contraception: Vaginal ring prior to pregnancy.

Review of Systems

- No cold or heat intolerance
- No diarrhea or constipation
- No skin or hair changes
- No headaches, no fever
- No nausea or vomiting
- No urinary symptoms
- *Vaccines*: up to date (hepatitis B vaccine series, MMR booster, annual flu shot)
- *Past medical history*: No previous illness, no neck radiation
- *Past surgical history*: None
- *Medications*: None/prenatal vitamins (PNV)
- *Allergies*: No known drug allergies

- *Social history*: No smoking, no ETOH, no drug abuse
- *Family history*: Mother—70 years, treated for thyroid cancer when she was 48 years old; currently on thyroid replacement therapy. Father died from diabetes complications at age of 72.

Physical Examination

- *Vital signs*: T 36.8°C oral, BP 110/75, P 80
- *Neck examination*: Right thyroid nodule (moves with swallowing) firm, non-tender, around 4 × 2 cm
- No lymphadenopathy
- *Cardiac examination*: No murmurs or gallops
- *Chest examination*: Clear lungs
- *Extremities*: No edema
- Gravid uterus, fetal movements present
- *Pelvic examination*: No vaginal bleeding, cervix is closed
- *Laboratory findings*: TSH and free T4 within normal range (TSH: 3 mU/L, free T4: 1.6 ng/dL).

■ CLINICAL QUESTIONS

1. What is the next step for the diagnosis and management of this patient?

Ans. Neck ultrasound is cost effective imaging modality to image the thyroid gland in pregnant and nonpregnant patients. Figures 58.1 and 58.2 demonstrate heterogeneous solid nodule containing microcalcifications. Figure 58.3 illustrates marked intrinsic vascularity demonstrated by color Doppler ultrasound.

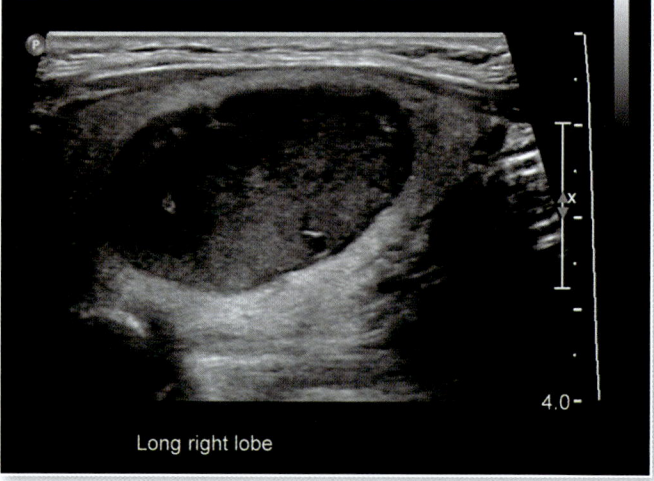

Figure 58.1: A 4 × 2.5 cm solid nodule in the right thyroid lobe containing microcalcifications

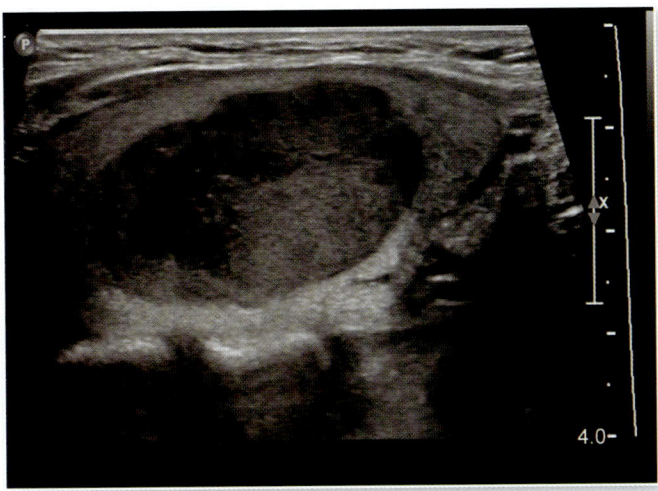

Figure 58.2: Solid right thyroid nodule with microcalcifications and irregular cystic component

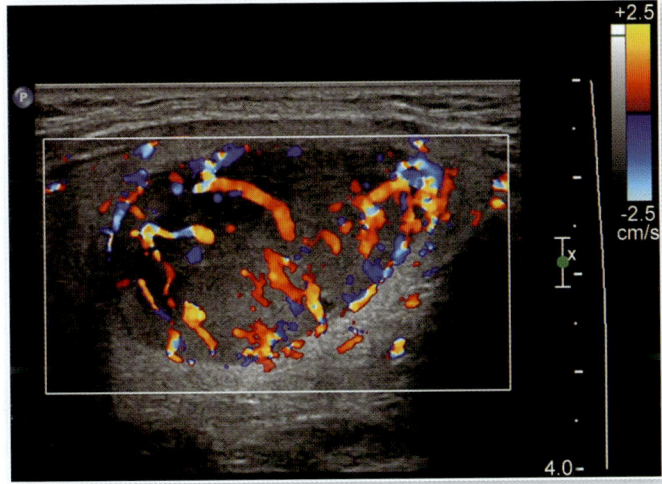

Figure 58.3: Color Doppler shows diffuse vascularity of a thyroid nodule

2. What are the indications for fine needle aspiration (FNA) of a thyroid nodule during pregnancy?

Ans.
- Ultrasonographic features of malignancy
  - >1cm nodule
  - Positive family history of thyroid cancer
  - Presence of cervical adenopathy
  - History of neck radiotherapy
  - Rapidly growing nodule
    - Both US and FNA are safe during pregnancy.

3. What are the main ultrasonographic features suggesting malignancy of a thyroid nodule?
Ans. Irregularity, hetero and/or hypo-echogenicity, increased intra-nodular vascularization, absent peripheral nodular halo, microcalcifications, and the presence of cervical lymphadenopathy.

■ TAKE-HOME MESSAGES

- The prevalence of thyroid cancer in pregnant women with nodules ranges between 12 and 43%. Thyroid function tests are usually normal in patients with thyroid cancer.[1]
- Presence of ultrasonographic features suggestive of malignancy such as irregularity, hetero and/or hypo-echogenicity, increased intra-nodular vascularization, absent peripheral nodular halo, microcalcifications, presence of cervical lymphadenopathy, presence of extra-capsular growth or metastatic lymph nodes warrant FNA evaluation. Otherwise, FNA of nodules that appear benign on ultrasound can be deferred until postpartum.[1,2]
- Differentiated thyroid cancer is the second leading malignant tumor during pregnancy after breast cancer, with a prevalence of 14 per 100,000 births.[3]
- Radioactive iodine (RAI) uptake is absolutely contraindicated during pregnancy and lactation because of the risk of transfer of radioactive iodine to the fetal thyroid gland causing its suppression.[4]
- Thyroidectomy can be delayed until after delivery due to high complication rates associated with thyroid surgery.[5]
- Exogenous administration of thyroid hormone is recommended to achieve a suppressed TSH level when surgical treatment for well-differentiated thyroid carcinoma is delayed until the postpartum period to maintain a serum TSH level between 0.1 and 1.5 mIU/L.[5,6]
- Second trimester thyroidectomy should be considered if the patient has lymph node involvement, rapid tumor growth, doubtful FNA results, anaplastic or poorly differentiated carcinoma, severe compressive symptoms, and significant growth of a malignant nodule (>50% in volume or >20% in diameter in two dimensions).[3,7]
- No evidence suggests that a thyroid cancer prognosis is worse if diagnosed during pregnancy. In most observational studies, there is no difference in overall prognosis in pregnant women with thyroid cancer compared with nonpregnant women.[8,9]
- Multidisciplinary care involving the obstetrician, endocrinologist, and oncologist is essential in managing patients with history of thyroid cancer or those with thyroid cancer diagnosed during pregnancy.[10]

■ REFERENCES

1. Stagnaro-Green A, Abalovich M, Alexander E, et al. Guidelines of the American Thyroid Association for the diagnosis and management of thyroid disease during pregnancy and postpartum. Thyroid. 2011;21(10):1081-125.
2. Kratky J, Vitkova H, Bartakova, et al. Thyroid Nodules: Pathophysiological insight on oncogenesis and novel diagnostic techniques. Physiol Res. 2014;63 (Suppl. 2):S263-75.
3. Galofréa JC, Riesco-Eizaguirreb G, Alvarez-Escola C, et al. Clinical guidelines for management of thyroid nodule and cancer during pregnancy. Endocrinol Nutr. 2014;61(3):130-8.
4. Cynthia F, Yazbeck S, Sullivan D. Thyroid disorders during pregnancy. Med Clin N Am. 2012;96(2):235-56.
5. Popoveniuc G, Jonklaas J. Thyroid Nodules. Med Clin N Am. 2012;96(2):329-49.
6. Lansdown A, Rees DA. Endocrine oncology in pregnancy. Best Pract Res Clin Endocrinol Metab. 2011;25(6):911-26.
7. Cabezón CA, Carrizo C, Costanzo PR. Evolution of differentiated thyroid cancer during pregnancy in a community University Hospital in Buenos Aires, Argentina. Arq Bras Endocrinol Metab. 2013;57(4):307-11.
8. Ahmad S, Geraci SA, Koch CA. Thyroid Disease in Pregnancy. South Med J. 2013;106(9):532-8.
9. Alves GV, Santin AP, Furlanetto TW. Prognosis of thyroid cancer related to pregnancy: a systematic review. J Thyroid Res 2011;2011:691719.
10. Fitzpatrick DL, Russell MA. Diagnosis and management of thyroid disease in pregnancy. Obstet Gynecol Clin North Am. 2010;37(2):173-93.

CHAPTER

Gestational Trophoblastic Disease

59

Sanja Kupesic Plavsic

■ CLINICAL CASE

ST is a 41-year-old G2P1 Chinese woman at 17 weeks gestation, who presents to ER with vaginal bleeding. She constantly feels nauseous, and complains of vomiting at least 4–6 times per day. Her morning sickness is worse than in the first trimester of pregnancy, and abdominal discomfort has worsened during the course of last few weeks. She also states she has chest palpitations and shortness of breath, which did not occur previous to her pregnancy. On physical examination, her temperature is 37.0°C (98.6°F), heart rate is 125 beats per minute, and blood pressure is 150/95. Abdominal and pelvic examination confirms a 22-week sized uterus with blood in the vaginal vault. Quantitative beta-hCG was 165,000 mIU/mL. TSH was low and further thyroid testing detected mild hyperthyroidism. Laboratory tests revealed anemia. Fetal Doppler tones are not auscultated. Ultrasound assessment of the uterus demonstrates multiple internal echoes consistent with a "snow storm" appearance in the uterus (Figs 59.1 and 59.2). Fetal pole is not visualized. Ultrasound assessment reveals bilaterally enlarged ovaries with multi-loculated theca lutein cysts.

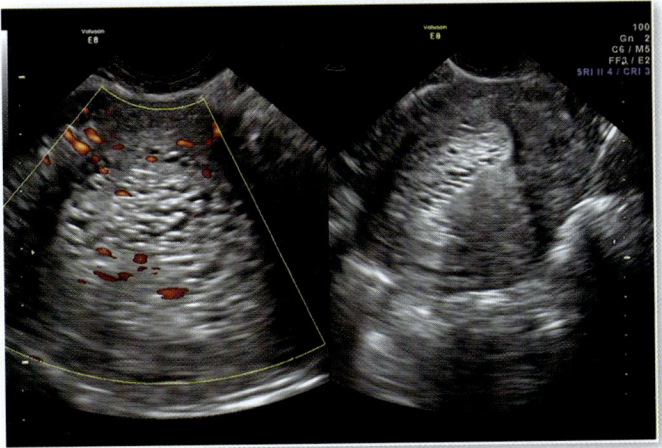

Figure 59.1: Transvaginal ultrasound (right) and color Doppler (left) images demonstrate snow storm appearance of the uterus. Fetal pole is not visualized

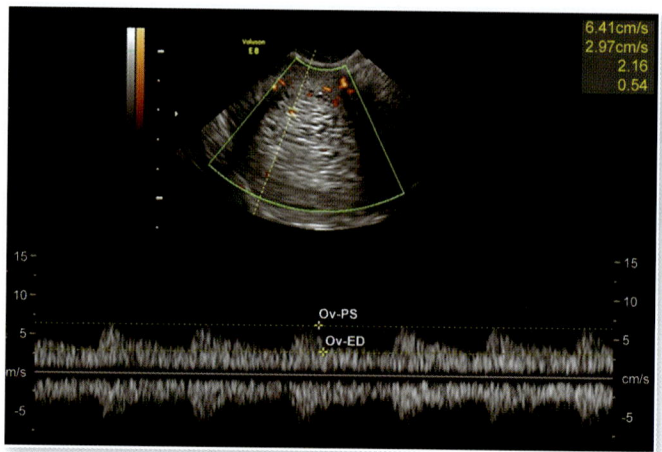

Figure 59.2: Pulsed Doppler ultrasound depicts low impedance blood flow signals from the honeycombed area within the uterus. Sonographic and Doppler findings are consistent with complete mole

Menarche: At age 12.

Menses: 28/4–5 days, regular.

LMP: 19 weeks ago.

Pregnancies/deliveries: One uncomplicated vaginal delivery at term 11 years ago.

Sexual history: Two male partners over her lifetime. For 13 years she is in a monogamous relationship with her husband.

Review of Systems

- Complains of headaches; no problems with vision
- No history of blood clots, DVT or PE. She complains of chest palpitations and shortness of breath, which did not occur previous to her pregnancy
- Positive for abdominal discomfort, nausea and vomiting (3 times today). No constipation and/or diarrhea
- Decreased urination noticed
- *Past medical history*: None, no hospitalizations
- *Vaccination*: Up to date (hepatitis B vaccine series, and MMR booster; flu shot past winter)
- *Past surgical history*: None
- *Medications*: Prenatal vitamins
- *Allergies*: None known drug allergies
- *Social history*: ST is a housewife; denies smoking, denies drugs, occasionally has a drink once in two weeks
- *Family history*: Mother—65 years with history of diabetes mellitus; father—72 years old, healthy. No family history of uterine, breast, ovarian, or colon cancer.

Physical Examination

- *Vital signs*: T 37.0°C oral, BP 150/95; P 125; BMI 24
- *Abdominal examination*: Uterus feels larger than would be expected for the gestational age
- *Pelvic examination*: Speculum examination revealed blood in the vagina. Doughy enlarged uterus (corresponding to 22 weeks) and bilaterally enlarged adnexa were detected by bimanual pelvic examination.

■ CLINICAL QUESTIONS

1. What evaluation is needed to make a final diagnosis?

Ans. Although clinical presentation, laboratory and ultrasound findings can diagnose gestational trophoblastic disease (GTD), pathology is needed to confirm the diagnosis and rule out malignant changes. A chest X-ray is recommended prior to uterine evacuation to diagnose the likelihood of metastatic disease.[1]

2. Why this patient is at risk for GTD?

Ans. Molar pregnancy is more likely to occur in women older than 40 years and younger than 15 years.[1-3] Asian women are almost twice as likely to develop GTD than women of other ethnic groups. GTD is frequently associated with hyperthyroidism due to the release of a thyrotropin-like compound by the molar tissue.[4]

3. What is your management plan?

Ans. First, the patient should be transfused for anemia. The primary treatment of this patient is suction evacuation of the uterus. Pathology examination and genetic analysis of the evacuated tissue need to be performed. The patient has to be monitored for bleeding, and post-procedural serial beta-hCG is required to rule out the development of malignant disease. The patient should not attempt subsequent pregnancy for at least one year follow-up period. Reliable contraception use (e.g. combined oral contraception) needs to be discussed and implemented.[3-5] Thyroid function should be followed until normalized.[4,6,7] Chest X-ray and pelvic ultrasound should be repeated to rule out malignant transformation and document the resolution of the ovarian cysts.[1,5]

■ TAKE-HOME MESSAGES

- A complete hydatidiform mole occurs after fertilization of an egg that is devoid of DNA. The genetic material is completely paternally derived, and around 90% will have a 46,XX diploid pattern resulting from the duplication of genes from a single sperm (androgenesis).[2,3] The other 10% will exhibit a 46,XX and 46,XY pattern that stemmed from fertilization of an empty egg by two sperm. A complete mole represents excessive hyperplasia of the trophoblast and edema of chorionic villi. The gross appearance is often described as a grapelike mass of edematous villi.[5]
- Partial moles are thought to result from the fertilization of an egg by two sperms. The karyotype of these molar pregnancies may be triploid (e.g. 69XXX) or even occasionally tetraploid (e.g., 92, XXXY).[2,3,5] Partial moles can also appear as a grape-like mass, but unlike complete moles are associated with the presence of fetal parts (Figs 59.3 to 59.5).

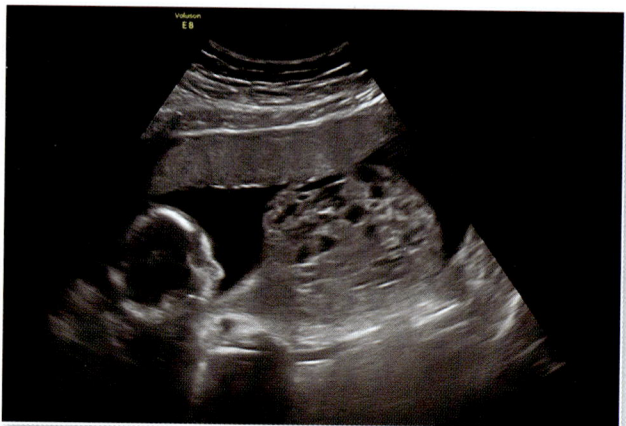

Figure 59.3: Transabdominal ultrasound image of a patient presenting with painless vaginal bleeding in second trimester. Hydropic changes of the placenta and fetal pole with absent cardiac activity are visualized

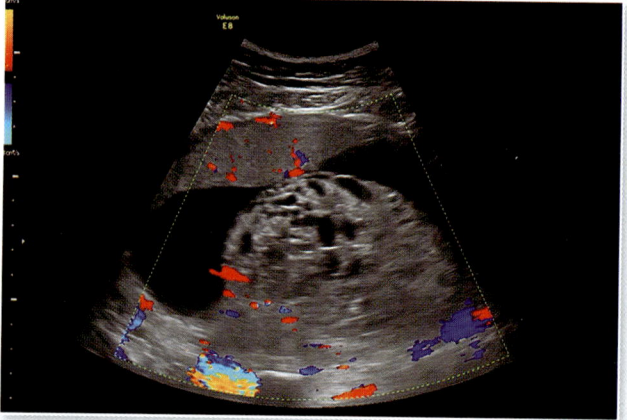

Figure 59.4: Transabdominal color Doppler image of the same patient

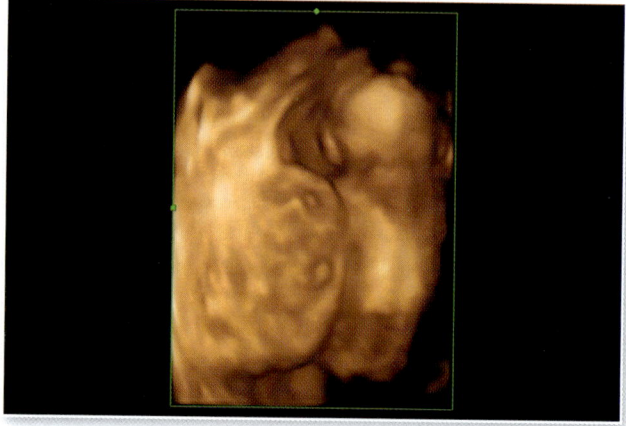

Figure 59.5: Three-dimensional ultrasound of the partial mole. Note fetal pole and surface rendering of the hydropic changes of the placenta

- Symptoms of GTD include vaginal bleeding, severe morning sickness, abdominal pain from ovarian cysts, and symptoms consistent with hyperthyroidism, if the beta-hCG levels become sufficiently elevated.[2] Signs may include a uterus that is larger than would be expected for the gestational age, a doughy rather than firm uterus, anemia, moderately to severely elevated serum and urine beta-hCG, and early-onset pre-eclampsia.[5,6]
- Hydatidiform moles are thought to occur in around 1 in 1,000 pregnancies in North America and Europe. For reasons that are currently poorly understood, the incidence of complete moles is much higher in Asia, with a peak incidence of 1 in 100 pregnancies in Indonesia.[2,3] The risk of developing a hydatidiform mole is greatest at the extremes of reproductive life; in teenagers and between the ages of 40 and 50 years.[2,3,5] Malignant gestational trophoblastic neoplasia occur in 2.5–7.5% of the patients with a partial mole as compared to 6.8–20% of patients with a complete mole.
- Choriocarcinoma is a rare, highly malignant neoplasm of trophoblastic cells typically derived from a previous normal or abnormal pregnancy. Rarely, choriocarcinoma originates as an ovarian or testicular germ cell tumor differentiating in the direction of trophoblastic structures admixed with other neoplastic germ cell elements. Choriocarcinoma arises in 1 in 20,000 to 30,000 pregnancies in the United States, but is much more common in the Far East and some African countries.[2-4] Before the era of chemotherapy for gestational disease became established, around 50% of choriocarcinomas would follow a molar pregnancy, 30% occurred after a miscarriage, and around 20% would follow a normal pregnancy.[8-10] However with the success achieved in managing molar pregnancies and use of ultrasound follow-up in recent years there has been a marked reduction in the percentage of choriocarcinomas following such pregnancies.[11]
- Choriocarcinoma can be remarkably invasive, metastasizing widely via lymphatics and hematogenous spread. Frequent sites of metastases, in descending order of occurrence, are the lungs, vagina, brain, liver, and kidney. Uterine bleeding is the most common symptom of the disease, but patients may present with symptoms related to metastases (e.g. intracranial bleeding, hemoptysis, hematemesis, or skin lesions).[3] Fortunately, gestational choriocarcinoma is sensitive to cytotoxic drugs and is now curable in many patients, even in the face of widespread metastasis.
- To monitor GTD after treatment, weekly monitoring of β-hCG in the absence of worsening clinical symptoms is sufficient. As long as levels are consistently dropping, no other intervention is necessary. Levels return to normal on average in 8–12 weeks.[2,3] Remission is defined as less than 5 mIU/mL of β-hCG in three consecutive tests. After remission is achieved, levels are measured monthly for one year.[12-14]
- Combined oral contraception is the preferred method of prevention of pregnancy during the one year follow-up period.[2] OCP has a low failure rate and low incidence of breakthrough bleeding, both of which can complicate the clinical picture. IUD is not the contraceptive of choice due to the risk of perforation. Reliable contraception is required because of increased risk of fetal anomalies during the first six months after treatment initiation of a chemotherapy regimen in patients who become pregnant.[12]
- The most serious complication of GTD is malignant transformation. Other serious complications include uterine perforation, hemorrhage, DIC and trophoblastic embolism.[2,3] The patients should be educated to seek an immediate care if they experience atypical pain, extensive bleeding, dyspnea and/or neurologic symptoms.[15]

■ REFERENCES

1. APGO Medical Student Educational Objectives. Educational Topic 50: Gestational Trophoblastic Neoplasia. *https://www.apgo.org/binary/TC50.pdf*. Published. 2014.
2. Kupesic Plavsic S (Ed). Step by Step Case Studies in Obstetrics and Gynecology. New Delhi, London, Philadelphia, Panama: Jaypee Brothers Medical Publisher. 2014. pp. 407-23.
3. Kumar V, Abul AK, Fausto N, Aster J. The female genital tract. In: Robbins, Cotran (Eds). Pathologic basis of disease. 8th ed. Philadelphia: Saunders. 2010. pp.1006-61.
4. Walkington L, Webster J, Hancock BW, et al. Hyperthyroidism and human chorionic gonadotrophin production in gestational trophoblastic disease. Br J Cancer. 2011;104(11):1665-9.
5. Fox H, Sebire NJ. Pathology of the Placenta. 3rd ed. Philadelphia: Saunders; 2007. pp. 431-72.

6. Kimura M, Amino N, Tamaki H, et al. Gestational thyrotoxicosis and hyperemesis gravidarum: possible role of hCG with higher stimulating activity. Clin Endocrinol .1993;38(4):345-50.
7. Goodwin TM, Montoro M, Mestman JH, et al. The role of chorionic gonadotropin in transient hyperthyroidism of hyperemesis gravidarum. J Clin Endocrinol Metab. 1992;75(5):1333-7.
8. Cavaliere A, Ermito S, Dinatale A, Pedata R. Management of molar pregnancy. J Prenat Med. 2009;3(1):15-7.
9. Seckl MJ, Sebire NJ, Berkowitz RS. Gestational trophoblastic disease. Lancet. 2010;376(9742):717-29.
10. Sasaki S. Clinical presentation and management of molar pregnancy. Best Prac Res Clin Obstet Gynaecol. 2003;17(6):885-92.
11. Tie W, Tajnert K, Kupesic Plavsic S. Ultrasound imaging of Gestational Trophoblastic Disease. Donald School Journal Ultrasound Obstet Gynecol. 2012;7(1):1-8.
12. Newlands ES, Holden L, Seckl MJ, et al. Management of brain metastases in patients with high-risk gestational trophoblastic tumors. J Reprod Med. 2002;47(6):465-71.
13. Tse KY, Ngan HY. Gestational trophoblastic disease. Best Pract Res Clin Obstet Gynaecol. 2012;26(3):357-70.
14. Shih IeM. Gestational trophoblastic neoplasia—pathogenesis and potential therapeutic targets. Lancet Oncol. 2007;8(7):642-50.
15. Kupesic Plavsic S, Kurjak A, Baston K. Gestational Trophoblastic Disease. In: Kupesic Plavsic S (Ed). Color Doppler, 3D & 4D Ultrasound in Gynecology, Infertility and Obstetrics. Jaypee Brothers Medical Publishers. 2011. pp. 243-51.

CHAPTER 60

Postpartum Tubal Ligation

Melissa D Mendez, Kathleen Green, Robert W Vera

■ CLINICAL CASE

A 38-year-old G4P3 presents to OB triage at 39 weeks by LMP and 10 weeks sonogram. She is in active labor at 5 cm dilation. The fetus is in vertex presentation. She has had three prior vaginal deliveries, and her last one was complicated by a postpartum hemorrhage. Her largest baby weighed 7.9 pounds. The patient is requesting an epidural. She greatly desires a postpartum tubal ligation after her birth and signed the appropriate consent forms.

Past gynecologic history: No abnormal Pap smears; has a history of *Chlamydia* 10 years ago that was treated.

Menarche: Age 10; normal cycle, every month. She is sure about her last menstrual period.

Past OB history: Three previous spontaneous vaginal deliveries. The first two without complications; the last one complicated with postpartum hemorrhage due to uterine atony; required two liters of packed red blood cells.

Review of Systems

- Her present pregnancy is without complications, all prenatal laboratory tests have been negative and her cell free DNA screening exam for chromosomal abnormalities is also negative. She feels the baby moving in between her contractions
- *Past medical history*: Noncontributory
- *Past surgical history*: Noncontributory
- *Social history*: Denies tobacco, drugs or alcohol. She is a high school science teacher.

Physical Examination

- *Vital signs*: T 37.1°C oral; P 90; BP 120/85
- *General*: Alert and oriented to place, time and date. Mild distress with each contraction
- *CV*: Mild 2/6 diastolic flow murmur
- *Lungs*: Clear to auscultation bilaterally
- *Abdomen*: Gravid, non-tender without contraction, vertex by Leopolds'
- *Extremities*: 1+ pedal edema, no calf tenderness bilaterally

- *Fetal heart Tracing*: Baseline 140's reassuring, category 1- positive accelerations, no decelerations noted
- *Toco*: Contractions noted every 4–5 minutes
- *Sterile vaginal examination (SVE)*: 5 cm /90%/-1
- The patient received epidural anesthesia. Amniotomy is performed, and clear fluid noted. At that time, she is 7 cm/100%/-1. She progresses quickly and has an uneventful spontaneous delivery. Given her previous history of uterine atony, you start Pitocin infusion before the placenta delivers and prophylactically give her misoprostol rectally to help with uterine contractions. Upon inspection, you do not see any perineal lacerations. You let her recover on Labor and Delivery for 2 hours and then decide to proceed with postpartum tubal ligation
- Figures 60.1 to 60.3 demonstrate different types of postpartum tubal ligation. In Figure 60.1 postpartum tubal ligation is being done at the time of a CS, while in Figures 60.2 and 60.3 postpartum tubal ligation is done after a vaginal delivery.

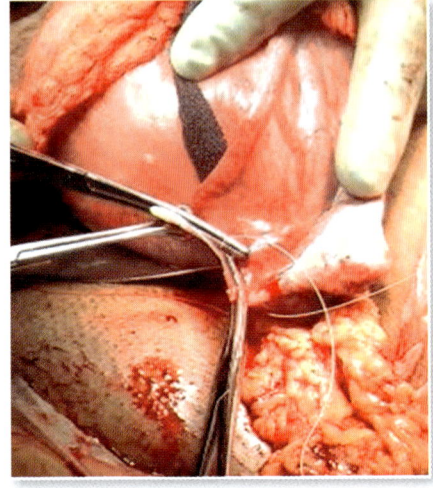

Figure 60.1: Partial salpingectomy at the time of cesarean section. The distal portion of the tube and the fimbria have been removed and sutures are placed for hemostasis

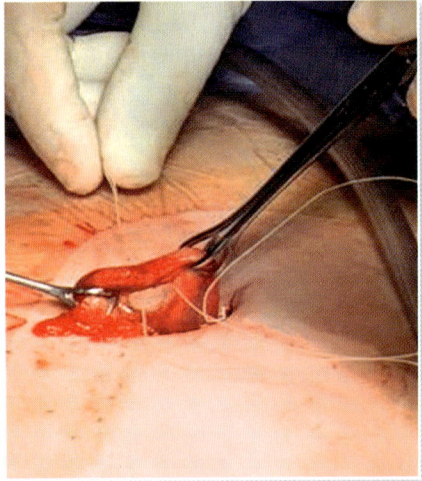

Figure 60.2: Parkland method postpartum tubal ligation. An infraumbilical incision was made. The tube is identified and gently pulled up through the incision with Babcock forceps. The tube is then ligated on each side with chromic or polyglactin (Vicryl) sutures. The tubal segment is then cut with scissors

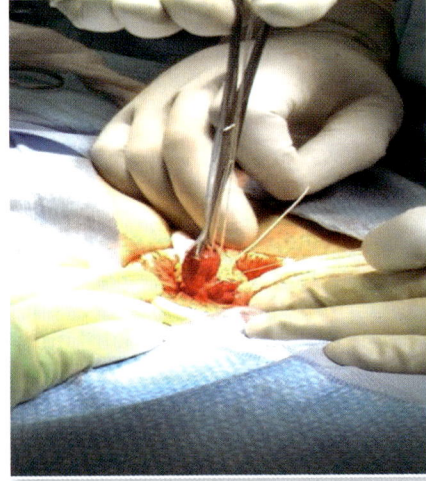

Figure 60.3: Pomeroy method postpartum tubal ligation. An infraumbilical incision was made. The tube is identified and gently pulled up through the incision with babcock forceps. A loop is created and the loop is then tied twice with chromic or polyglactin (Vicryl) sutures. The loop is then cut with sharp scissors

CLINICAL QUESTIONS

1. What types of postpartum tubal ligation exist?

Ans. Female sterilization is the most popular method of pregnancy prevention in the United States. About 50% of all tubal occlusions occur during the postpartum period.[1] There are several types of postpartum tubal ligation available after a spontaneous vaginal delivery or at the time of CS. Female sterilization is achieved with tubal blockage, ligation or removal. Tubal ligation and excision include the Pomeroy and the Parkland techniques. When excision is used, the tubal segments should be sent to pathology to confirm a complete transection.[1] Tubal blockage includes spring loaded clip placement or silicon band placement. Tubal removal includes partial salpingectomy and total salpingectomy (removal of the tube), which may be used in cases of abnormal tubes, such as hydrosalpinx (Fig. 60.1). Tubes can also be coagulated using electrical current.[1]

Probably the most used technique is the Pomeroy technique which includes placement of a free tie around a loop of the fallopian tube which is then excised. Usually, the mechanical methods of occlusion are used with the laparoscopic approach as an interval tubal ligation.[2-4] Sterilization can also be achieved hysteroscopically as an outpatient procedure 4–6 weeks postpartum.[4] Any surgical or mechanical technique can be used at the time of a postpartum tubal ligation via mini laparotomy or at the time of CS.[2,4]

2. Which type of tubal ligation is most effective?

Ans. The failure rate for all types of procedures is low. The lifetime risk of failure is estimated to be 18.5/1,000 according to the Collaborative Review of Sterilization (CREST) study.[4] A partial salpingectomy according to the CREST study has the lowest failure rate.[4,5] The Pomeroy technique and a partial salpingectomy appear to have a lower failure rate than titanium clips.[2-4] There is some evidence that laparoscopic tubal ligation with silicone rubber band and bipolar cautery has a lower failure rate than hysteroscopic tubal occlusion.[5] Failure rates of postpartum tubal ligation appears to be comparable to IUDs' (0.8% failure rate for copper IUD and 0.2% failure rate for the levonorgestrel IUD) and the etonorgestrel implant (0.05%).[1,6,7]

3. What are the risks associated with postpartum tubal ligation?

Ans. Common risks are bleeding, infection, damage to other internal organs, risk of failure and risk of subsequent ectopic pregnancy if the woman does become pregnant.[1] Risks of laparoscopic tubal ligation are less than 1%.[1] General anesthesia carries its own risks, separate from the procedure. Women with a failed tubal ligation have an increased risk for ectopic pregnancy, although an absolute risk is lower than in nonsterilized female population. There is some evidence that use of electrocautery can cause a higher incidence ectopic pregnancy than other methods.[2] Failure usually occurs due to incomplete occlusion, slippage of the occlusion device or suture, and/or placement on the wrong anatomical structure.[2]

4. What alternatives to postpartum tubal ligation are available?

Ans. Female sterilization is the most popular method of pregnancy prevention in the United States.[3] The second most popular method is male sterilization. Twenty percent of couples use oral contraceptives, 15% use male condoms and 7% use IUDs.[4] These are all considered alternatives to permanent female sterilization. Other long-acting reversible contraception such as IUDs and implantable devices can be used as alternatives to tubal ligation, however are underutilized.[5,8] Compared to abdominal approaches to female sterilization, a vasectomy is safer, more effective and less expensive.[1]

5. Who is at risk for regret?

Ans. Ideally, the consent process begins during prenatal care. Insurance coverage varies as well as state laws and regulations regarding Medicaid coverage so it is important to familiarize yourself with these laws. Counseling should also include other methods of sterilization such as hysteroscopy or male sterilization as well as other methods of contraception. Women who are of young age (less than 30), in unstable relationships or have a low parity may have a higher rate of regret later in life.[9,10] Women should also be counseled that the procedure is permanent and is not intended to be reversible.[9,10]

6. What are some barriers women may encounter while trying to obtain sterilization?

Ans. Women also face barriers to postpartum contraception and access to any birth control postpartum due to insurance barriers.[8,9] Women from low-income and racial/ethnic minorities face the greatest barriers in obtaining desired sterilization, especially due to federal policies through medicaid services.[9,10] These restrictive policies may place a woman at risk for an unintended pregnancy.[10]

■ TAKE-HOME MESSAGES

- Female sterilization is the most popular method of pregnancy prevention in the United States. The second most popular method is male sterilization.[1,3] Twenty percent of couples use oral contraceptives, 15% use male condoms and 7% use IUDs.
- Compared to abdominal approaches to female sterilization, a vasectomy is safer, more effective, and less expensive.[1]
- There are several techniques to achieve a postpartum tubal ligation, either after a vaginal delivery or at the time of CS. These include the Pomeroy, Parkland, Urshida, Filshie clips or tubal removal.[2]
- Probably the most used technique is the Pomeroy technique which includes placement of a free tie around a loop of the fallopian tube which is then excised.[2]
- Failure rate for all types of female sterilization are 18.5/1,000 according to the CREST study.[5,6] A partial salpingectomy according to the CREST study has a the lowest failure rate.[4,6]
- Women who are of young age (less than 30), in unstable relationships or have a low parity may have a higher rate of regret later in life.[1] Women should also be counseled that the procedure is permanent and is not intended to be reversible.[1]
- Women from low-income and racial/ethnic minorities face the greatest barriers in obtaining desired sterilization, especially due to federal policies through Medicaid services. [9,10] These restrictive policies may place a woman at risk for an unintended pregnancy.[10]

■ REFERENCES

1. American College of Obstetrics and Gynecology. Benefits and Risks of Sterilization. ACOG Practice Bulletin Number 133. Obstet Gynecol. 2013;121(2):392-404.
2. Oligobo N, Revicky V, Udeh R. Pomeroy technique or Filshie clips for postpartum sterilization? Retrospective study on comparison between Pomeroy procedure and Filshie clips for a tubal occlusion at the time of Caesarean section. Arch Gynecol Obstet. 2010;281:1073-5.

3. Rodriguez MI, Seuc A, Sokal DC. Comparative efficacy of postpartum sterilization with the titanium clip versus partial salpingectomy: a randomized controlled trial. BJOG. 2013;120(1):108-12.
4. Peterson HB, Xia Z, Hughes JM, Wilcox LS, Tyler LR, Trussell J . The risk of pregnancy after tubal sterilization: findings from the US collaborative review of sterilization. Am J Obstet Gynecol. 1996;174:1161-8.
5. Gariepy AM, Creinin MD, Smith KJ, Xu X. Probability of pregnancy after sterilization: a comparison of hysteroscopic versus laparoscopic sterilization. Contraception. 2014;90:174-81.
6. Trussell J. Contraceptive failure in the United States. Contraception. 2004;70:89-96.
7. Whiteman MK, Cox S, Tepper NK, Curtis KM, Jamieson DJ, Penman-Aguilar A, et al. Postpartum intrauterine device insertion and postpartum tubal sterilization in the United States. Am J Obstet Gynecol. 2012;206(2):127 e1-7. doi: 10.1016/j.ajog.2011.08.004. Epub 2011.
8. White K, Teal S, Potter J. Contraception after delivery and short interpregnancy intervals among women in the Unites States. Obstet Gynecol. 2015;125(6):1471-7.
9. White K, Potter JE. Reconsidering racial/ethnic difference in sterilization in the United States. Contraception. 2014;89(6):550-6.
10. Borrero S, Zite N, Potter JE, Trussel J. Medicaid Policy on Sterilization- Anachronistic or still relevant? NEJM. 2014;370:102-4.

Index

Page numbers followed by *f* refer to figure

A

Abdomen 42
Abdominal
    cavity 10*f*
    circumference 210*f*
    discomfort 141, 169
    distension 51, 52
    wall, right 149*f*
Acute pelvic inflammatory disease 35*f*, 46
Adenocarcinoma, endometrial 81, 88*f*
Adenomyosis 42, 156
Adhesiolysis 43
Adhesions 37
Adnexa 80
Adnexal malignancy 39
Adnexal mass 30, 109, 254*f*, 266
    complex 37
Adnexal torsion 125
Adult respiratory distress syndrome 54
Alendronate 64
Amenorrhea
    obstructive cause of 172
    primary 169, 171, 172
    secondary 18, 20, 21
American College of Obstetrics and Gynecology 4
American Society for Colposcopy and Cervical Pathology 5
American Society for Reproductive Medicine 11
Amniotic fluid 218, 219, 253*f*, 256
    index 219, 231
    role of 218
Ampulla of Vater 286
Angiotensin converting enzyme inhibitors 220
Anhydramnios 219
Antenatal corticosteroids 202
Antiestrogen 16
Antihypertensive therapy 84
Anti-Müllerian hormone 55
Antral follicle count 55
Anuria 54
Aortic valve replacement 279
Apgar score 220
Appendectomy 30, 141, 147
    laparoscopic 275
Appendiceal wall 274*f*
Appendicitis 115, 122, 272
Arcuate arterial calcifications 61*f*
Arcuate uterus, development of 25
Arcuate veins 127*f*
Arterial blood flow 128*f*
Artery, ovarian 123*f*
Asherman's syndrome 20
    prevalence of 21
Assisted reproductive technology 206
Asymptomatic adnexal mass 262
Atrophic endometrial glands 70*f*
Atrophic endometrium 81
Attention deficit hyperactivity disorder 169
Autosomal recessive polycystic kidney disease 220
Avascular intrauterine adhesions 20*f*

B

Babcock forceps 308*f*
Bacterial vaginosis 46
Bacteroides 48
Bagel sign 118*f*
Bicornuate
    bicollis 25
    uterus 25, 27
Bicuspid stenotic aortic valve 277*f*, 278*f*
Bilateral multicystic dysplastic kidney 220
Biliary pancreatitis 286
Bimanual pelvic examination 154
Biophysical profile score 213
Biopsy, endometrial 67, 70, 87, 91
Bladder peritoneum 104
Blood
    count, complete 63, 192
    flow
        peripheral 112*f*
        venous 128*f*
Body mass index 5, 187
Bone mineral density 62, 62*f*, 138
Borderline ovarian tumor 102, 105

Brachytherapy 89
Breast cancer 84
Breath, shortness of 3
Breech presentation 232
Bumpy lesions 164

C

Calcium 84
Cancer
    endometrial 71, 88
    ovarian 100
Carbohydrate diet, low 252
Carcinoma 87
    endometrial 84, 87-89
Cardiac disease 278
Caudal regression syndrome 252, 256
Celebrex 90
Centers for disease control and prevention 48, 167
Cephalohematoma 243
Cerebral
    artery 237f
        middle 208
    vein thrombosis 282
Cervical
    canal 197f
    cancer 5
        screening 5
    dysplasia 158
    fibroids 37
    insufficiency 200, 202, 203
    intraepithelial neoplasm 160f
        low-grade 161f
    length 202
    motion 129
    tenderness 47
Cervix 80
    progressive shortening of 197f
Cesarean
    delivery 250
    hysterectomy 228, 229
    section 132, 245
Chemotherapy 92
Chills 118, 284
Chlamydia 23, 29, 42, 56, 102, 117, 119, 127, 141, 147, 158, 307
    salpingitis 35
    test 15, 18, 153, 262
    trachomatis 48
Chlamydial infection 41, 42, 44, 45
    treatment of 42

Chocolate cyst 137f, 138f
Cholangitis 286
Cholecystectomy 66, 280, 287
Cholecystitis 286, 287f, 288
Choledocholithiasis 288
Cholestasis, intrahepatic 291, 292
Cholesterol 3, 13
Choriocarcinoma 305
Chorionic villi 193f, 227f
Chorionicity 206
Chromopertubation, laparoscopic 10f, 12
Circle of Willis 237f
Cirrhosis 148
Clindamycin penetrates neutrophils 49
Clomiphene citrate 16, 53
Coital issues 11
Colonoscopy 90
Complete adnexal torsion 268f
Comprehensive metabolic profile 63
Conception, residual products of 190, 192
Condylomata acuminata 164-167
    typical appearance of 165
Constipation 3, 224
Contraception 3, 23, 36, 56
Controlled ovarian stimulation 55
Copper intrauterine device 221
Corpus luteum 118f
Cramping 202
Crinkled paper appearance 180
Crohn's disease 115
Crown-rump length 186f
Cryotherapy 162, 167
Cul-de-sac 38f, 53f, 104, 149f, 170f
Cyst
    complex 107f
    ovarian 73, 112f, 125f
    rupture 109
Cystadenocarcinomas 105
Cystadenomas 105
Cystectomy, ovarian 110
Cystic inclusions, multiple 66f
Cystic lesion 133f
    heterogeneous appearance of 123f
Cystic teratomas 110
Cytotrophoblastic cells 193f

D

Deep dyspareunia 47
Deep venous thrombosis 280
Depression 41, 90

Dermoid cyst 108f, 109, 125, 263f, 264
    ovarian 109
Diabetes mellitus 13, 15, 36, 45, 252
Diarrhea 3, 224
Dichorionic diamniotic twin gestation 206f, 207f
Didelphys uterus 25, 27
Disseminated intravascular coagulopathy 228
Distal tubal occlusion 38f
Dizziness 51, 118
Doxycycline plus metronidazole 48
Duplex ultrasound 282
Didelphys 25
Dysmenorrhea 7, 23, 42, 127, 129, 130, 136, 138, 139, 141, 147, 148, 151
    primary 138
    secondary 136, 139
Dyspareunia 7, 60, 127, 129, 130, 136f, 147, 148, 151, 153
Dysuria 3, 141, 147

E

Eclampsia 292
Ectopic pregnancy 45, 114f, 117, 117f, 118f, 119, 120
    medical treatment of 120
    persistent 120
Eczema 180
Edema 123f
Embryo transfer 16
Embryonic flow 187f
Endocervical canal 25f, 26f, 159f
Endocervical polyp 76, 77
Endocervix 5
Endometrial biopsy, limitations of 70
Endometrial polyp
    histologic appearance of 76f
    large 75f
    tamoxifen associated 70f
Endometrioma 134f, 138, 151
    ovarian 114f
    ultrasonographic features of 139
Endometriosis 11, 37, 42, 129, 136, 139, 147-149, 151, 156f
    detection of 148
    diagnosis of 151
    laparoscopic treatment of 139
Endometriotic lesions 149f
Endometritis 21, 194f
Endometrium 10f, 19f, 29f, 57f, 61, 191f
    honey-comb appearance of 71f
    non-polypoid 70f
    proliferative 133
    surface of 68f
    thick avascular 14f
Endoscopic retrograde cholangiopancreatogram 287
Epidermal growth factor 53
Epidural anesthesia 246f
Epithelial cell thickness 160f
Epithelial ovarian cancer 100
Escherichia coli 48
Estrogen-progestin withdrawal test 19
External beam radiotherapy 89
External cephalic version 231, 232
External genitalia 52, 57, 80, 119, 129
Extraparenchymal venous congestion 128f

F

Fallopian tube 10f, 11, 38f, 49, 119f, 124f
Fasting glucose 13
Fatty liver, acute 286, 288, 292
Female sterilization 310
Femoral vein 282f
Fertility 120
    evaluation 12
Fetal
    chest, abnormal shape of 253f
    circulation 253f
    face, surface rendering of 255f
    head, delivery of 248f
    heart tracing 308
    hydronephrosis 257, 260
    intrauterine growth restriction 212
    kidneys 218
    malpresentation 230
    scalp
        hematomas 243
        lacerations 243
    urine 219
Fever 45, 47, 284
    low grade 118
Fibroids 32, 129
    submucosal 31, 32f, 33, 148f
Fibromyalgia 129
Fitz-Hugh-Curtis syndrome 38f
Fluid-filled endometrial cavity 81
Free fluid surrounding cyst 114f
Frozen pelvis 37

G

Gallbladder
    mucosa 287f
    wall thickening 285f
Gallstone 284, 288
    disease, complicated 288
Gamma-glutamyl transpeptidase 290
Gastritis 90
Genital
    tract injury 250
    tuberculosis 20
    warts 165
Gestational
    hypertensive disorders 234, 238
    sac 186f
    trophoblastic disease 301, 303
Gestations, multiple 207
Gland, endometrial 68, 81
Glucophage 7
Glucose tolerance test 13
Gonadal dysgenesis 172
Gonadotropin
    releasing hormone 53, 151
    therapy 52f
Gonorrhea 42
    tests 23, 29, 56, 102, 127, 141, 147

H

Headache 234
    premenstrual 147
Heart 80
    disease 45
        congenital 276
    shaped uterus 25
HELLP syndrome 292
Hematocrit 192, 268
Hematometra 79, 80f, 81, 170f
    treatment of 82
Hematuria 3, 141, 147
Hemoglobin 192
Hemoperitoneum 119f
Hemorrhage 54, 93f, 123f
    postpartum 20, 243, 250, 307
    retinal 243
Hemorrhagic cyst 109, 111, 113, 113f, 114f, 115, 115f
    complex 113, 114f
    rupture of 113, 114f
Hemorrhagic ovarian cysts
    appearance of 113
    typical sonographic appearance of 113

Hepatitis 289
    B vaccine 23, 30, 147, 257, 273, 289, 297
    test 253
HIV test 253
Hormonal replacement therapy 60, 65
Horseshoe kidney 256
Human chorionic gonadotropin 192
Human papilloma virus 162
Hydatidiform mole, complete 303
Hydrochlorothiazide 132
Hydrosalpingeal fluid, transvaginal aspiration of 40
Hydrosalpinges 39
Hymen 170
Hymenectomy 170
    surgical 172
Hyperandrogenemia 16
Hyperemesis gravidarum 292
Hypergonadotropic hypogonadism 173
Hyperinsulinemia 16
Hyperkeratosis 180
Hyperplasia 70f, 71
    endometrial 156
Hypertension 15, 36, 41, 73, 81, 84, 90, 132, 174, 192, 201, 238
Hypertensive disorders 238
Hypertrophy 176
Hypocalcemia 64
Hypoechoic masses 31
Hypomenorrhea 19f, 21
Hypoplasia, bilateral 256
Hypotension 54
Hypothyroidism 178
Hypoxemia 237f
Hysterectomy 146, 225
    total laparoscopic 37
Hysterosalpingogram 11, 12, 21, 22
Hysterosalpingography 27
Hysteroscopy 21, 22, 27, 32, 81
    diagnostic 67
    therapeutic 19, 22
Hysterosonography 67

I

Iatrogenic ureteral injury 37
Ibuprofen 30, 136, 141, 147
Iliac lymphatic nodes 37
Imiquimod 167
Immature teratoma 109
Imperforate hymen 170f, 172
    treatment of 172
In vitro fertilization 16

Incisional endometriosis 132
Incomplete abortion 20
Infertility 11, 21
    assessment 7
    secondary 23
Inflammatory cells, acute 193*f*, 194*f*
Insulin 84
International Pelvic Pain Society 42, 44
Intestinal serosa 105
Intra-amniotic infection 286
Intracavitary fluid 170*f*
Intraendometrial vessels 67*f*
Intramural fibroid 145*f*
Intraovarian vascularity 14*f*
Intrauterine
    adhesions 10*f*, 18-21
        management of 21
        prevalence of 21
        thick partial 9*f*
    contraceptive device 82
    gestation 117*f*
    growth restriction 200, 210*f*, 213*f*, 217*f*
        causes of 212
        management of 213
Intravenous ceftriaxone 48
Iron deficiency anemia 29, 142, 156
Isolated aortic stenosis murmur 277

K

Kidney stones 295
Kocher clamps 247*f*

L

Labia majora 176
Labia minora 174-176
Labial fusion 169
Labial hypertrophy 176
Labiaplasty 176
Lacerations 243
Langerhans histiocytosis 174
Laparoscopic surgery 37, 104
Laparoscopy 27, 269
Laparotomy 269
Laser ablation 162
Leiomyomas 42, 144
Leiomyosarcoma 90, 92, 93*f*, 94*f*
    metastatic 92
Letrozole 53
Levonorgestrel 153

Lichen planus 180
Lichen sclerosus 178, 179*f*, 180
    hourglass appearance of 179*f*
Lisinopril 73
Liver
    disease 289
    function tests 141
Loop electrosurgical excision procedure 159, 161
Losartan 90
Low molecular weight heparin 283
Lower uterine segment, high degree of 57
Lugol's solution, application of 159*f*
Lumbar and sacral spine 253*f*
Lumpectomy 66
Luteinized cysts, multiple 270*f*
Lymph node metastases 87

M

Malignant neoplasms 37
Malignant teratoma 109
Manual vacuum extraction 188
Mature cystic teratoma 109, 110
Medroxyprogesterone acetate 151
Megacystis microcolon intestinal hypoperistalsis syndrome 220
Membranes, preterm premature rupture of 195, 295
Menarche 117
Meningocele 176
Menopause 60
Menorrhagia 47
Metaplasia 71
Metformin 7, 16, 90, 252
Methotrexate 45, 51, 117
Mirena IUD 3
Miscarriage 193
Missed abortion 18, 23, 188
Molar pregnancy 303
Monochorionic diamniotic twin gestation 205
Monodermal teratoma 109
Müllerian abnormalities 172
Müllerian agenesis 173
Müllerian anomalies 172
Müllerian duct 25, 81, 82
Multicystic dysplastic kidney, contralateral 220
Multifetal gestation 205
Multifocal vulvar lesions 164, 165*f*
Multiple gestation, prevalence of 206
Multivitamin 4
Mycoplasma genitalium 48
Myelomeningocele 176

Myomectomy 21, 146
  hysteroscopic 33
  laparoscopic 149
Myometrial lesion 91
Myometrium 31, 33, 61f, 86f
Myxoid degeneration 145f

N

National Osteoporosis Foundation 63
Nausea 35, 45, 51, 126, 185, 224, 284
Necrotic chorionic villi 193f
Necrotic decidua 194f
Neisseria gonorrheae 48
Neoplasia, endometrial 86f
Nephrolithiasis 174, 295
Nephrolithotomy, percutaneous 295
Nonsteroidal anti-inflammatory drugs 220
Nonstress test 213
Normal spontaneous vaginal deliveries 45, 117

O

Office hysteroscopy 21, 22
Old knife cone biopsy 162
Oligoasthenozoospermia 56, 105
Oligohydramnios 216, 218-220, 256
  causes of 218
  severe 217f
Oligomenorrhea 7
Oliguria 54
Omentum 105
Omeprazole 90
Operative vaginal delivery 243, 244
  contraindications for 244
Oral contraception
  combined 303
  pills 42, 136, 195
Osteopenia 62f, 63
Osteoporosis 62f, 63
  development of 62
  diagnosis of 62f
  prevention 84
Ovarian
  borderline serous tumors 105f
  cyst, complex 103, 112
  dermoid, malignant degeneration of 109
  drilling, laparoscopic 16
  fossa, left 149f
  hyperstimulation syndrome 51, 52
    clinical features of 54
    development of 54
    management of 54
    pathophysiology of 53
    three-dimensional ultrasound of 52f
  injury, mechanism of 125
  torsion 109, 122, 125
    complete 123f
    mechanism of 125
Ovary 49
  epithelial tumors of 105
Ovulation induction 16, 51, 56
Oxytocin infusion 250

P

Pain 178
  abdominal 35, 51, 52, 79, 90, 115, 117, 118, 126, 136f, 153, 266
  acute 145f
  back 141, 147, 148, 202
  chest 3
  chronic 42
  lower abdominal 45, 79, 90, 136
  musculoskeletal 64
  pelvic 41-44, 127, 129, 130, 136, 146-148, 151
Pancreatitis 288
Pap smear 3, 6, 15, 18, 23, 29, 41, 51, 79, 84, 147, 153, 158, 262, 307
Para-aortic lymph node 88
Parkland method postpartum tubal ligation 308f
Partial mole, three-dimensional ultrasound of 304f
Partial salpingectomy 308f
Pedunculated fibroid 150f
  ligation of 150f
  morcellation of 151f
  removal of 150
Pelvic
  adhesions 41, 130
  congestion syndrome 127, 130, 139
  discomfort 169
  examination 130
  floor, infiltrative endometriosis of 37
  inflammatory disease 21, 37, 45, 129
    acute episodes of 156
  masses, large 37
  pain 7, 35, 41, 42, 45, 51, 79, 90, 115, 118, 136, 136f, 141, 153, 266
  peritoneum 104
  pressure 200, 202
  tumors 37
  ultrasound 8, 19, 190, 268

varices 130
wall 104
   left lateral 149f
Pelvi-calyceal systems 258f
Penicillin 132
Percocet 136
Perianal itching 178
Periovarian adhesions 38f
Peripheral cysts, multiple small 13f
Peripheral vessels 143f
Peritoneal lavage 104
Peritoneum, abdominal 104
Peritonitis, acute 109, 281f
Peritubal adhesions, severe 38f
Pfannenstiel incision 246f
Pfannenstiel scar 133
Placenta
   accreta 225, 225f, 227, 228
   percreta 221-225, 225f, 228, 232
Podophyllotoxin 167
Polycystic kidneys 219
Polycystic ovarian
   appearance 9f
   syndrome 7, 13, 51
Polyp
   endometrial 31, 32f, 68f, 71, 73, 74f, 76, 76f, 77, 87, 211
   glandulocystic appearance of 70f
   removal of 77
Polypoid endometrium 70f
Pomeroy method postpartum tubal ligation 308f
Pre-eclampsia 238, 239, 292
Pregnancy 3, 15, 288
   loss
      early 185
      recurrent 21
      spontaneous 193
   test 19, 46, 159
Preoperative ureteral catheter placement 37
Preterm labor, prevalence of 198
Prostate cancer 102
Psoriasis 180
Pubic hair distribution 170

Q

Quad screen blood test 255

R

Radiation therapy 37, 89
Raloxifen 64

Renal agenesis 172, 219, 220
   unilateral 220, 256
Renal function tests 141
Renal pelvic diameter 260
Retroperitoneal lymph nodes 105
Risendronate 64
Rokitansky nodule 107f, 263f
Rokitansky protuberance 109

S

Saline fibrotic band 19f
Saline infusion
   sonography 8, 27, 57, 58f, 87
      advantages of 31, 69
   sonohysterography 11, 19
Salpingectomy 39f, 119
   bilateral 39f
Salpingostomy 120
Scar endometriosis 133f, 135
Sepsis 243
Septate uterus 23, 25, 26f
Sexually transmitted disease 7, 23, 30, 56, 65, 73, 90, 147, 185, 195, 224, 231, 234
Simple ovarian cyst 123f
Simvastatin 90
Single umbilical artery 256
Sirenomelia 256, 256
Smooth muscle cells 144f
Snow storm appearance 301, 301f
Solid right thyroid nodule 299f
Sperm analysis 23
Spina bifida 176
Spindle cells 144f
Spontaneous abortion 158
   management of 21
Sprintec 7
Stroma 68f
Stromal fibrosis 70f
Stromal vessels, ovarian 14f
Syphilis test 253

T

Tamoxifen 66, 71, 84
Tanner stage 175
Thrombocytopenia, heparin-induced 283
Thromboembolism 54
   venous 282
Thrombosis 282f
Thyroid nodule 297, 299f
   fine needle aspiration of 299
   malignancy of 300

Tocolytic therapy 198
Tonsillectomy 23, 147
Torsed hyperstimulated ovary 268f, 269f
Transabdominal aspiration 49
Transcatheter embolization 130
Transperineal sonography 81
Transvaginal aspiration 49
Trauma, endometrial 20
Trichomonas 158
Triglycerides 13
Tubal damage, severe 39f
Tubal hyperemia 48
Tubal ligation 309
    bilateral 141
    postpartum 307, 309
    types of 309
Tubal obstruction 11
Tubal occlusion, hysteroscopic 40
Tuberculosis 20
Tubo-ovarian abscess 45, 46
Turner syndrome 172

U

Umbilical artery 213, 236f, 256
    Doppler waveforms 211f
Ureteral injury 37
Ureterocele 258f
Ureteropelvic junction 259
Uretrocele 258f
Urinary tract infection 36, 169
Ursodeoxycholic acid 291
Uterine anomalies
    assessment of 25
    congenital 27, 28
Uterine artery 235f
    embolization 34
Uterine bleeding 87
    abnormal 211
Uterine cavity 19f, 24f, 26f, 31, 190f
    division of 25f
    lumen of 32
    three-dimensional reconstruction of 25f
Uterine fibroid 141, 142, 144, 144f, 156
Uterine leiomyosarcoma
    diagnosis of 92
    FIGO staging system for 93

Uterine lesion 92f
Uterine lower segment thickness 57
Uterine rupture 58, 286
Uterine thickness 57
Uterosacral ligaments 149f
Uterotonic medications 250
Uterus 14f
    after hysterectomy 76f
    didelphys 26
        gross anatomy of 26f
    palpable 91
    snow storm appearance of 301f
    three-dimensional ultrasound of 85f
    transvaginal ultrasound of 61f

V

Vagina 80
Vaginal bleeding 192
    postmenopausal 65
Vaginal delivery 250
    spontaneous 79, 230
Vaginal discharge 48, 147
    abnormal 79
Vaginal dryness 60
Vaginal progesterone 51
Vaginal spotting 117, 153
Vein compression ultrasonography 282
Venous thromboembolism, incidence of 282
Vitamin D 63, 84, 90
    supplementation 84
Vitiligo 178, 180
Vomiting 35, 126, 185, 224, 284
Vulvovaginal candidiasis, chronic 180

W

Wet mount 29, 147
White blood cell 192
    counts 268
White homogenous uterine mass 144f
Wound
    disruption 250
    hematoma 250
    infection 250